Contents

Acknowledgements

This book has taken four years to come to fruition and involved tremendous hard work and support from many people. Starting at the very beginning, I would like to thank my parents for supporting me financially through further and higher education and for encouraging me to be my best. Thanks also to the staff of the beauty therapy department at North Lindsey College (1987–1990) for providing the best possible start to my career. My high standards are due to theirs.

Colleagues and students in the beauty therapy department of the London College of Fashion have been a source of inspiration and frustration in almost equal measures over the past six years. Implementing the new National Diploma in Beauty Therapy Sciences and guiding students through their first IVA has been a challenge but one I have learnt from and enjoyed. LCF also provided the backdrop for the photo shoot – a very enjoyable day. Thank you to the team from Heinemann and also to the models who provided an invaluable student's perspective on each shot: Amreet, Olivia, Leila, Sarah and my mum. Thanks also to Karen whose door is always open when I need support and who had the great suggestion of a book launch.

My wonderful friends have doled out encouragement, praise, advice and dinners and kept me in good spirits when times have been hard. Much love and appreciation to them.

It was a great honour to have Sheila and Gill on board, two brave, bright and clever ladies. Thanks also to Tom Yeo for his expert help with 'Scientific Principles'.

And finally, this book would never have grown from an idea in my head to the finished product if it were not for Pen Gresford at Heinemann who believed in both my ideas and my ability from the start. Also thanks to Camilla who had the (I think) painstaking task of editing the enormous manuscript which landed on her desk and turning it into this fabulous book. Thanks to them, my vision is now a reality.

Jeanine Connor

I would like to thank the following for their help and contributions:

⏮ Moira Paulusz – Health and Beauty Salon
⏭ Dawn Ward – vice-principal of Warwickshire College
⏭ Janice Brown – House of Famuir
⏭ Kaye Johnson

Sheila Godfrey

Photo acknowledgements

The authors and publishers would like to thank the following individuals and organisations for permission to reproduce photographs:

Camilla Abbot page 14;
Carlton pages 12 (right), 197, 200, 205, 206 (bottom), 234 and 235 (left);
Corbis page 107 (right) and 248;
Getty Images UK/Photodisc page 107 (middle);
Guinot page 199;
Harcourt Education Ltd/Peter Morris pages 156–7;
Julia Conway page 173 (right column);
Science Photo Library pages 18, 19, 32, 70, 103, 107 (left), 113–4, 117, 118, 122, 123 and cover;
Bridal photo page 171 Sara Greenfield;
Evening make-up page 173 Emma Fairfield.

All other photos by **Harcourt Education Ltd/Gareth Boden.**

The artwork in Unit 13:Aromatherapy (pages 285–298) was created by **Gill Milsom**.

Every effort has been made to contact copyright holders of material reproduced in this book. Any omissions will be rectified in subsequent printings if notice is given to the publishers.

Introduction

About this book

The purpose of this book is to offer support as you work towards a nationally recognised qualification in beauty therapy. The book is structured around the BTEC National Diploma in Beauty Therapy Sciences but also includes guidance for mapping other qualifications such as NVQs and Technical Certificates. Guidance is offered for mapping Key Skills units in Communication and Application of Number at level 2 and/or level 3.

This book is for you! It includes lots of colour illustrations including diagrams, tables, photographs and drawings as visual aids to learning. There are many pointers for linking topics between and within chapters to avoid repetition and to encourage you to make connections between theory and practice.

As well as assessment tasks and revision questions there are 'thinking and doing' activities in each chapter to allow you to check and consolidate your learning and to encourage independent study.

BTEC National Diploma in Beauty Therapy Sciences

As the title suggests, the BTEC National Diploma course in Beauty Therapy has a high science content which reflects the needs and nature of the industry. It is, of course, a vocational and a practical qualification, but potential candidates are often surprised by the amount of theory included. From the outset you will be made aware of the importance of underpinning scientific, legislative and theoretical knowledge related to beauty therapy. The reason for this is to enable you to:

▸▸ carry out beauty therapy procedures safely and effectively
▸▸ understand how and why treatments work as they do
▸▸ assess clients' needs and suitability for therapy.

In addition, a substantial amount of your time will be spent studying the human body: the structure and function of the skin, skeleton, muscles and internal systems as well as investigating some of the more common diseases and disorders which affect the systems of the body. Also, of course, you will learn how to provide a wide range of beauty therapy treatments, both manually and using electrical or mechanical equipment, to a high commercial standard.

Successful completion of the BTEC National Diploma in Beauty Therapy Sciences will equip you with the knowledge, understanding and practical skills necessary to gain employment in beauty therapy or related industries, or for entry into higher education (foundation and/or undergraduate degree).

The course consists of eleven mandatory core units and this book also explores two of the most popular specialist units: Aromatherapy and Indian head massage.

BTEC National in Beauty Therapy Sciences:

Practical skills and theory	Scientific studies	Business studies
Basic skills in beauty therapy	Scientific principles for beauty therapy	
Facial therapy	Human physiology	
Body massage	Anatomy	Organisational practices and procedures
Body therapy	Dermatology and microbiology	
Electrical epilation		
Aromatherapy		
Indian head massage		

Integrated Vocational Assignment (IVA)

What is the IVA?

The National Certificate and the National Diploma in Beauty Therapy Sciences consist of units, most of which are internally assessed by your subject tutors. There are two externally assessed units which form the Integrated Vocational Assignment (IVA).

This is set by the awarding body and is a compulsory part of your course. Failure to complete the IVA will mean that you will not achieve your qualification. The IVA is designed to assess your practical skills and theoretical knowledge of **Unit 8: Facial therapy** and **Unit 10: Body therapy**. Your work will be assessed internally in the first instance by your subject tutors using a national marking scheme, and then it will be assessed externally by the awarding body. The awarding body will confirm your final grade once re-marking has been completed. Marks will be awarded for the quality rather than the quantity of your written work according to how well you meet the criteria for a pass, merit or distinction for each unit. Assessment criteria are summarised in general terms below:

Assessment criteria:

Pass	Merit	Distinction
▶▶ learning outcomes are met	▶▶ learning outcomes are met	▶▶ learning outcomes are met
▶▶ little detail is included	▶▶ some detail is included	▶▶ lots of detail is included
▶▶ a descriptive style is used	▶▶ an explanatory style is used	▶▶ an evaluative and/or analytic style is used
▶▶ basic treatment applications	▶▶ good treatment applications	▶▶ professional treatment applications
	▶▶ comparisons are made between treatments	▶▶ a constructive critique of treatments is made

Requirements of the IVA

The IVA requires that you apply the knowledge and skills from your course to a realistic work-based situation. It will provide the full assessment requirements for Unit 8: Facial Therapy and Unit 10: Body Therapy. The IVA is based on a number of tasks which relate to your practical work with clients in a work-based setting and as such informs potential employers of your abilities. Practical work will be assessed by your subject tutors who will mark off each treatment when you can 'consistently achieve the standard required'. A record of practical work for Units 8 and 10 must be submitted with your assignment as it forms a mandatory part of the IVA. Your written work should be professionally presented, ideally word processed, in a coherent and structured format. It should be accompanied by an Assignment Coversheet (Form IVA L1) which fully references your work.

IVA tasks

An exemplar IVA is included below for reference, although the exact format will change slightly from year to year. A summary of the work you must submit to your tutor is also included on pages 4 and 5. Marks are included in brackets (total 150) and full details of the assessment criteria are included at the end of this section, on page 5. The evidence that you present must meet the learning outcomes and assessment criteria for Unit 8: Facial Therapy and Unit 10: Body Therapy.

Task 1 (total: 18 marks)

Complete all the practical work in Unit 8: Facial Therapy and Unit 10: Body Therapy and the record provided. You must be able to demonstrate that you can carry out all the treatments listed in each category to a safe, professional and commercial standard.

Manual facial treatments (2)
cleansing
exfoliation
extraction
face masks
toning
moisturisation

Manual facial massage (2)
effleurage
petrissage
tapotement

Mechanical facial treatments (2)
vapour
brush cleansing
lymphatic drainage

Electrical facial treatments (2)
direct high frequency
indirect high frequency
galvanic desincrustation
galvanic iontophoresis
electrical muscle stimulation (EMS)
microcurrent

Mechanical body treatments (2)
gyratory vibration
ultrasound
vacuum suction

Electrical body treatments (2)
faradism (EMS)
galvanism

Hair treatments (2)
radiant heat
infra-red

Light irradiation and self-tanning treatments (2)
sunbeds
self-tanning

All the treatments must be carried out with due regard to health and safety and to indications and contra-indications. (2)

Tasks 2–4

You must demonstrate facial treatments and body treatments in a realistic working environment. All the tasks will be based on real clients who have received treatment as part of your practical assessment activities. You must devise two treatment plans for two different clients selected because of their need for electrical and mechanical facial and body treatments.

Task 2 (total: 18 marks)

Explain the treatment proposed for each client. Consider the benefits to the client and how the benefits and effectiveness of your selected techniques compare to the others that are available. Draw up a facial treatment plan taking the needs of the client into account. Show that for each client you have considered the range of possible facial treatments available. For each client show:

➡ a description of each of the chosen techniques, the health and safety aspects for the client and the therapist, and the reasons for that choice of facial treatment (10) the benefits to and expected outcomes of each of the chosen treatments for each client (including physical, physiological and psychological effects) (**8**)

Task 3 (total: 24 marks)

Carry out a figure and posture analysis for each of the two clients and identify the figure and postural problems that they have:

- identification of the main figure and posture problems and the implications for the client (**8**)
- the benefits and expected outcomes of each mechanical body treatment for each client (including physical, physiological and psychological effects) (**8**)
- the benefits and expected outcomes of each electrical body treatment for each client (including physical, physiological and psychological effects). (**8**)

Task 4 (total: 32 marks)

Record the pre-treatment activities that you carry out for the facial treatment of each client. Take into account the following:

- pre-treatment preparation procedures and the health and safety aspects of these preparation procedures for each facial treatment (**8**)
- issues around contra-indications and indications to the facial treatments. (**8**)

Record the pre-treatment activities that you carry out for the body treatment of each client. Take into account the following:

- pre-treatment preparation procedures and the health and safety aspects of these preparation procedures for each body treatment (**8**)
- issues around contra-indications and indications to the body treatments. (**8**)

Task 5 (total: 24 marks)

Maintain a record card of the facial treatment for each client; you may devise your own or use one with which you are familiar. You will also need to provide a description of issues about:

- the selection and preparation of tools, materials and equipment and the health and safety issues related to these (**8**)
- the functions of each of the products you have chosen for the clients (**8**)
- the retail opportunities provided by each of the clients and the home aftercare advice you would give to each client. (**8**)

Task 6 (total: 24 marks)

Maintain a record card of the body treatment for each client; you may devise your own or use one with which you are familiar. You will also need to provide a description of issues about:

- the selection and preparation of tools, materials and equipment and the health and safety issues related to these (**8**)
- the functions of each of the products you have chosen for the clients (**8**)
- the retail opportunities provided by each of the clients and the home aftercare advice you would give to each client. (**8**)

Task 7 (total: 10 marks)

Light irradiation treatments remain popular within beauty salons and health spas, despite health warnings in the press and by the health authorities. It is important that the therapist has a thorough understanding of the benefits, risks and effects of light irradiation treatments, so that their use in the salon can be evaluated and sound advice given to clients.

Light irradiation provides for infra-red, radiant heat, sun-tanning equipment and self-tanning applications. For light irradiation, consider the benefits and hazards to clients. Describe when and with what frequency their use would be indicated in the salon. (**10**)

Always do your best work and aim for the highest possible mark. If you just try to scrape through with the minimum amount of work, chances are you will fall short and fail the IVA. If you aim for the moon, you might land somewhere in the stars!

Evidence to be submitted for IVA

Task 1 (total: 18 marks)

A completed **record card** showing that you have carried out all the treatments listed for Units 8 and 10. Each treatment must be dated and signed off by your assessor.

Task 2 (total: 18 marks)

Two **treatment plans** showing facial treatment programmes. These must include a description and justification of the facial treatment techniques selected and an explanation of the benefits of the treatments for each of the two clients.

Task 3 (total: 24 marks)

Two **treatment plans** for body treatments and postural defects. These must include a description and justification of the body treatment techniques selected and an explanation of the benefits of the treatments for each of the two clients.

Task 4 (total: 32 marks)

Present information that shows clearly which **pre-treatment activities** are required for each of the two clients. The information provided should show that you have considered all issues relating to the chosen treatments.

Task 5 (total: 24 marks)

You should complete a **record card** of the facial treatment for each client. For each client you should include information about the functions of the products you have chosen, the retail opportunities that are available, and the aftercare advice you would provide.

Task 6 (total: 24 marks)

You should complete a **record card** of the body treatment for each client. For each client you should include information about the functions of the products you have chosen, the retail opportunities that are available, and the aftercare advice you would provide.

Task 7 (total: 10 marks)

You must present a **report** on the effects of light irradiation treatment. You must describe each of the treatments and conditions clearly and concisely. Remember to label your report clearly so that the marker knows which part of the assignment you are completing.

Assessment criteria

Decoding assessment criteria

The language used in the grading criteria for assessment might seem a little complicated at first. The following guidelines have been designed to help differentiate between a pass, merit and distinction, to enable you to achieve the best possible grade.

Language used in assessment criteria:

Command	Explanation	Grade
Appropriate	True but basic information	Pass
Clear and coherent	Makes sense and is in a useful format with some detail	Merit
Accurate, precise and reliable	Lots of specific detail and justification with comparative reflection	Distinction
Describe	Make recognisable with little detail	Pass
Describe with attention to detail	Explain more fully with specific consideration	Merit
Analyse	Explain and evaluate in detail	Distinction
Evaluate	Offer a value judgement, positive and negative	Distinction
Adequate	Just enough, basic information	Pass
Demonstrate awareness	Show that you have thought about something and have a view	Merit
Justify	Give reasons for, with attention to detail	Distinction
Compare and contrast	Consider the similarities and differences between two or more things	Merit/distinction

A final note from the authors

Remember that potential employers will be interested in your grades when you apply for jobs …

Aim to achieve a distinction, that way if you miss out you will still achieve a merit.

Aim to pass and miss out and your qualification and career is at stake.

I wish you the very best of luck with your course in beauty therapy and with the IVA. I hope that you find it an enjoyable and rewarding experience. I hope also that you continue to find this book a valuable source of information and guidance both now and throughout a long and fulfilling career in beauty therapy. Enjoy!

Jeanine Connor, Sheila Godfrey and Gill Milsom

SECTION 1:
Professional basics for beauty therapy

This section examines the skills that are common to all practical treatments and which must be performed in order to ensure safe working practice to a commercial standard. It includes the whys and hows of preliminary client consultation, including a list of generic **contra-indications**, as well as guidelines for health, safety and hygiene procedures in the working environment. Consultation for specific practical treatments as well as special considerations are investigated further in the subject chapters.

Preliminary consultation

A consultation is a two-way discussion between client and therapist which takes place prior to treatment of any kind. It involves a sharing of information and its purpose is to establish a professional relationship with the client and gain a clear and coherent picture about the client's requirements and constraints. The beauty professional must assess the client **holistically** by examining all aspects of his or her physical and mental wellbeing and lifestyle in order to gain as much information as possible. While assessment involves making informed judgements, it is important not to assume too much based on your own experience or expectations. Each client must be treated as an individual with individual needs and aspirations. Never suppose that you know already why the client has come to the salon or how the client is feeling without first conducting a thorough consultation. As well as discussing the client's concerns and requirements, the preliminary consultation is a time to assess the client's medical history. Certain conditions or prescribed drugs may be the cause of the client's skin problem, or the client may have an allergy or other conditions which may contra-indicate treatment. Consulting with the client also gives you an opportunity to provide treatment and product recommendations, as well as general advice according to the client's requirements and constraints, and the treatment plan you have agreed together.

While consultation for different practical treatments requires some specialist information, there are some general things which the therapist needs to establish prior to all practical work. Personal details will enable better lines of communication between you and the client; lifestyle factors will help to establish the cause of any client concerns; and a detailed medical history will enable you to decide on safe and effective treatment plans.

Purpose of the consultation

personal details   ⟶   effective communication

lifestyle factors   ⟶   establish causes of client concerns

medical history   ⟶   prescribe safe and effective treatments

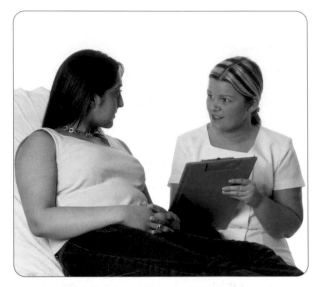

A consultation between client and therapist.

Personal details

You will need the client's name, address and telephone number for the salon database so that the client can be contacted in the future. This information might also be stored electronically on a computer. It can be used to confirm or cancel an appointment, or for marketing purposes to inform clients about promotional events. It is also necessary to record the contact details of the client's doctor, to be used in case of an emergency. This information is confidential to the salon. Sharing information stored on record cards will undermine the professional relationship you have with your clients. Furthermore, the **Data Protection Act (1998)** exists to protect information stored on computer and breaking confidentiality can lead to prosecution.

Lifestyle

A discussion about lifestyle can include factors as diverse as occupation, hobbies, number of children, diet, exercise, sleep patterns, alcohol consumption, UV exposure or smoking – anything which will help you to make informed decisions about the causal factors of your client's problems and appropriate recommendations for treatment. The spacing of treatments, home care and retail advice can also be tailored to the individual, considering the time and finances your client has available. You might also wish to include on the record card reminders about other things you have talked about with your client, such as forthcoming holidays, other special events, recent stress or bad news. This will help to prompt

your discussion the next time you see the client for a follow-on treatment.

Medical history

You will need to establish the client's general health and wellbeing, both physical and emotional, by asking general questions about how he or she is feeling. You also need information about any current medical conditions or medication as this might affect treatment. Historical conditions should be taken into account, such as major or recent operations, and you need to establish any allergies since these will inform product choice and retail recommendations. The presence of certain medical conditions means that treatment cannot safely proceed; these are known as non-treatable conditions or contra-indications. Some of these conditions mean that treatment cannot proceed at all, whereas others which are more localised indicate that a particular area should be avoided. Experience and common sense will help you to decide.

▸▸ **Practice point:** Remember that even the most experienced beauty therapist is not a doctor. You should never diagnose a medical condition or interfere with the advice given to a client by his or her doctor. Remember also that you cannot be expected to know the names and characteristics of all the medical conditions and/or medication you hear about. If you are unsure, it is much more professional to ask for clarification from the client and/or assistance from a manager than risk making a dangerous mistake.

Other conditions should alert the therapist to the fact that extra caution or further information is required, perhaps from the client's doctor, before treatment can safely commence. There are some contra-indications specific to different practical treatments but many conditions should be treated with caution in all practical areas. Some of the more common ones have been included in the table on page 9 and divided into four sections, to help you remember them: skin diseases/disorders, systems diseases/disorders, anatomical diseases/disorders and specific considerations for female clients. These lists are by no means exhaustive and you should add to them as your knowledge of treatments and of the human body develops.

An important skill which you will learn is how to differentiate between treatable and non-treatable conditions.

Contra-indications:

Skin	Systems	Anatomy	Female
cuts	diabetes	broken bones	pregnancy
bruises	epilepsy	sprains	lactation
abrasions	asthma	operations	menstrual problems
inflammation	digestive problems		menopause
recent scar tissue	high/low blood pressure		operations
infectious disease	high fever		

If faced with a novel situation try asking yourself these three questions:

▸ Will beauty therapy treatment make the condition worse?
▸ Will beauty therapy treatment cause discomfort to the client?
▸ Will beauty therapy treatment put me or my colleagues in danger of cross-infection?

If you answer 'yes' to one or more of the questions, do not proceed with treatment. If you remain unsure, ask for a second opinion from a colleague, manager or medical specialist.

Record cards

Beauty therapists record client's details on a record card, which becomes an important source of reference. In the beginning there is a lot of information for trainees to remember when they are conducting consultations and the record card can act as a prompt. Recording information in this way also means that you have a reminder of the client's personal details for the next meeting. If another therapist treats the client next time, he or she will also have an idea of the client's medical, lifestyle and treatment history. Even if the client has previously completed a record card at your salon, it

---

BEAUTY RECORD CARD

Name: Francesca Rushby   Age: 23   Tel. No.: 07957 373727

Address: 29, Stanmore Lane, Belton

PERSONAL DOCTOR	DETAILS OF PRESCRIBED DRUGS
Name: Dr. Matthews Address: The Surgery Belton Lane Tel. No.: 01257 314982	none

MEDICAL HISTORY

Details of Operations: none

Other Comments: Allergy to penicillin and sticking plaster

Date	Treatment	Remarks
12 May 04	Deep cleansing facial	Getting married, Jan 06
30 Jun 04	Deep cleansing facial	
27 Jul 04	Pedicure	Jessica – 'Merlot'
19 Nov 04	Deep cleansing facial	
17 Dec 04	Manicure, mini facial	French paint

Beauty therapy record card.

it is important to check that the information is up to date, because things do change. However, the consultation will usually be a much quicker process on subsequent visits.

Another way that record cards are used as a point of reference is when any post-treatment problems arise. Salon managers or supervisors can use the record card to check the name of the practitioner, the treatment given and the products used. This information can then be used to establish the cause of any adverse reactions or client concerns. It is a good idea for both the beauty therapist and the client to sign and date the record card, which then forms an agreement between them that the information it contains is accurate. It should be made clear that client records are confidential and that any data contained in them is only to be used for the purposes of ensuring safe and effective salon treatment and/or in-house marketing. It goes without saying that anything you discuss with a client throughout the course of the visit is strictly confidential.

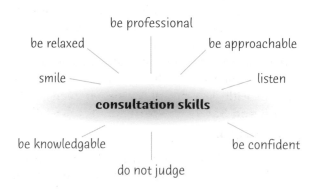

▸▸ **Practice point:** The best way to develop your consultation skills is to practise them repeatedly with friends and colleagues before you come into contact with a 'real' client. It can be a daunting experience at first with so much to remember, but the more relaxed you are the more confident and professional you will appear.

Health, safety and hygiene

It is imperative to ensure the safety of yourself, your colleagues and your clients at all times by adhering to strict codes of professional practice set out by official government guidelines. However, before embarking on any area of practical treatment there are some basic 'housekeeping' rules which must be acknowledged. Much of this chapter is common sense and hopefully will become second nature to you from the very beginning of your development in beauty therapy. Habits are hard to break so make sure that you form good ones!

Personal considerations

Most beauty professionals have an innate interest in personal appearance and skin hygiene. It is important to maintain your appearance and hygiene to the highest possible standard in order to portray a pleasing, pleasant and professional image to anyone whom you come into contact with during the course of your work. Remember that you are a walking advertisement for the organisation you work for before you ever administer a treatment to a member of the public.

Personal appearance

Most salons and colleges have a uniform or colour scheme which identifies therapists as belonging to a particular organisation. Many opt for the traditional salon dress or tunic and trousers, usually in a neutral colour such as white. Whatever uniform you wear, it must always be in pristine condition: freshly laundered, ironed and smelling clean. Footwear should be appropriate for the physical nature of your work. Flatter style shoes are best for working, with a small heel for women and non-slip sole to give support. Backless shoes or open toes are not really practical due to the potential safety hazards which are present in a salon environment. Additional protective clothing should be worn where appropriate; for example, a plastic apron for waxing. Jewellery should be discreet and kept to a minimum.

Personal hygiene

Hair should be clean, neat and tidy. Long hair must be tied back to avoid it hanging onto the client or into products. Fingernails should be clipped short and filed neatly, to avoid scratching or cross-infection, with no traces of nail enamel. Hands should be washed with an anti-bacterial cleanser before and after each treatment, as well as after eating, drinking, coughing or blowing your nose, to avoid cross-infection. Teeth should be cleaned after eating strong-smelling food or drink, but ideally these should be avoided during working hours. Any beauty therapist who cannot avoid smoking during break times must go to great lengths to remove the smell of cigarette smoke from his or her hands, breath, hair and clothing before returning to the salon.

Professional conduct

The world of beauty therapy is an intimate one, where professionals and clients are in close contact and share personal details. Discretion and confidentiality have already been mentioned but the absolute importance of professional conduct must be stressed. Clients are often self-conscious about visiting a salon, particularly the first time, for a number of reasons. They may be embarrassed about their size, shape, age, skin condition, superfluous hair, or a host of other things which may or may not be immediately apparent to you, and these feelings may manifest as either introvert or aggressive behaviour. Your job is to make clients feel comfortable and confident that you will treat them with the utmost respect during their visit. Never judge; never interfere with medical advice; never gossip to friends, colleagues or other clients about what you have seen or heard at work. Gossip tends to travel fast, become distorted and find its way back to the source. In the real world the customer may not always be right but the client must always be your top priority. If you aim to treat each client as a welcome guest you will both benefit from the experience.

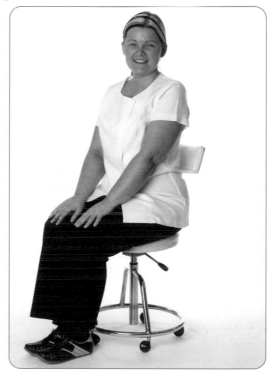

A high standard of professional appearance is important at work.

Salon considerations

Your place of work is likely to be a bright, warm, busy environment with lots of different people coming and going all the time. It is the ideal breeding ground for disease-causing **micro-organisms**, as well as being a place where potentially dangerous chemicals and equipment are stored and used. You must uphold strict standards in order to minimise health and safety risks and to conform with government legislation such as the **Health and Safety at Work etc. Act (1974)**.

Salon health

The health of the salon depends on stringent procedures for **sterilisation** and **sanitation** being carried out by *all* people at *all* times. Half measures are not good enough. Trainee therapists often grumble about the amount of cleaning involved in their job; however, if it is carried out regularly and as an integral part of every treatment, it will not become a chore. All trolleys, equipment and work areas should be wiped with an anti-bacterial cleaning solution before and after use. Fresh towels, capes and couch roll should be used for every client. Product containers should be wiped clean and stored safely. Small items, such as manicure equipment and tweezers, should be sterilised between clients; brushes and sponges should be sanitised; and items such as cotton wool and tissues should be disposed of. The salon should have appropriate methods of disposal for **clinical waste** such as used needles and **micro-lances**. Before each client arrives it is your responsibility to make sure your that your work area has been sanitised and prepared neatly with all the products and sterilised equipment you need. This will ensure the health, safety and efficiency of the treatment.

Salon sterilisation

Sterilisation is the complete destruction of all living micro-organisms to help prevent the spread of disease. Sanitation is the partial destruction of some micro-organisms, which can help prevent cross-infection. In a salon environment, where tools and equipment are used on a number of different individuals, it is vital to maintain high standards of sterilisation. This can be done in a number of ways.

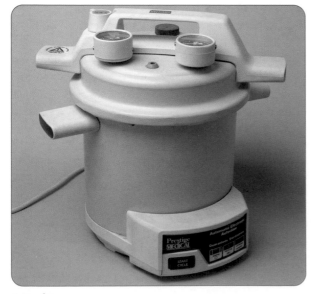

Autoclave.

Autoclave

The autoclave resembles a pressure cooker. It works by changing a reservoir of distilled water to steam at temperatures of between 121–134 degrees Celsius. Small metal and glass items can be sterilised in this way although it is not suitable for plastic items which would melt at such extreme temperatures. The autoclave takes about 15 minutes to reach optimum temperature for sterilisation; different models have different programmes lasting about 15 to 20 minutes.

Glass bead sterilisers

The glass bead steriliser is an electrically-operated metal container about the size of a tumbler, which contains thousands of tiny glass beads. It reaches temperatures of between 190–300 degree Celsius, which must be maintained for 30 to 60 minutes prior to use for optimum sterilisation to occur. This method has limited use because it is only suitable for small metal equipment. It is commonly used by electrologysts and facialists for the fast sterilisation of tweezers.

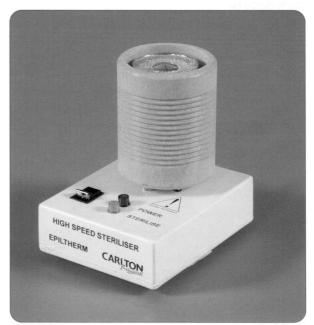

Glass bead steriliser.

Chemical sterilisers

Chemical methods of sterilisation vary according to the product used. Some chemical agents fully sterilise equipment while others merely sanitise it; always check the manufacturer's instructions. A common chemical steriliser for salon use is bactericide, which kills bacteria and can be used for all small equipment.

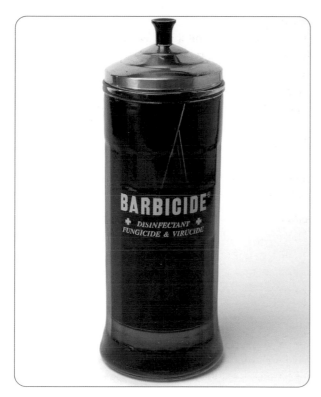

Bactericide jar.

Ultraviolet cabinets

Direct exposure to UV light will inactivate bacteria; however, this is difficult to achieve. The strength of UV in cabinets varies according to position of the equipment in the cabinet and any shaded areas; for example, the blades of scissors or the underside of equipment receives limited exposure. UV cabinets are therefore generally used for storing equipment that has been sterilised by other methods or for sanitising items such as brushes and sponges.

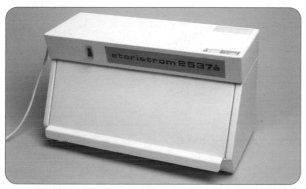

UV cabinet.

Salon safety

How many people come and go in your salon every day? Ten; twenty; more? If all of these people rushed around without due care and attention, not putting things away and ignoring hazards, it would be a very dangerous place to work or visit. Salon safety is basic common sense because you put people at risk if you ignore the rules. Your own personal effects should be stored away, ideally in a locker or staff room. Anything valuable belonging to the client, such as jewellery, which has to be removed, should be returned for safe keeping, clothes, shoes and bags should be stored out of the way in a locker or under the treatment couch. You should also be aware of other trip hazards, such as stools and electrical cable. Spillages should be wiped up immediately and faulty equipment should be labelled for repair.

Salon stock and equipment

Even the smallest of salons will contain thousands of pounds worth of stock and equipment which must be treated with respect. All products must be labelled and stored correctly according to government legislation for the **Control of Substances Hazardous to Health 2003 (Amendment) Regulations (COSHH)** and the **Cosmetic Products (Safety) Regulations (1996)**, to avoid careless mistakes or accidents. Equipment must be checked regularly and any faults reported and repaired. Stock and equipment can be divided into:

▸ consumables, which are disposable items or things that are 'used up'
▸ semi-consumables, which are not disposable but do occasionally need to be replaced
▸ non-consumables, which is small equipment such as personal tools and large equipment such as specialist machinery and furniture.

Consumables	Semi-consumables	Non-consumables
all products	towels	furniture
cotton wool	blankets	equipment
tissues	uniforms	small tools
wooden spatulas	plastic spatulas	couch
couch roll	headbands	
micro-lances	gowns	
needles	sponges	
wax strips	face cloths	
	turbans	

Theory into practice

Occasionally, things go wrong no matter what you do. However, being prepared can prevent a small mistake from turning into a major crisis. Knowing how to cope is a skill acquired through knowledge and experience.

▸▸ How will you avoid potential dangers in the salon?
▸▸ Think about how you would react if things went wrong.

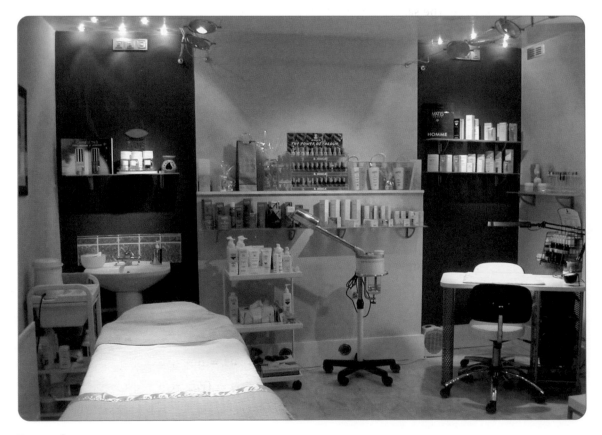

Beauty therapy treatment area.

Scientific principles for beauty therapy

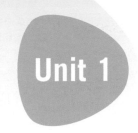

Unit 1

This unit introduces you to the basic scientific principles which are relevant to the study of beauty therapy. The knowledge of biological and physical principles gained here will help you to understand the scientific basis of the treatments and equipment used. This information will also alert you to some of the potential health and safety hazards in beauty therapy.

The first part of the unit explores biological principles: the structure and function of proteins, lipids and carbohydrates, and the structure and function of cells. The second part covers the physical principles associated with electricity and the electromagnetic spectra.

In order to achieve Unit 1 in Scientific principles for beauty therapy you must complete the following learning outcomes:

LEARNING OUTCOMES

1. Review the structure and functions of the major biological chemicals.

2. Analyse the structure and function of cells.

3. Describe the properties and applications of the main regions of the electromagnetic spectra.

4. Investigate the safe use of electricity.

The structure and functions of biological chemicals

There is a link between the study of biological chemicals and the process of digestion which is discussed in Unit 2: Human physiology. You should refer to Unit 2 (pages 15–52) for sources and functions of carbohydrates, proteins and lipids as well as a detailed discussion of metabolism.

Structure of carbohydrates

Carbohydrates, as their name suggests, are made up of carbon, hydrogen and oxygen and have the general formula $(CH_2O)n$. They can be divided into and sourced from sugars, starch and cellulose. The simplest form of carbohydrates are simple sugars known as **monosaccharides**. These include glucose, fructose (from fruit) and galactose (from milk). These monosaccharides share the same formula, which has six carbon atoms in each molecule: $C_6H_{12}O_6$, but the arrangement of atoms varies between the different molecules; for example:

$$CHO - CHOH - CHOH - CHOH - CHOH - CH_2OH = glucose$$

$$CH_2OH - CO - CHOH - CHOH - CHOH - CH_2OH = fructose$$

Monosaccharides can combine to form more complex carbohydrates called **disaccharides**. Disaccharides are formed when two monosaccharide molecules join together under certain conditions (which are reversible). Disaccharides are insoluble but can be converted back into monosaccharides and transported in the body to release energy. Examples of disaccharides are maltose, sucrose and lactose.

When many monosaccharides combine they form large molecules called **polysaccharides**; for example, starch and cellulose are both polysaccharides made from glucose. Starch is obtained from foods which provide 'bulk', such as bread, rice and cereals. Glycogen is also a **polymer** of glucose and is the form in which carbohydrates are stored in the liver and muscles, to be later released as energy. Cellulose, or fibre, is a complex carbohydrate which is indigestible in the human body but is necessary to maintain the health of the digestive tract. It is obtained from green vegetables, cereals and dried and fresh fruits.

Function of carbohydrates

The chief function of carbohydrates is to provide energy. The process of cellular respiration **oxidises** starch and sugar to release energy in the form of **adenosine triphosphate** (ATP, see page 18). Respiration is the opposite process of **photosynthesis** whereby plants use energy obtained from sunlight to manufacture glucose. Energy is trapped in the carbon–hydrogen bonds of the glucose molecules which the body obtains from food and can break down to release energy. Energy is measured in calories but these units are so small that what we accurately use for measuring energy are kilocalories.

Structure of proteins

Proteins are made up of long chains of **amino acids** of which there are 23 different types. Thirteen of these can be manufactured by the human body in sufficient quantities while the remaining ten must be obtained from a balanced diet. The essential amino acids are obtained from animal proteins such as milk, cheese and eggs, and are called first class or complete proteins. Vegetable proteins are of low biological value because they lack some of the essential amino acids and are therefore called incomplete or second class proteins. Proteins in the diet are broken down into their constituent amino acids, which are then used to manufacture different types of proteins in to a source that can be used by the body, e.g. enzymes.

There are two types of protein. Fibrous proteins contain insoluble filaments and therefore have mainly structural roles, e.g. **collagen** in connective tissue and **keratin** in skin. Globular proteins are more soluble and are therefore able to take part in chemical reactions in the body, e.g. **haemoglobin** in blood and enzymes such as salivary amylase.

Theory into practice

Study the list of amino acids below. Do you recognise any of their names? Can you remember (or work out) the function of those you recognise?

Amino Acids

can be manufactured:	cannot be manufactured:
alanine	arginine*
aspartic acid	histidine*
cysteine	isoleucine
cystine	leucine
diiodotyrosine	lysine
glutamic acid	methionine
glycine	phenylalanine
hydroxylysine	threonine
hdroxproline	tryptophane
proline	valinethyroxine
tyrosine	
serine	(*can be made in small quantities)

Function of proteins

Proteins are responsible for a variety of functions in the human body associated with support, transport and protection. Their main function is to build tissue, and protein is a chief component of plasma membrane. It is therefore imperative that the body

Function of proteins:

Type of protein	Name of protein	Function
▸▸ support	▸▸ collagen and elastin	▸▸ provides strength and elastic qualities in connective tissue
▸▸ enzymes	▸▸ pepsin	▸▸ digests protein
	▸▸ lipase	▸▸ digests lipids (fats)
▸▸ hormones	▸▸ insulin	▸▸ regulates blood glucose levels
	▸▸ thyroxin	▸▸ regulates metabolism
▸▸ globular proteins	▸▸ haemoglobin	▸▸ transports oxygen in the form of oxyhaemoglobin
▸▸ contractile proteins	▸▸ actin and myosin	▸▸ contract muscle as one protein 'walks over' the other
▸▸ protection	▸▸ fibrinogen	▸▸ involved in blood clotting

has adequate supplies of protein during times when new cells and tissues are being manufactured, such as infancy, adolescence and pregnancy.

Structure of lipids

Lipids are solid fats and liquid fats or oils which are insoluble in water. They contain carbon, hydrogen and oxygen, like carbohydrates, but the ratio of oxygen to carbon and hydrogen is lower in lipids. As with carbohydrates, lipids also take different forms: monoglycerides, diglycerides and **triglycerides**. Lipids in foods are mostly triglycerides, which are the combination of one unit of glycerol and three units of fatty acid. When fats are broken down during the process of digestion they are split into their constituent parts – glycerol and fatty acid – which can be absorbed into the cells.

You may be familiar with the terms saturated and unsaturated in association with fats but unfamiliar with their definitions. One molecule of lipid fully saturated with hydrogen atoms is said to be a saturated lipid; if it is not saturated with hydrogen it is described as an unsaturated lipid. We require unsaturated fats, called essential fatty acids, which have a role in the formation of plasma membranes, the manufacture of hormones and immunity. Good dietary sources are fish and vegetable or seed oils.

Function of lipids:

Function of lipids	Detail
Storage and release of energy	Sourced from triglycerides in the diet and stored as adipose tissue. Fat is dense and insoluble which makes it a good store for energy.
Insulation	The subcutaneous 'fatty layer' lies beneath the dermis. The properties which make fat a good area for storing energy also mean it offers good insulation.
Protection	The subcutaneous layer protects the bones from knocks and bangs. Lipids also surround, insulate and protect the internal organs.
Transport	Triglycerides are liquid at body temperature and carry the fat soluble vitamins (A,D,E,K) to the small intestine as well as aiding their absorption.

Assessment task 1.1

Describe the structure and function of carbohydrates, proteins and lipids. (M)

Metabolism

Metabolism is the collective term given to all physical and chemical changes that take place in tissues and cells. **Catabolism** refers to all processes whereby larger molecules are broken down into smaller ones and energy is released, such as the digestion of food. **Anabolism** refers to all processes whereby smaller molecules are built up into larger ones, which requires the addition of energy. The functions of metabolism can be summarised as the provision of energy in the form of adenosine triphosphate (ATP) and the exchange of carbon between molecules. Every process which uses energy is dependent on the functions of metabolism, such as digestion, which breaks down molecules into more usable substances for energy and raw materials. **Glycolysis** is the metabolic process of breaking down glucose to produce pyruvic acid and ATP. Lipids are broken down into fatty acids and then, during glycolysis, are broken down further to produce carbon dioxide, water and ATP. Amino acids, produced during the synthesis of proteins, can also be broken down to produce energy.

Fact file

Sources of energy
1g of carbohydrate = 4.3 kcal
1g of protein = 4.3 kcal
1g of fat = 9.3 kcal

The structure and function of cells

The cell is the basic building block of all life forms. There are many types of cell in the human body which vary in size, structure and function – there is no such thing as a 'typical cell'. However, cells do share certain structural characteristics.

Fact file

Prefix cyt = cells
cytology – the study of cells
cytolosis – the destruction of cells
cytoplasm – the protoplasm within cells

Structure of cells

Cells are minute structures which can only be studied using specialist viewing equipment called microscopes. There are two types of microscope: light microscopes use light beams and are useful for viewing tissues and larger cells; electron microscopes use beams of electrons and provide much greater magnification in order to study the interior of human cells.

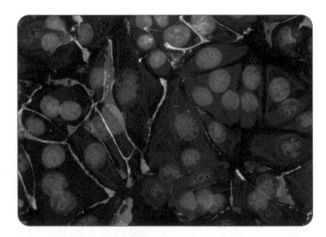

Cells viewed under a light microscope (x300).

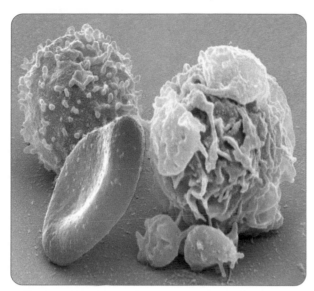

Before the first electron microscopes, in the 1940s, the interior of human cells was described by scientists as a structureless soup. Since then, greater magnification has highlighted the specific structure of cells and the complex reactions that take place within them. The structure of cells viewed through electron microscopes is sometimes called the ultra-structure, to emphasise the high levels of magnification required. Different parts of the ultra-structure are known collectively as **organelles**.

Theory into practice

Try to think of the names of some specific cells of the human body and their functions.

Cells viewed under an electron microscope (x1000).

Structure and function of cell organelles:

Cell organelle	Structure	Function
Plasma/cell membrane	Outer or cell membrane: layer of lipids sandwiched between two layers of larger protein molecules.	Allows selective permeability, the passive transport of fat soluble substances, and the active transport of charged particles.
Mitochondria	Rod shaped with double membrane: outer membrane is similar to plasma membrane; inner membrane is folded into ridges.	Contains enzymes which convert ADP into ATP to provide energy. Mitochondria are more abundant in high energy cells such as muscle and liver cells.
Ribosomes	Some attached to rough ER, some remain free in cytoplasm; contain ribonucleic acid (RNA).	Manufactures enzymes and proteins both for export and for use within the cell.
Endoplastic reticulum (ER)	Network of branches; similar structure to and continuous with plasma membrane. Rough ER is studded with ribosomes.	Contributes to cell support and channels transport materials within the cell. Rough ER with ribosomes produces proteins and enzymes; smooth ER produces phospholipids and steroids.
Gogli apparatus	Similar to smooth ER with vesicles that contain proteins and enzymes, lipids, collagen and mucus.	Produces collagen and mucus and keeps all secretions away from cytoplasm. Is best developed in secretory cells such as those in the pancreas and salivary glands.
Lysosomes	Powerful enzyme produced as vesicles from the Gogli apparatus.	Breaks down bacteria and destroys damaged cell structures and extracellular matter, e.g. osteoclasts in bone formation.
Nucleus	Largest cell structure, containing a double layered membrane continous with the ER. Contains a tangled mass of chromatin made up of DNA and protein.	Controls all cellular activities. Contains genetic material and nucleic acids (DNA and RNA).

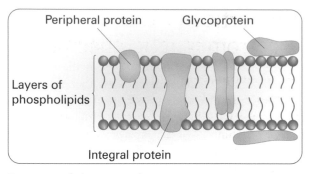

Structure of plasma membrane.

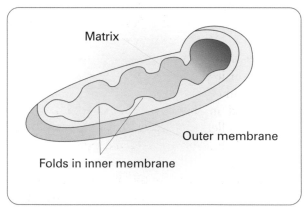

Structure of mitochondria.

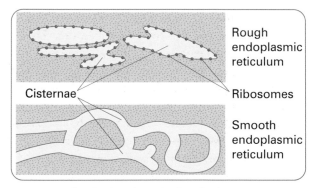

Structure of endoplasmic reticulum (ER).

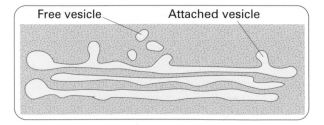

Structure of Gogli apparatus.

Assessment task 1.2

Identify and describe the basic structure and function of cells and cell organelles. (M)

Transport in cells

As you have learnt, cells export some materials out of the cell body and also receive substances from outside. There are three methods of transport in cells: diffusion, osmosis and active transport.

Diffusion

Diffusion is the mixing together of molecules of a liquid or gas so that they become equally distributed between two regions. Molecules are in a constant state of movement. In solids this is more of a vibration in order that the substance remains fixed; however, in liquids and especially gases the molecules move freely within the structure or apparatus which contains them. In order for diffusion to take place there must be a difference in levels of concentration, known as the concentration gradient, and a permeable barrier (or no barrier at all). Molecules in an area of high concentration pass through the barrier to an area of lower concentration, thus balancing the numbers of molecules on each side and creating equilibrium. The state of equilibrium stops further diffusion but the molecules still move around freely in their own region. The rate of diffusion is affected by body temperature and the surface area of the barrier between the two areas of different levels of concentration: the higher the temperature and the larger the surface area, the greater the rate of diffusion.

The process of diffusion can be illustrated by gaseous exchange, which takes place during respiration: high levels of oxygen in the alveoli diffuse into the low levels of oxygen in the veins. Meanwhile, carbon dioxide diffuses from a region of high concentration in the blood vessels to a region of low concentration in the alveoli. (Respiration is discussed in detail in Unit 2: Human physiology, pages 57–9). The transport of gases in the bloodstream is a continuous process so the state of equilibrium is not desirable. A high concentration of oxygen in the lungs is constantly 'topped up' as we inhale more air, and carbon dioxide levels in the blood are replenished by the removal of waste products from all areas of the body.

Osmosis

Osmosis is a particular kind of diffusion that involves the transport of a liquid from an area of *low* concentration to an area of *high*er concentration through a semi-permeable membrane. A simple illustration is the passage of water from a weak sugar solution to a strong sugar solution through a semi-permeable membrane. The molecules of sugar are too big to pass through the membrane but the smaller water molecules are not. The strong sugar solution therefore becomes diluted and the two solutions are of equal concentration.

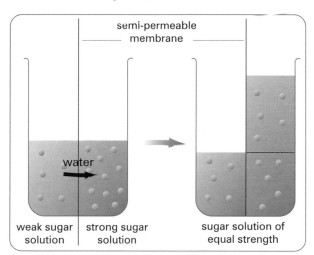

Osmosis.

Active transport

The transport of solid matter from an area of *low* concentration to an area of *higher* concentration through a semi-permeable membrane cannot be explained by diffusion or osmosis and is known as active transport. Transporting material against a concentration gradient requires energy and so only occurs in cells which contain a store of energy in the form of adenosine triphosphate (ATP). Factors that affect the rate of active transport include the quantity of energy available, the surface area to be covered and the concentration gradient. The movement of glucose across the lining of the digestive tract is one example of active transport. (Digestion is discussed in detail in Unit 2: Human physiology, pages 44–52.)

Theory into practice

Return to this section after you have studied Unit 2: Human Physiology and provide further examples of diffusion, osmosis and active transport which occur in the body.

Assessment task 1.3

Describe in detail how the structure and function of cells and cell organelles relates to their function. (D)

Properties of the electromagnetic spectra

Wave properties

Light and sound are both waves; however, it's hard to imagine what light and sound waves are like. It's easier to think of water waves when we want to understand the properties of light and sound.

Imagine that you are in a swimming pool that has a wave machine. When the wave machine is switched off, the water will be flat (no swimmers are allowed in this pool!). Now switch the wave machine on. Waves will move across the pool. As the waves move, the water will be higher in some places than it was with the machine switched off, and lower in other places.

We could measure the *speed* of the waves (in metres travelled each second). Water waves travel quite slowly but sound waves and light waves travel much faster.

We could also measure the distance between the top of one wave and the top of the wave next to it. This is called the *wavelength* of the waves (and is measured in metres).

Now let's measure how high the tops of the waves are above the starting level of the water. This is called the *wave amplitude* and is also measured in metres. Bigger waves have larger amplitudes and will be more powerful. The amplitude of a wave is a measure of its power.

How long does it take for one wave to be replaced by the next wave? This is the *periodic time* (and will be measured in seconds). For water waves the periodic time may be one or two seconds but for sound and light waves the value will be a lot less.

Finally, how many waves pass you in one second? This is the *frequency* and is measured in hertz (one hertz means one wave per second). For water waves, this will be a small number (it may be less than one

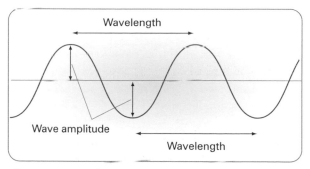

The properties of a wave.

hertz) but for sound and water waves, the frequencies can be very high. For example, ultraviolet light has a frequency of about 15000 million million hertz!

An important equation

If we multiply the *frequency* of the waves by the *wavelength*, we will find that the answer is the same as the *speed* of the wave:

Wave speed = frequency × wavelength

Using the following symbols: *ws* for wave speed; *f* for frequency; and λ for wavelength, the equation is **ws = f × λ**.

This equation can be used to calculate the value of one of the three things provided that we know the values of the other two. You may have used triangles to help you with this type of calculation.

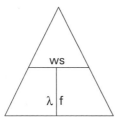

Suppose we know the speed of a wave to be 340 m/s (this is about the speed of sound in air) and the frequency to be 3400 hertz (*hertz* means the same as *per second*). We need to calculate the wavelength (λ). Put your finger over the λ symbol in the triangle. The triangle tells us to divide the speed (ws) by the frequency (f) to get the value of the wavelength.

Try it! You should get a value of 0.1 metre (or 10 cm). This might seem quite small but the wavelengths of light are very much smaller than this. To be able to use this method for parts of the electromagnetic spectrum, you will have to be able to work with very large and very small numbers. For example, the speed of light is 3,000,000 metres per second, often written as 3×10^8 m/s.

Two types of wave

As we said above, both light and sound are waves. However, they are different types of wave. Sound is a longitudinal wave while light is a transverse wave.

Sound and light are different in a number of other ways, which are described below.

⟩⟩ *Speed*

Sound travels quite fast in air, about 330 metres per second. Compare this with a car travelling at

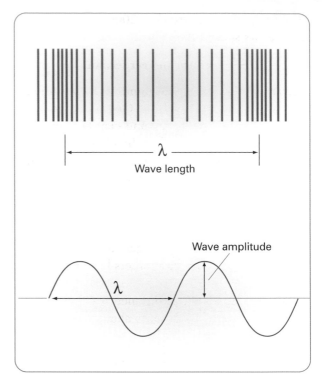

Longitudinal and transverse waves.

70 miles per hour, which is about 12 metres per second. Sound travels even faster in solids, at up to 5000 metres per second. However these values are really slow compared with the speed of light, which is 3,000,000 metres per second in a vacuum. Note that all parts of the electromagnetic spectrum travel at this speed. The fact that we see a firework explode before we hear it is explained by the differences in the speed of light and sound.

⟩⟩ *Medium*

Sound can travel through gases (such as air), liquids (such as water) and solids. However, it cannot travel through a vacuum. Sound needs a *medium* to travel through; in other words, a gas, liquid or solid. Light, on the other hand, does not need a medium and can travel through a vacuum. This must be the case since light has to travel through the vacuum of space to get from the sun to us.

Measuring the speed of light and sound

Calculating the speed of a car is not difficult. All we have to remember is that speed is given by dividing the distance travelled by the time taken. The equation is:

$$\text{speed} = \frac{\text{distance}}{\text{time}}.$$

Therefore, if a car travels 2000 metres in 40 seconds, its speed is:

$$\frac{2000}{40} = 50 \text{ metres per second.}$$

Measuring the speed of sound is more difficult because sound travels so fast. One way is to stand 50 metres away from a wall and clap two pieces of wood together. The sound of the clap will travel to the wall and bounce back. When the echo reaches you it will have travelled 100 metres.

If you clap again exactly when the echo reaches you, the sound again goes to the wall and back. The total distance is now 200 metres. Keep repeating, clapping exactly as the echo gets to you each time (some people find this easy, others have no sense of rhythm!).

Do this until the total distance is 3000 metres. You should find that this takes about 9 seconds. In other words:

$$\text{speed} = \frac{\text{distance}}{\text{time}} = \frac{3000}{9} = 333 \text{ metres per second}$$

Measuring the speed of light is, of course, more difficult again because light is much faster than sound. Special equipment is needed although this is available in many schools and colleges. The basic idea is the same: find the time taken to travel a certain distance and use the equation:

$$\text{speed} = \frac{\text{distance}}{\text{time}}.$$

The electromagnetic spectrum

Take a CD disk and hold it up to a bright light. As you turn it, you will see the colours of the visible spectrum. The white light that falls onto the disk splits into the colours of the rainbow (often given as red, yellow, green, blue, indigo and violet).

The visible spectrum is only a small part of what is known as the electromagnetic spectrum (the ems), which also includes ultraviolet (UV), infrared (IR) and microwaves.

All parts of the ems travel at the same speed in a vacuum but have different wavelengths and frequencies. All parts of the ems carry energy, but those with shorter wavelengths are more energetic. Wavelengths shorter than those in the blue region of the ems can cause chemical reactions whereas those with longer wavelengths do not. Ultraviolet, gamma rays and X-rays may be dangerous because of this. However, microwaves can be dangerous because they can heat body tissues up.

Assessment task 1.4

Describe the main regions of the electromagnetic spectrum in terms of the associated radiation. (P)

The ultraviolet spectrum

The ultraviolet (UV) spectrum is the part of the ems that has wavelengths between 10 and 400 nanometres. UV rays come from the sun and, of course, sun beds. It is usual to divide the UV spectrum into three regions: UVA, UVB and UVC, where UVC has the smallest wavelengths and the highest energy.

▸▸ UVA is the least energetic form of UV. Unlike UVB, these rays are present all the year round and can penetrate deep into the dermis of the skin. As a result, prolonged exposure over a number of years may increase the chance of skin cancer and lead to skin aging. (A is for ageing.)

▸▸ UVB is a stronger form of UV and causes sunburn (or even sunstroke) if we are exposed to too much sunlight at one time. Very little UVB is present during the winter in Britain and it does

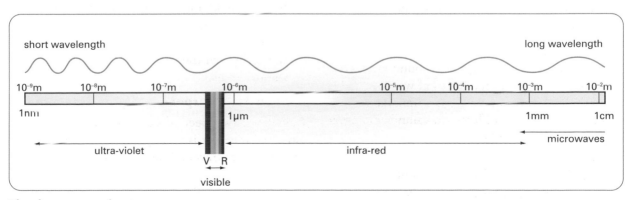

The electromagnetic spectrum.

not penetrate very far into our skin. However, it can easily cause burning. (B is for burning.)

» UVC is the highest energy form of UV and is dangerous. Fortunately, UVC from the Sun is stopped by the ozone layer at the top of the atmosphere. Some lamps designed to kill germs produce high-energy UV rays and would be dangerous to human tissue. However, these lamps should have safety devices to ensure that this does not happen.

The benefits and hazards of UV:

Benefits	Hazards
When UV irradiates skin, it produces vitamin D that is needed for good health	Skin ageing (mainly UVA)
UVB and higher energy UVA trigger melanin production in the skin, which leads to tanning	Sunburn and sunstroke (mainly UVB)
	Skin cancer
	Eye damage

UV protection

» Eyes should be protected with good quality sunglasses. Eye protection is particularly important for sunbed users. Poor quality sunglasses, which are dark but give poor UV absorption, can be dangerous, especially for young children. These glasses will cause eye-dilation because they are dark and allow more UV to enter the eye as a result.

» Skin can be protected by use of sunscreens. These have a SPF rating (sun protection factor) that shows how effective they are against UVB. UVA protection is now included in many products and this is shown by the Star Rating System.

Electricity

Electrical terminology

Everyone who uses electricity (and that is nearly everybody) must use it safely. The dangers of electricity are described in the section on Electrical safety (see pages 25–6). To use electricity correctly, we need to know what is happening in electrical appliances and some of the electrical terms used.

Electricity is a very convenient way of moving energy from one place to another, so that it can be used. Mains electricity is generated in power stations that may be a long distance from the places where we will use the energy, i.e. where we live and work. Simply by plugging appliances into the mains sockets, the energy is available for us to use in various forms.

The diagram below shows a simple circuit, which you may have seen at school or college. Energy is stored in the battery. When an electric current flows in the wires, energy is carried by the current to the bulb. The bulb uses the energy to get hot.

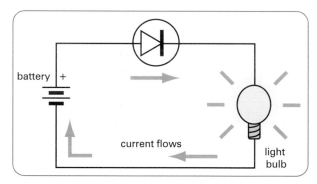

A simple circuit.

The following terms are used to describe what happens in electrical circuits:

» **Current** is the flow of electricity. We measure currents in amperes (usually shortened to amps or abbreviated to A). We can compare the current in a circuit to the flow of water in pipes.

» **Direct current (dc)** means that the current always flows in the same direction. This is what happens in the circuit shown above, and also when a mobile phone is recharged.

» **Alternating current (ac):** the electricity from the mains is ac, meaning that the direction of the current is always reversing (alternating). In Europe, the frequency of the ac supply is 50 Hz (which means that the direction of the current is reversed 100 times a second).

- **Potential difference (or voltage):** this can be thought of as the push that makes the current flow. It is usually called the voltage and is measured in volts. The voltage from the mains is about 230 volts. If we increase the potential difference across an appliance, the current will increase.
- **Resistance (ohms):** all electrical circuits have resistance. This is a measure of how hard it is for the current to flow around the circuit; high resistances will mean small currents. Resistance is measured in ohms.
- **Power (watts):** this is how we measure how much energy an appliance uses each second. We measure power in watts. For example, a lightbulb may be labelled as 60 watts while a kettle may be labelled as 2200 watts (or 2.2 kilowatts – 'kilo' means 'thousand'). The potential difference (voltage) will be the same for the lightbulb and the kettle at 230 volts. As we might expect, the kettle will require a larger current flowing though it (about 9.5 amps) than the bulb (about ¼ amp).

Ohm's law and electrical circuits

Ohm's law states that the current which flows though a circuit will vary in direct proportion to the potential difference, and in inverse proportion to the resistance. Therefore, if the potential difference increases, so does the current; but if the resistance increases, the current decreases.

> **Fact** file
>
> The equation for Ohm's law is:
>
> $$\text{current (amps)} = \frac{\text{potential difference (volts)}}{\text{resistance (ohms)}}$$
>
> This formula can be remembered by using a triangle (as with wavelengths).

Electrical safety

The electrical appliances we use at home and at work can be dangerous if not used correctly. The hazards include:

- **Electrocution:** the mains supply (at 230 volts) can deliver a large enough current through our bodies to injure or kill us. A fatal current can be as low as 0.1 amps.

- **Electrical fires:** faulty appliances and overloaded adaptors can lead to overheating and fires.
- **Explosions:** electrical switches can give the spark needed for a gas leak to explode.
- **Tripping:** badly positioned appliances can lead to people falling over them or tripping over the wires.

Both employers and employees have responsibilities under the **Electricity at Work Regulations (1989)** to ensure that electrical equipment is used safely. The following rules should be observed:

- Store equipment in the correct place when not in use, with all the wires and attachments securely fixed.
- Equipment with twisted, worn or frayed wires or with cracked or loose plugs should not be used.
- Do not overload plug sockets by using multiple adaptors. Check that plugs have the correct fuse.
- When using equipment, make sure that it is on a stable surface, away from water and that the leads cannot be tripped over.
- Keep your hands dry when touching equipment or plugs.
- Read and follow the manufacturers' instructions.

Safety features

Modern electrical appliances have a number of features designed to ensure safe use:

Fuses

All 3-pin plugs have fuses fitted. Some appliances may have other fuses fitted to them. A fuse is a deliberate weak spot in a circuit that is designed to 'blow' if the current flowing through it is too large.

Replace blown fuses with a fuse of the correct rating. If fuses keep blowing, the appliance is faulty and should be checked by an expert before further use. Note that fuses by themselves do not protect against electrocution, but do offer protection from overheating.

Earthing

The largest pin on a 3-pin plug is known as the earth pin. No current flows through this pin if the appliance is working correctly. When certain types of fault occur, current flows through the earth pin and allows the fuse to blow. The earth pin and the connections to it are important safety features since they give protection against electrocution.

Metal water pipes should also be earthed. This is done using wires with green and yellow striped plastic coating. This helps to prevent electrocution; if a live wire happens to touch a pipe, the pipe will be dangerous. If the pipe is connected to earth, current will flow to earth through the wires and the fuse will blow.

Double insulated appliances

Some appliances such as hairdryers are double insulated. As the name implies, this means that the electrical mechanisms are protected by two layers of insulated material and are not earthed.

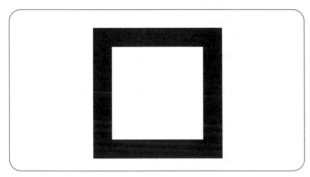

This symbol appears on double insulated appliances.

Double insulated appliances do not need earthing. They may have a plug with a rigid plastic pin rather than a metal one.

Residual current circuit breaker

The two smaller pins on a 3-pin plug are called the *live* pin and the *neutral* pin. If the appliance is working correctly, the current flowing in the two pins will be equal. If a fault develops and current starts to flow through you, less current will be coming out of the appliance through the neutral pin than is going into the appliance through the live pin (because some is going out through you!). A residual current circuit breaker is designed to detect that the currents flowing in the two pins are not equal and switch off the circuit before you are electrocuted.

Assessment task 1.6

Consider the risk involved in using facial and body electrotherapy equipment. As a beauty therapist, what precautions would you take to ensure the electrical safety of you and your clients?

Cost of electricity

We pay for the electrical energy we use. This is measured in kilowatt–hours (sometimes called units). To calculate the cost of running an appliance, multiply the power of the appliance (measured in kilowatts) by the length of time of use (measured in hours). This gives the number of units used. Multiply this figure by the cost of each unit to get the total cost. For example, if we run a 3-kilowatt electric fire for six hours we will have used $3 \times 6 = 12$ kilowatt-hours. If the cost of one unit is 8p, then this will cost $12 \times 8 = 96$p.

Theory into practice

Calculate the cost of operating a 5kw sunbed for 1 week if I unit = 8p:
▶▶ Monday = 4 hours
▶▶ Tuesday = 6 hours
▶▶ Wednesday = 6 hours
▶▶ Thursday = 4 hours
▶▶ Friday = 10 hours
▶▶ Saturday = 10 hours.
The salon charges £6 for a 15-minute session on the sunbed. How much profit will be made from the bookings shown above?

Knowledge check

1 Explain the difference between monosaccharides, disaccharides and polysaccharides.

2 Define metabolism.

3 State the equation for respiration and explain its function in cells.

4 Illustrate and explain the methods of transport in cells.

5 Explain the differences between sound waves and electromagnetic waves.

6 Illustrate the main regions of the electromagnetic spectrum.

7 Describe Ohm's law.

8 Give the unit of measurement for current, potential difference, resistance and power.

9 Explain the features of the Electricity at Work Regulations Act (1989).

10 Present a diagam to illustrate the safe wiring of a 3-pin plug.

Human physiology

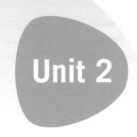

Unit 2

This unit introduces you to the functions or 'physiology' or the human body. You will investigate the biological organisation of cells, tissues, organs and organ systems. The principle of homeostasis and its role in maintaining an optimum internal environment is explored. You will study the regulation and co-ordination of the body systems by examining the nervous and endocrine systems.

Also in this unit you will investigate the structure and function of the body's systems of transport and digestion by examining the digestive, cardiovascular, respiratory, urinary and reproductive systems. This unit has links with Unit 5: Anatomy.

In order to achieve Unit 2 in Human physiology you must complete the following learning outcomes:

LEARNING OUTCOMES

1 Recognise the structure and function of tissues and organ systems.

2 Demonstrate understanding of the importance of homeostasis by examining the roles of the nervous and endocrine systems in the regulation and co-ordination of the body.

3 Explain the role of the digestive, cardiovascular, lymphatic, respiratory and urinary systems in transport in the body.

4 Explain the physiological basis of reproduction.

Tissues and organ systems

Biological organisation

In order to understand how the human body functions, we must first explore the different levels of biological organisation which are arranged in a hierarchy of structures. If any 'thing', biological or not, is broken down into its smallest individual particles, we would be left with a cluster of atoms. The name **atom** is derived from a Greek word meaning 'indivisible' and is used to describe a particle of matter which cannot be broken down any further. Atoms are so minuscule that it would take twenty million of even the largest atoms to stretch to just one centimetre.

Fact file

The human body consists of:
- ▸▸ 65% oxygen (O)
- ▸▸ 18.5% carbon (C)
- ▸▸ 9.5% hydrogen (H)
- ▸▸ 3.2% nitrogen (N)
- ▸▸ 3.8% trace elements – calcium, zinc, iron (Ca, Zn, Fe)

A substance which consists of only one type of atom is called an **element**. Most living organisms consist of the four elements hydrogen, carbon, nitrogen and oxygen. The human body contains 65 per cent oxygen (O), mostly in the form of water; 18.5 per cent carbon (C), which is found in all living things; 9.5 per cent hydrogen (H), which is a constituent of water and all food stuffs; and 3.2 per cent nitrogen (N), which is a component of proteins. You may have noticed that these four elements total 96.2 per cent of total body mass. The remaining 3.8 per cent comes from what are known as the *trace elements*. These are required by the body in very small amounts and include elements such as calcium (Ca), zinc (Zn) and iron (Fe), which the body acquires from food or food supplements.

Dissimilar atoms, when joined together, are known as **molecules**. The water molecule (H_2O) is a compound of the elements hydrogen and oxygen and is considered to be the basic ingredient for all life forms. Certain biological molecules contain hundreds of thousands of atoms and these structures are called **macromolecules**. All biological macromolecules contain the element carbon and these particles of living matter are sometimes known as **organic**. Carbon atoms can form many more different types of structure than any other element, and these organic structures are the building blocks of human life.

The types of food we eat, such as carbohydrates, fats and proteins, are examples of macromolecules. Despite containing so many hundreds of thousands

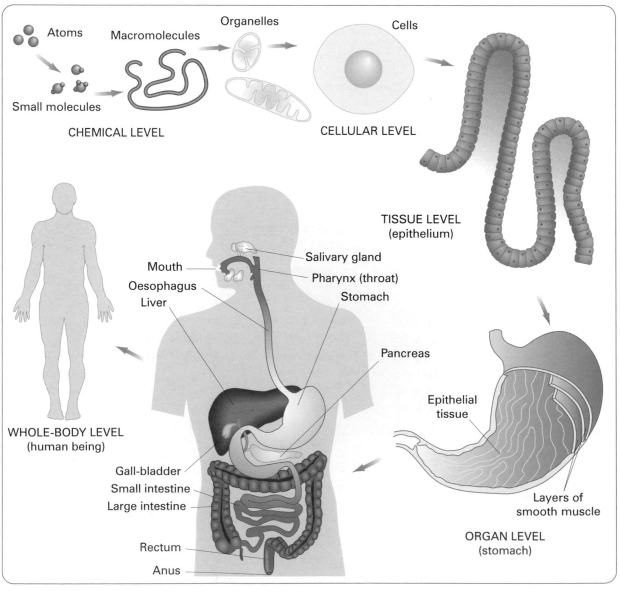

Levels of biological organisation.

of atoms, these structures are still minute. Even the very largest macromolecules are only just visible through the most powerful microscopes.

The smallest biological structure which is able to exist independently is the **cell**. A cell consists of dissolved macromolecules and other cellular structures called organelles, meaning 'little organs'. Many different types of cell make up the human body and each group of cells has its own distinct structure and function. For example, cells called melanocytes, which are found in the deepest layers of the skin, are responsible for producing the colour pigment melanin.

Fact file

Cells are microscopic structures that are so small that the finger of a newborn baby contains about ten billion individual cells.

Groups of cells with a shared structure and function are called **tissues**, of which the human body contains many types. For example, muscular tissue constructs muscle, connective tissue holds everything together, and blood is an example of a fluid tissue.

An **organ**, such as the heart, kidneys or skin, is a specialised structure which consists of different types of tissues organised in a specific way. Each organ has a particular and unique function. For example, the heart pumps blood around the body and to the lungs while the kidneys filter the blood to remove harmful waste substances.

The uppermost level of organisation is the **organ system**. This term is used to refer to a group of organs that work together. For example, in the circulatory or cardiovascular system, the heart works in conjunction with the vast network of blood vessels to pump blood around the body. In this way, the hierarchy of biological organisation, from the atom to the organ system, makes up the human body to produce a living, breathing, eating, reproducing and fully functioning person.

Tissues

A group of cells that all perform the same function is called a tissue. After fertilisation, cells multiply rapidly and form into different types of tissue in a process called **differentiation**. Some cells have more than one function and can therefore be classified as more than one type of tissue; for example, some cells of the immune system are also blood cells. Tissues can be classified into four main groups: epithelial, connective, muscular and nervous.

Epithelial tissue

Epithelial tissue (epithelium) provides the lining for surfaces inside and outside the body, protecting it from wear and tear and continually renewing itself as required. Epithelial tissue is also the tissue from which glands are developed. Lining epithelia can be sub-divided according to its structure; the various types are summarised in the table below and overleaf.

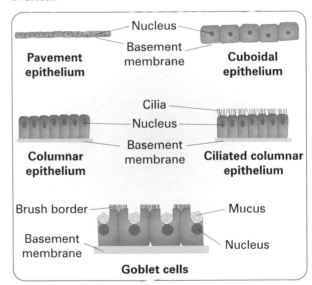

Types of epithelial tissue.

A summary of the structure and location of epithelial tissue:

Type of epithelial tissue	Structure	Location in the body
Simple pavement epithelium	Simple flat cells form a smooth lining	Lining the blood vessels
Simple cuboidal epithelium	Simple cube-shaped cells	Covering the ovaries
Simple columnar epithelium	Tall, column-shaped cells on a basement membrane, that provide greater protection against wear and tear	Lining the stomach and intestines

A summary of the structure and location of epithelial tissue (cont.):

Type of epithelial tissue	Structure	Location in the body
Ciliated columnar epithelium	Has hair-like projections which move mucus and other substances	Lining the respiratory tract
Stratified epithelium	Many layers of cells, flattened surface – process of keratinisation where surface epithelium is dry	Skin
Stratified epithelium	Flattened surface cells found in moist areas; cells survive longer and keratin is not formed	Lining of the mouth
Transitional epithelium	Similar to stratified epithelium but with rounded surface cells which adapt to expanding, waterproof organs	Bladder

Glands

Glands develop from epithelial tissue and can be classified as **exocrine** or **endocrine**. Endocrine glands secrete hormones directly into the bloodstream and are investigated later in this unit, pages 39–44. Exocrine glands pass their secretions through a single duct (simple glands; below) or through several secretory ducts (compound glands; see page 31). Many of these secretions contain enzymes, which produce chemical changes in specific substances but remain unchanged by the reaction. Exocrine glands are summarised in the table below.

A summary of the location and secretions of exocrine glands:

Type of exocrine gland	Location in the body	Secretions
Simple tubular glands	Walls of small intestine, stomach	Secrete substances which aid digestion
Simple coiled glands	Sweat glands in skin	Secrete sweat to control body temperature
Simple saccular glands	Sebaceous glands in skin	Secrete sebum which lubricates skin and hair
Compound tubular glands	Duodenum	Secrete substances which aid digestion
Compound saccular glands	Salivary glands in mouth	Secrete substances which aid digestion

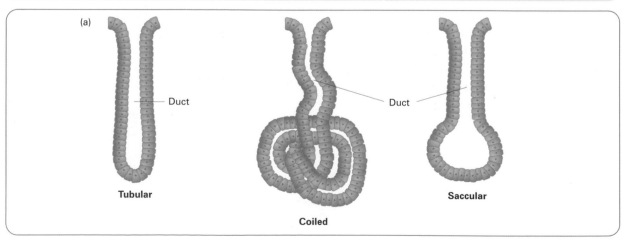

(a)

Tubular   Coiled   Saccular

Simple glands.

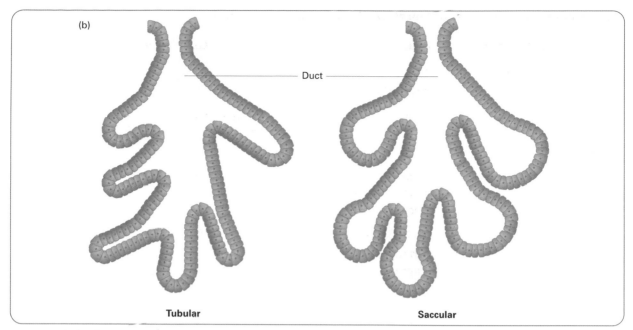

Duct

Tubular

Saccular

Compound glands.

Connective tissue

As the name suggests, connective tissue connects and supports all other types of tissue. It consists of living cells as well as non-living matrix and fibres. There are two types of fibres – collagenous and elastic. Collagenous fibres develop from cells called fibroblasts which secrete collagen, the main supporting cells of the body. These form coarse fibres that are formed into bundles. Elastic fibres allow for the stretchy or elastic properties required in some areas of the body, such as tendons and internal organs. There are five types of connective tissue which are summarised in the table at the top of the next page.

the table at the top of the next page.

Theory into practice

You will have explored some types of connective tissue in your studies of the skin and of the skeletal system. Try to remember the structures and functions of those you have learnt and then return to the relevant units to check your learning.

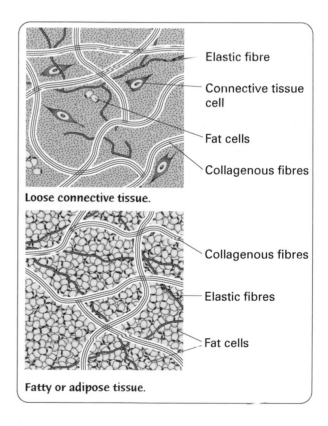

Elastic fibre

Connective tissue cell

Fat cells

Collagenous fibres

Loose connective tissue.

Collagenous fibres

Elastic fibres

Fat cells

Fatty or adipose tissue.

A summary of the five types of connective tissue:

Type of connective tissue	Structure	Location in the body
Loose connective tissue or areolar tissue	Loose network of collagenous and elastic fibres; few blood cells and nerves, some fat cells.	Forms tough, transparent lining between and within organs.
Fatty tissue or adipose tissue	Similar to areolar tissue but with network of fat cells which provides food reserves for the body and insulates against heat loss.	Protects delicate organs such as the kidneys.
Dense connective tissue or fibrous tissue	Bundles of strong collagenous fibres and fibroblasts arranged regularly or irregularly.	Regular bundles in tendons and ligaments, irregular arrangement in fascia surrounding muscles.
Cartilage	Cells called cohndrocytes separated by fibres; no blood vessels, tough and elastic.	Intervertebral discs
Bone tissue	Specialised type of cartilage which has undergone ossification; collagenous fibres provide strength and mineral salts provide rigidity; has a rich blood supply.	Bones of the human skeleton.

Assessment task 2.1

Identify the different types of tissues from the photograph below. (M)

Muscle tissue

Muscle cells, often called muscle fibres, are long and thin so that contraction produces skeletal movement. Muscle tissue can contract without firstly being stretched, unlike elastic connective tissue fibres. There are three types of muscular tissue, as summarised in the table overleaf.

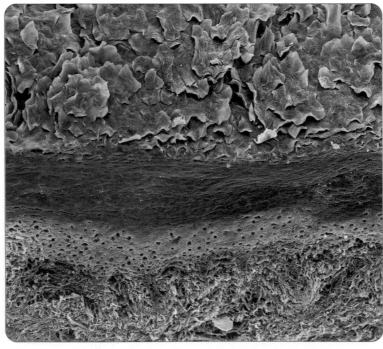

Skin tissue.

A summary of the three types of muscle tissue:

Type of muscle tissue	Structure	Function
Skeletal muscle (also known as voluntary muscle or striped muscle)	Long muscle cells/fibres containing striped myofibrils of actin and myosin bound together by connective tissue; rich blood supply provided by capillaried running between muscle cells.	Contracts strongly when stimulated to provide voluntary movement.
Smooth muscle or unstriped muscle	Spindle-shaped cells bound together by connective tissue, supplied by automatic nerves. Contracts automatically without conscious control to provide slow contractions over long periods of time.	Forms walls of blood vessels and internal organs including uterus, stomach and intestines.
Cardiac muscle	Short, cylindrical branched, with fibres bound together by connective tissue to allow nerve impulses to spread from one to another and along the muscle. Involuntary and irregularly striped. Contractions are rhythmic, controlled by nerves and occur automatically throughout life.	In the heart wall only.

Nervous tissue

Fact file

> The prefix *neu-* relates to the nervous system: neurology, neurones, neuroglia, neuralgia, neuritis, and so on.

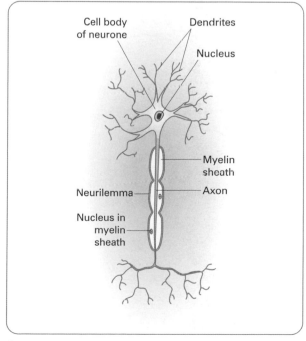

A neurone.

Nervous tissue consists of nerve cells called **neurones** and a supporting network called **neuroglia**. Neurones have a large cell body containing a nucleus as well as several short projections called **dendrites** and one long projection called an **axon**. The function of nervous tissue is to transmit messages or nervous impulses from inside or outside the body to other tissues in a process of communication. The dendrites import nervous impulses from other cells and tissues while the axon exports nervous impulses away from the cell body to other structures. You could think of dendrites as taking incoming calls and axons as making outgoing calls from a single neurone! The nervous system is explored in more detail later in this unit (see pages 33–9).

Theory into practice

> Try to find the definition of each of the prefix *neu-* words listed in this section. Can you find any other *neu-* words not listed here?

Assessment task 2.2

> Relate the structure of different types of connective tissue, muscle tissue and nervous tissue to its function. (D)

Organs and organ systems

A group of tissues functioning together is called an **organ**. The skin is an example of an organ which consists of epithelial tissue, connective tissue and muscular tissue. Organs can be classified as tubular or compact, and while each type shares some common structures, none are identical. All organs contain a blood supply.

One or more organs functioning together is called an **organ system**. The skeletal and muscular systems, sometimes known collectively as the skeletomuscular system, are discussed in Unit 5: Anatomy. The systems of the human body are explored later in this unit while a summary of the structure and role of each organ system is included in the table below.

Organs:

Type of organ	Structure	Example
Tubular organs	Three common layers: outer epithelium, middle muscular layer, inner endothelium, plus unique layers associated with its individual function and a space called a lumen.	Heart, small intestine
Compact organs	Superficial layers called the cortex, deeper layers called the medulla, no lumen.	Liver, kidney

A summary of the structure and role of the organ systems:

Organ system	Structure	Role
Circulatory system	Blood, heart and blood vessels: arteries, veins, arterioles, venules and capillaries	Transports oxygen and nutrients to the tissues in blood and carries waste away
Respiratory system	Mouth, nasal cavities, trachea, bronchii, bronchioles, lungs	Facilitates gaseous exchange (oxygen and carbon dioxide) between body and environment
Lymphatic system	Lymph, lymphatic vessels, lymph nodes, spleen	Filters and eliminates harmful bacteria and waste, produces lymphocytes which fight infection
Digestive system	Mouth, oesophagus, pancreas, liver, gall bladder, stomach, small and large intestines	Breaks down food and facilitates the absorption of nutrients and elimination of waste
Urinary system	Kidneys, bladder, ureter, urethra	Main excretory system, storage and elimination of urine
Nervous system	Central nervous system: brain and spinal cord, peripheral nervous system and sense organs	System of communication within body and between the body and the environment
Endocrine system	Endocrine glands: hypothalamus, pituitary, thyroid, adrenals, gonads and pancreas	Produces hormones which control many functions and facilitate homeostatic regulation
Skeletal system	Axial and appendicular skeleton, joints, cartilage and tendons	Supporting framework which provides protection and facilitates movement
Muscular system	Skeletal muscles	Facilitates movement in conjunction with skeletal system
Reproductive system	Male: penis, testis, epididymis, scrotum, sperm duct; female: ovaries, uterus, vagina, mammary glands	Hormonal regulation, menstrual cycle, fertilisation, pregnancy, birth, lactation, continuation of the species

Regulation and co-ordination of the body

Principles of homeostasis

Homeostasis is explored in other chapters of this book which are concerned with the functioning of the human body. Unit 5: Anatomy investigates bone homeostasis as well as homeostatic imbalances that affect bone tissue and homeostatic disorders of joints. Unit 6: Dermatology and Microbiology explores homeostasis in relation to the functions of the skin and wound healing.

Homeostasis is a key principle in physiology. It is concerned with maintaining the constancy of the internal environment despite changes in the external environment. Homeostasis is controlled by the various organs and organ systems which maintain stability or restore the normal internal state once it has been disturbed. For example, the urinary system is concerned with maintaining body water levels and salt concentration and, together with the respiratory system, it works to maintain the pH of blood. Bone remodelling is an example of homeostasis that involves the replacement of old, worn-out bone tissue with new tissue. Similarly, the constant process of renewal which takes place in the dermis, as hair, muscle cells, vascular tissue and collagen and elastin fibres are renewed, is a further example of homeostasis.

Fact file

Constancy in the internal environment was first described by French physiologists as *milieu interier*. Homeostasis comes from a Greek word meaning 'staying the same'.

In every cell there are thousands of different reactions occurring simultaneously which are catalysed by enzymes. As you have discovered, cells have specialised functions and therefore have sets of enzymes and reactions that are specific only to that cell. As well as these cell specific reactions, there are a set of so called 'housekeeping' reactions, which are core reactions that occur in every cell. An example of a core reaction is the regulation of other cell reactions and the production of the cell's energy in the form of ATP. The rate of each cell reaction must be regulated to ensure that the right amount of product, either a hormone or other secretion, is produced at the right time, and also that the amount of ATP produced is appropriate. These core reactions are concerned with maintaining a constant internal environment and are further illustrations of homeostasis.

Negative and positive feedback

As with the control of many physiological processes, the regulation of reactions occurring in cells is possible by means of a **negative feedback** mechanism. This mechanism is also known as 'end-product inhibition', which may give you a clue about how it works.

When a particular level of concentration has been exceeded, an enzyme earlier in the process becomes inhibited or switched off, so preventing further production of the end product.

Fact file

Negative feedback:
(–) ENZYME < X < X < EXCESS END PRODUCT

As a consequence, the end product will decline as it is used up in other processes. This instigates a further process known as **positive feedback**, which is a reverse of end product inhibition. The switching off mechanism is relieved and this allows the enzyme to start functioning again and to produce more of the end product.

Fact file

Positive feedback:
END PRODUCT DECLINES > X > X > (+) ENZYME

Theory into practice

Replace ENZYME and END PRODUCT in the equations above using examples you have come across in your course so far.

Homeostasis depends on communication between different parts of the body to allow for its regulation and co-ordination. Communication and control are the functions of two organ systems which you will now begin to investigate: the nervous system and the endocrine system. These two systems also have an effect on behaviour, although the degree to which the psychological can alter the physical, and vice versa, is a contentious subject that is greatly debated by psychologists interested in behaviour.

Try to think of some personal examples where physical and psychological processes have been linked. Have physical symptoms affected your mood or has your state of mind triggered a physical response?

Organisation of the nervous system

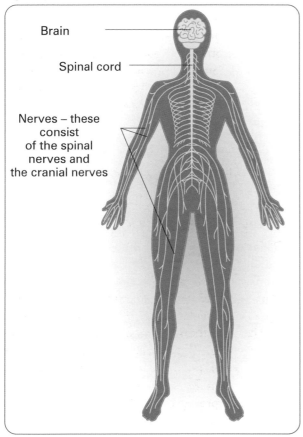

Brain

Spinal cord

Nerves – these consist of the spinal nerves and the cranial nerves

The nervous system.

The nervous system is is a collection of millions of nerve cells or **neurones**, which are the basic tissue of the nervous system, and **neuroglia**, which is a type of connective tissue found only in the nervous system. The nervous system is made up of the **central nervous system** (CNS), which is the brain and spinal cord, and the **peripheral nervous system**, which is the remainder of the nervous system (*periphery* meaning 'around the edge'). The nervous system provides an organised network of communication between different areas of the body and also acts as a receptor for information from the external environment, which is transmitted in the form of sensations.

The **autonomic nervous system** (ANS), which supplies the internal organs, is so called because these organs function without conscious effort, that is, their functions are *automatic*. The autonomic nervous system is mainly constituted of **efferent** nerve fibres, which run outwards from the organs including the stomach, bladder, heart and blood vessels. There are relatively few **afferent** (inwards running) nerve fibres running towards the organs.

There are two parts to the ANS: the sympathetic nervous system and the parasympathetic nervous system. The **sympathetic** nervous system has nerves that supply the internal organs and run back to the spinal nerves, as well as nerves which supply the blood vessels, sweat and sebaceous glands and the arrector pili muscle in the dermis. The **parasympathetic** nervous system has branches which run to all of the internal organs. So, each organ has a double nerve supply which provides opposing actions.

Fact file

The functioning of the autonomic nervous system resembles the pedals of a car – an accelerator pedal to increase the working speed of the car in opposition to the brake pedal which slows the engine down.

The sympathetic nervous system is so called because it is stimulated by strong emotions such as fear, anger and excitement. It stimulates the cardiovascular and respiratory systems while checking (or slowing) the activity of the digestive system so that the body has the ability to respond to emotional situations. Muscles are provided with a better supply of oxygen-rich blood enabling the body to fight or flee, while the digestive system reacts by emptying its organs, via vomiting or bowel movements, which are characteristic of bodily reactions to highly emotional situations.

Fact file

The sympathetic nervous system works closely with the adrenal glands, which it stimulates. The adrenals secrete the hormone **adrenalin** which is known as the 'fight or flight hormone'.

The parasympathetic nervous system is responsible for actions opposite to those described. It stimulates the digestive system to produce more gastric secretions and increases peristaltic action, while blood circulation and respiration are slowed down. These nerves are stimulated by pleasant emotions. The famous psychological experiments involving Pavlov's dogs, who salivated at the sound of a dinner bell, can be said to illustrate the action of the parasympathetic nervous system. Hasn't your mouth ever watered at the sight or smell of delicious, well-presented food or the sound of someone calling you to dinner?

Theory into practice

Consider some personal examples of emotional effects on the nervous system. Try to think of instances where you felt excited, anxious, afraid or angry and the physiological changes that resulted from sympathetic nervous activity. What illustrations of parasympathetic nervous activity can you think of?

Structure of a neurone

Neurones constitute the grey matter of the brain and spinal cord. They have a relatively large cell body which contains the nucleus of the cell. Shape and size varies according to the position and function of each neurone. Information is received via short, branched processes called **dendrites** and information is carried away from the cell body along nerve fibres or **axons**. It is these nerve processes and fibres that make up the white matter of the brain and spinal cord. A neurone with many processes attached to the cell body is a *multi*polar neurone. Other types, called *uni*polar neurones, have one process attached to the cell body which divides into two branches. One branch receives messages from the organs while the other branch, the axon, transmits impulses towards the CNS. A third type of nerve cell, the *bi*polar neurone, has one branch from each end of the cell. The axon carries impulses away from the cell while the dendrite carries impulses towards it.

Axons, and some dendrites, are protected by a fatty sheath of myelin between the cell and the connective tissue. The **myelin sheath** acts to insulate the nerve fibre so that impulses are not

Fact file

Remember: Axons Away!
Axons carry impulses Away from the cell body;
Dendrites carry impulses towards the cell body.

transmitted along it to adjacent nerves. It also protects the fibres from pressure and injury. The myelin sheath is grooved which enables contact with surrounding tissue fluid, necessary for the exchange of nutrients and waste matter. The fibrils which form an axon have tiny expanded ends which lie very close to, but do not touch, the cell body or dendrites of other neurones. This minute space is the point of communication between neurones and is called a **synapse** or reflex arc. It allows for the transmission of impulses in *one direction only*.

Fact file

Transmission of nervous impulses from cell to cell:
cell body of neurone 1 > axon > synapse > dendrite > cell body of neurone 2 > axon > synapse

An example of the simplest circuit in the CNS involves a single sensory neurone which forms a synapse with a motor neurone in the brain or spinal cord. This then transmits an impulse to a muscle or gland, causing a reaction. Some reflex actions involve several neurones, such as the knee-jerk reflex and the reflex action of the pupil in response to light. The presence of reflex actions is used to indicate the condition of the nervous system.

Nerves

A collection of neurones within the peripheral nervous system is referred to as a **nerve**. Some, known as **afferent** or sensory nerves, carry information towards the CNS from the sensory organs. Others carry information away from the CNS and are called **efferent** or motor nerves, since they initiate movement. The neurones which make up a nerve are all the same length and lie alongside each other, a bit like individual wires within a cable. The diagram of the nervous system (page 36) illustrates a section of a nerve within the peripheral nervous system.

Illustrate the actions of efferent and afferent nerves by describing what would happen if you accidentally touched a hot lightbulb.

Sensation from the left side of the body is interpreted by the right side of the brain.

Sense organs

The sense organs are the eyes, ears, nose, mouth and skin, and their function is to interpret the many impulses that are continually stimulating them. They receive sensory impulses from the external environment and transmit information to the CNS via nerves, which stimulate a physical or a psychological reaction. All sensory neurones form a synapse in the thalamus of the brain where sensory information is interpreted. This is like the main 'sorting office' of our internal communication network. The thalamus then distributes the information between the cerebral cortex and other areas of the brain which deal with particular kinds of sensory information. Some impulses are dealt with by the CNS automatically without conscious effort, such as the rate of heartbeat or the contraction of muscles in the digestive system. A sensory nerve fibre which teminates in a muscle, gland or organ and stimulates a particular action is called an effector. More obvious illustrations of sensory impulses are those of sight, sound, smell, taste and touch, which are summarised in the table below.

A summary of the sensory impulses:

Sensory impulse	Path from sense organ to CNS	Point of interpretation
Sight	Optic nerve (2nd cranial nerve)	Interpreted in the visual areas of the occipital lobes.
Hearing	Vestibulococlear nerve (8th cranial nerve)	Interpreted in auditory areas of temporal lobes.
Smell	Olfactory nerve (1st cranial nerve)	Interpreted in the temporal lobe.
Taste	Facial nerve (7th cranial nerve) and glossopharyngeal nerve (9th cranial nerve)	Interpreted in the temporal lobe with the corresponding smell. Few tastes can be interpreted without corresponding sense of smell.
Pain, heat and cold	Nerve endings that transmit pain and temperature changes	Sensory nerve fibres …
Light touch	Nerve endings that transmit light touch	… run in the spinal nerves …
Firm pressure	Nerve endings that transmit firm pressure	… to the posterior nerve roots in the spinal cord.

Functions of the nervous system

The function of the nervous system is one of communication. The particular function of communication initiated by different structures within the nervous system are summarised in the table below.

Assessment task 2.3

Describe the functions of the nervous system in terms of the transmission of nerve impulses. (P)

A summary of how the CNS communicates:

Structure	Function	Illustration
Initiation of the nerve impulse	Initiates the process of communication	Stimulation of the nerve endings as a response to sound, sight, smell, taste or touch
Transmission of the nerve impulse	Allows for communication between neurones	The nerve impulse travels from the axon of one neurone to the dendrite or cell body of another
Afferent or sensory impulses	Impulses which travel towards the brain or spinal cord	Heat or cold received by touch sensors in the skin (afferent or sensory neurones)
Efferent or motor impulses	Impulses which travel outwards from the brain or spinal cord	Command from the brain to move a part of the body (sent via efferent or motor neurones)
Autonomic nervous system (sympathetic and parasympathetic)	Divided into sympathetic and parasympathetic nervous systems	Controls those functions that do not require conscious effort, e.g. heartbeat and secretions from glands
Sympathetic nervous system	Stimulates circulatory and respiratory system, slows digestive system	Responds to emotional situations which provoke anger, fear or excitement
Parasympathetic nervous system	Stimulates digestive system, slows circulatory and respiratory systems	Responds to emotional situations which promote feelings of happiness

Organisation of the endocrine system

The nervous and endocrine systems interact to regulate and co-ordinate the functions of the body. The sympathetic nervous system works in conjunction with the adrenal glands in times of high emotion. We shall now investigate the various glands which make up the endocrine system, the principle hormones produced by each gland and its function.

The endocrine system is often described as functioning like an orchestra, with the **hypothalamus** acting as band leader and the **pituitary gland** acting as the conductor. The pituitary is sometimes referred to as the 'master gland' because of its regulating function; however, as in an orchestra, all the components must work in synchrony with one another to produce harmony. If one gland is not working efficiently, the others must become more active to compensate and maintain homeostasis.

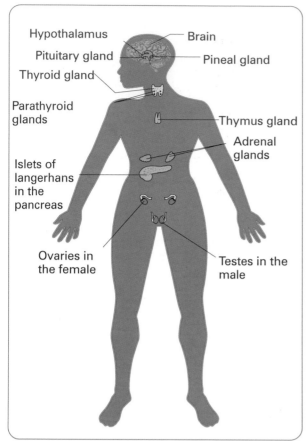

Location of endocrine glands.

Functions of the endocrine system

Endocrine glands could accurately be described as organs. They produce organic chemical compounds called **hormones**, which are mostly derivatives of proteins, although some are steroids. These hormones are secreted directly into the bloodstream and are carried to specific organs, glands or tissues in other parts of the body where they have a specific effect. Hormones are slow acting chemical messengers which control many of the body's functions, including growth, metabolism, sexual development and co-ordination. Endocrine glands continually secrete hormones although the level of secretion is altered to meet the body's needs. This control mechanism is known as homeostatic regulation and it relies upon a feedback mechanism like that described earlier in this section (page 35). If the amount of hormone (X) falls below a certain level, the hypothalamus sends a message to the pituitary gland to stimulate the (X)-producing gland, which responds by secreting more hormone, thus stabilising the levels of hormone (X). If glands over- or under-secrete hormones, the body reacts by displaying abnormal physical or physiological symptoms that are characteristic of certain homeostatic disorders. Disorders of the endocrine system are of concern to beauty therapists since they can contra-indicate certain treatments; alternatively, a client's concerns may point to the presence of an endocrinological disorder. While we, as beauty therapists, are not in a position to diagnose medical conditions, it is our duty to be aware of what our clients bring to the salon and to refer them for medical attention if necessary.

Assessment task 2.4

Explain the roles of the nervous and endocrine systems in the maintenance of homeostasis. (M)

Hypothalamus

The hypothalamus, or mid brain, is situated between the thalamus and the pituitary gland. It produces hormones which release or inhibit the actions of the pituitary gland and also produces two hormones, antidiuretic hormone (vasopressin) and oxytocin, which are stored in the posterior pituitary gland. The role of the hypothalamus is to control the endocrine and autonomic nervous systems and it therefore has an effect on many of the body's functions, including:

▸▸ emotion
▸▸ appetite
▸▸ body temperature
▸▸ sexual activity
▸▸ autonomic nervous system
▸▸ metabolism
▸▸ secretion of pituitary hormones
▸▸ water balance.

Pituitary gland

The pituitary, or master gland, is situated at the base of the skull. It is a small, round structure connected by a stalk to the hypothalamus. The pituitary gland is divided into two sections: anterior pituitary and posterior pituitary, each having different functions and secretions.

Secretions of the anterior pituitary gland:

Hormone	Target	Function
Thyroid stimulating hormone (TSH)	Thyroid gland	Regulation of metabolism, breakdown of fat, control of water content.
Adrenocorticotrophic hormone (ACTH)	Cortex of the suprarenal glands	Mobilisation of fats, increase in muscle glycogen, resistance to stress.
Somatrophic (growth) hormone	Hard tissues of the body	Increases rate of growth and maintains size in adulthood. Over-secretion in children can cause gigantism; under-secretion can cause dwarfism.
Follicle stimulating hormone (FSH)	Sexual organs	Controls maturation of ovarian follicles in females and sperm production in males.
Lutenizing hormone (LH)	Sexual organs	Formation of corpus luteum in ovaries; prepares breasts for lactation in pregnancy.
Lactogenic hormone (prolactin)	Breasts of females	Production of milk.

Secretions of the posterior pituitary gland:

Hormone	Target	Function
Oxytocin	Pregnant uterus, breasts	Contraction of smooth muscle.
Antidiuretic hormone (ADH) or vasopressin	Kidneys	Increase in absorption of water so less urine is excreted. Under-secretion can cause diabetes insipidus which is characterised by excess excretion of dilute urine.

Thyroid gland

The thyroid gland is situated in the neck, below the larynx. It is the largest endocrine gland and consists of two lobes joined by a narrow stalk which crosses the trachea. The thyroid gland produces two hormones, thyroxine and tri-iodothyronine, which are produced from the mineral iodine and the amino acid tyrosine. The parathyroid glands are pea-sized structures which lie behind the thyroid glands, usually two on either side. They produce the hormone parathormone.

Secretions of the thyroid and parathyroid glands:

Hormone	Target	Function
Thyroxine and tri-iodothyronine	Cells and tissues throughout the body.	Regulates metabolism in tissues, increases urine production, breaks down protein and increases uptake of glucose by cells.
Parathormone	Calcium and phosphorus stores in bone	Distribution and metabolism of calcium and phosphorus.

Homeostatic disorders of the thyroid gland:

Hormone	Under-secretion	Over-secretion
Thyroxine and tri-iodothyronine	**Hypothyroidism** – dry, coarse skin and hair, low metabolism, weight gain, low body temperature, cold	Hyperthyroidism – anxiety, high pulse rate, increased metabolism, weight loss, heat intolerance
Parathormone	Dry, brittle hair, muscle spasm (tetanus)	Brittle, porous bones; kidney stones

Pancreas

The pancreas is situated behind the stomach in the curve of the small intestine. It produces pancreatic enzymes which play a part in digestion and are described as an exocrine function of the pancreas.

The pancreas also has an endocrine function. An area called *the islets of Langerhans* produce two hormones from alpha and beta cells. The alpha cells produce glucagon and the beta cells produce insulin.

Secretions of the pancreas:

Hormone	Target	Function
Insulin	Blood sugar	Controls metabolism of carbohydrates; lowers blood sugar levels
Glucagon	Blood sugar	Releases glycogen stored in the liver to raise blood sugar levels

Diabetes mellitus is a condition which occurs when insulin levels are too low, thus raising the blood sugar levels. This condition is common during pregnancy and the menopause while some children who have diabetes in infancy outgrow the disorder. Clients who suffer from diabetes may require a doctor's note prior to certain treatments such as pedicures, due to poor skin healing and other symptoms listed below:

▸▸ increased thirst
▸▸ increased urination
▸▸ weight loss
▸▸ poor skin healing
▸▸ prone to skin infections
▸▸ likely to pick up infections
▸▸ low pain tolerance.

Theory into practice

Considering the symptoms of diabetes mellitus, explain which treatments would require special precautions and why.

Adrenal glands

The two adrenal glands are situated above and in front of each kidney. They are surrounded by fatty areolar tissue and actually consist of two separate endocrine glands, the **adrenal medulla** and the **adrenal cortex**, which have different functions. The adrenal medulla produces three types of hormones: mineralocorticoid, glucocorticoid and sex hormones. The adrenal cortex produces two hormones: adrenaline and noradrenaline.

Theory into practice

There are clues about the functions of these hormones in their names. Before you read on, try to work out the main function of the five named hormones:

▸▸ mineralocorticoid
▸▸ glucocorticoid
▸▸ sex hormones
▸▸ adrenaline
▸▸ noradrenaline.

Secretions of the adrenal glands:

Hormone	Target	Function
Mineralocorticoids, e.g. aldosterone	Water content of tissues	Regulate mineral content of body fluids, regulate salt and water balance.
Glucocorticoids, e.g. cortisone, cortisol, hydrocortisone	Blood sugar, liver	Regulate metabolism of carbohydrates and proteins; conversion of protein to glycogen for storage in the liver; increase blood sugar level by decreasing use of glucose.
Sex hormones (androgens and oestrogens) and steroids	Reproductive organs	Development and function of sex organs; physical characteristics in both sexes; psychological characteristics in both sexes.
Adrenaline	In conjunction with and stimulated by the sympathetic nervous system	Fight and flight mechanism increases heart rate and supply of glucose, blood and oxygen to muscles; digestion slows down.
Noradrenaline	Circulation	Contracts blood vessels and raises blood pressure.

Homeostatic disorders of the adrenal glands:

Hormone	Over-secretion	Under-secretion
Mineralocorticoids	Increased likelihood of ulcers; increased blood pressure	Excess water loss from the body; lowered pH of blood (**acidosis**)
Glucocorticoids	**Cushing's syndrome**: excess fatty tissue on trunk, oedema, male pattern hair growth, raised pH of blood (**alkalosis**)	Rare
Sex hormones	An **adrenal tumour** in females produces male characteristics: male pattern hair growth, deepening of the voice	Rare
Adrenaline and noradrenaline	Rare	**Addison's disease**: anaemia, low blood pressure, muscle wastage, hyper-pigmentation

Gonads

The gonads in females are the **ovaries**, which produce ova; in males the gonads are the **testes**, which produce sperm. Both male and female gonads are controlled by follicle stimulating hormone (FSH) and lutenizing hormone (LH), which are produced by the anterior pituitary gland. The gonads themselves produce the hormones oestrogen, progesterone and androgens, and so are classified as endocrine glands.

The ovaries are situated in the female pelvis on either side of the uterus and they resemble almonds in both shape and size. They produce the female hormones **oestrogen** and **progesterone** as well as small amounts of **androgens**. The testes are the endocrine glands in males. They are suspended in the scrotum and secrete androgens, which are steroid hormones; testosterone is an example.

Secretions of the gonads:

Hormone	Target	Function
Oestrogen	Secondary sexual characteristics in females	Development of female reproductive system, external genitalia, uterus and breasts; regulation of menstrual cycle
Progesterone	Structures involved in pregnancy	Maintenance of pregnancy; development of placenta; prepares breasts for lactation
Androgens	Secondary sexual characteristics in males	Development of male reproductive system, male hair growth pattern, voice deepening, muscle bulk

Homeostatic disorders of the ovaries

If the ovaries fail to respond to stimulation by the pituitary gland, the production of oestrogen and progesterone can be reduced or the secretion of androgens can increase. Homeostatic disorders of the ovaries produce similar effects and are usually characterised by a masculine pattern of hair growth in females, known as **hirsutism**. Primary hirsutism is caused by an increased sensitivity to normal levels of androgens in the blood, which usually begins during puberty and settles down during the thirties. Secondary or true hirsutism is caused by increased androgen production in the ovaries or adrenal glands and can begin just prior to or just after puberty.

Theory into practice

Explain why it is important to establish the cause of hair growth prior to methods of permanent hair removal.

Assessment task 2.5

Identify a common homeostatic disorder and describe the cause and treatment with reference to relevant physiological information. (D)

Digestion and transport in the body

Essential dietary components

Most people are aware, through education and the media, of the importance of eating a healthy diet, and that a poor diet can be responsible for disease and even fatality. We usually associate images of malnutrition with third world countries, but poverty is also one of the main reasons for malnutrition in the western world, albeit on a lesser scale. The World Health Organisation (WHO) began developing dietary recommendations in the UK in the early twentieth century as a way of educating individuals about the nutritional requirements needed to sustain a healthy body. The WHO introduced **'recommended daily allowances'** (RDAs) to show how much of each foodstuff we should consume each day. The current advice is that about one-third of our daily food intake should consist of fruit and vegetables, the ideal being at least five portions; one-third of our diet should be carbohydrate-based foods like potatoes, rice and bread; and the remaining one-third of our diet should be divided equally between protein foods, such as meat, fats and dairy produce (as shown in the illustration on page 45).

There are seven essential dietary components that the body needs for energy and maintenance. These are: carbohydrates, lipids, proteins, vitamins, minerals, dietary fibre and water. A diet that is deficient in any one of these components can lead to ill health. Fortunately, in the UK in the twenty-first century, many of the diseases associated with malnutrition are rare. However, for others facing poverty or a limited food supply they are a harsh reality.

The biological structure and function of carbohydrates, lipids and proteins is explored in Unit 1: Scientific Principles. A table is included overleaf for reference which summarises the main functions as well as the food source and RDA of each dietary component.

Recommended daily proportions of food:

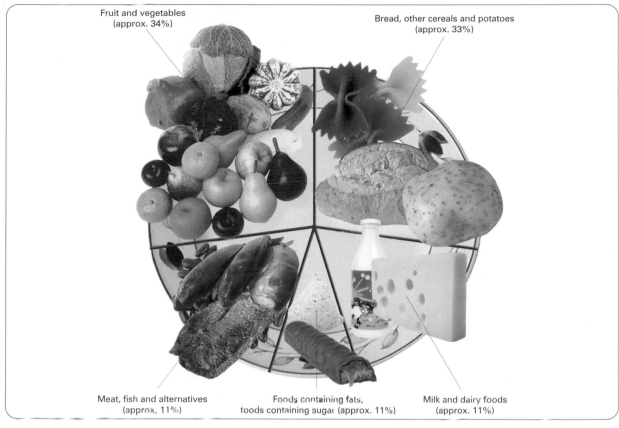

Fruit and vegetables
(approx. 34%)

Bread, other cereals and potatoes
(approx. 33%)

Meat, fish and alternatives
(approx. 11%)

Foods containing fats,
foods containing sugar (approx. 11%)

Milk and dairy foods
(approx. 11%)

Sources of dietary components:

Dietary component	Functions	Food source	Advice
Carbohydrates: starch sugar cellulose	Easily burnt in tissues to provide fuel and energy	Starch: potatoes, cereals, pulses; sugars: confectionery, sweet fruit & vegetables, milk, honey; cellulose: green leafy vegetables	Choose starches over sugars
Lipids: fats (solid) oils (liquid)	Energy store, insulation & protection of body & organs, transport of fat soluble vitamins (A,D,E,K)	Animal: red meat, oily fish, fish oils, cheese, butter, lard, suet; plant: nuts, soya beans, cereal, vegetable oils	Less than 30% of total calories
Proteins: animal vegetable	Transport of oxygen in blood; protection: anti-bodies, clotting; support: collagen & elastin in connective tissue	Animal: lean meat (myosin), milk (lactalbumin), eggs (albumin), cheese (casein); plant: wheat (gluten), pulses (legumin)	No more than 0.8g per kg of body weight
Fibre	Maintain functioning of the intestinal tract	Dried & fresh fruit, green vegetables, cereals	RDA 20–30g
Water	Body fluids, tissues, gastric secretions, excretion, temperature control	Fresh source, milk, cabbage	RDA 2–3 litres

- All food stuffs contain at least one of the seven essential dietary components.
- Vitamins have no use as body builders or sources of fuel but are essential as regulators of tissue activity.
- Some unlikely sources of water include:
  cabbage = 92% water
  milk = 87% water
  lean meat = 75% water.

List everything that you ate or drank yesterday and make a note of the dietary components of each item. Is your diet lacking in any areas? How well does your diet map onto the recommended proportions needed for a healthy diet? Compare your diet on a working day with a day at the weekend and note any differences.

Essential vitamins and minerals:

Name	Function	Food source	Deficiency
Vitamin A (retinol)	Vision, maintenance of epithelial tissue	Liver, dairy foods, green vegetables	Night blindness, dry skin
Vitamin B1 (thiamine)	Facilitates release of energy from food	Meat, vegetables, wholemeal bread	Nervous disorder: beri-beri
Vitamin B2 (riboflavine)	Facilitates release of energy from food	Milk	Rare
Vitamin B3 (nicotinic acid)	Facilitates release of energy from food	Meat, potatoes, wholemeal bread	Skin disease: pellagra
Vitamin B12	Synthesis of nuclear matter in cells	Liver, yeast extract	Anaemia
Vitamin C (ascorbic acid)	Maintains connective tissue	Citrus fruit, vegetables	Bleeding gums, scurvy
Vitamin D (calciferol)	Facilitates exchanges of calcium & phosphorus between blood & bones	Egg yolk, margarine, exposure to sunlight	Rickets
Vitamin E	Maintain cell membranes	Plant oils	Rare
Vitamin K	Blood clotting	Dark green leafy vegetables	Rare
Sodium	Transmission of nervous impulses, kidney function, tissue fluids	Salt, bread, cereals	Calcium loss in urine, raised blood pressure
Calcium	Growth/repair of bones & teeth, blood clotting, muscle contraction	Milk, cheese, bread	Osteoporosis, kidney stones, increased blood pressure
Phosphorus	Healthy bones & teeth, production of DNA & RNA, muscle contraction	Milk, cereals, bread	Loss of bone tissue (particularly post-menopause)
Potassium	Transmission of nervous impulses, cell metabolism	Fruit & fruit juices, vegetables, meat, milk	Increased blood pressure, reduced heart beat
Chloride	Tissue fluid & gastric secretions	Salt	Rare
Iron	Production of haemoglobin	Liver, watercress	Anaemia
Iodine	Production of thyroxine	Seafood, salt	Goitre

Structure of the digestive system

The digestive system, or **alimentary canal**, is made up of a number of organs and glands which facilitate the chewing, swallowing, digestion, absorption and elimination of food. It runs from the mouth, where food is ingested, to the rectum, where the waste products of food are expelled. Food is passed from one structure to another in a process which breaks it down into its component parts, ensuring that essential nutrients are absorbed into the bloodstream.

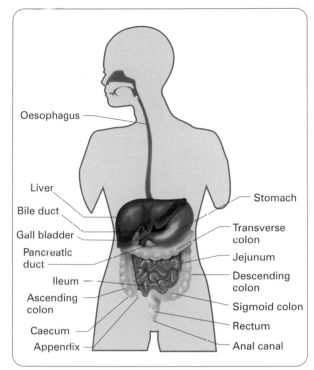

The human digestive system.

Structure of the digestive system:

Name	Structure and location
Mouth	Cavity bound by lips & cheeks consisting of the hard palate (palatine bones and maxillae) and soft palate. Contains the tongue and teeth which assist in mastication (chewing) and the salivary glands which produce saliva, the functions of which include softening food, digestion of carbohydrates and cleansing of the mouth and teeth.
Pharynx	Muscular flap of skin which prevents food entering the wind pipe.
Oesophagus	Muscular canal which extends from the pharynx to the stomach. It is located behind the trachea and in front of the vertebral column.
Stomach	J-shaped structure located below and to the left of the diaphragm. The upper opening from the oesophagus consists of a weak sphincter muscle, while the lower opening into the small intestine consists of a strong pyloric sphincter which prevents the regurgitation of food.
Pancreas	A gland approximately 12–15cm long which lies across the posterior abdominal wall behind the stomach.
Liver	Largest gland in the body. It is located in the upper right section of the abdominal cavity, beneath the diaphragm.
Gall bladder	A pear-shaped organ located near the right lobe of the liver. The cystic duct of the gall bladder joins the hepatic duct of the liver to form the bile duct.
Small intestine	Consists of the duodenum, jejunum and ileum and is a long tube (6 metres) extending from the pyloric sphincter to the large intestine. It is located in the central and lower abdominal cavity within the curves of the large intestine.
Large intestine	A tube approximately 1.5 metres in length which extends from the ileum to the anus and consists of seven sections: caecum, ascending colon, transverse colon, descending colon, sigmoid colon, rectum and anal canal.

Functions of the digestive system

Food provides the main building blocks of life, and this is a useful analogy when you are beginning to explore the functions of the digestive system. Imagine that the dietary components are actual building blocks and that each one is represented by a different colour: red for protein, yellow for lipids and blue for carbohydrates. An average meal of pasta with a meat and vegetable sauce contains each of these components in different proportions: green, blue and red building blocks which form a solid structure. When the meal is eaten, this structure is broken down into individual blocks: a pile of red, a pile of blue and a pile of yellow. During the process of digestion, the blocks are broken down further into even smaller pieces which can later be rebuilt to create a different type of structure from the one originally presented. This building, knocking down and rebuilding process is analogous to what happens during digestion. Specific enzymes act on carbohydrates, proteins and lipids to break them down into smaller molecules. These are then reassembled so that the nutrients are in a form which the body can use as raw materials or as a source of energy.

Food's journey

The journey of food along the alimentary canal begins in the mouth with the process known as **ingestion**. Food is broken down and softened by mastication (chewing) and becomes mixed with the enzyme **salivary amylase** which acts on cooked starch, breaking it down into maltose and dextrin. Already, both mechanical and chemical digestion have begun. Mechanical digestion is the term given to the physical breakdown of food in the form of biting and chewing. The churning of food in the stomach is also an illustration of mechanical digestion, which works a bit like a food processor, mashing food down and mixing it with digestive secretions. Chemical digestion involves the production of biological catalysts, or **enzymes**, which act on nutrients and break them down into smaller molecules. Enzymes are specific to the material which they break down; thus salivary amylase, for example, will only act on cooked starch and has no effect on the digestion of proteins or lipids. During the process of digestion, nutrients are broken down into small, soluble molecules which can be easily absorbed into the bloodstream and later used as raw materials for cells and tissues or as energy for respiration.

Digestion involves three interdependent phases. The **'cephalic phase'** stimulates the release of gastric juices and movement in the stomach which we recognise as 'rumbles'. This process can occur when we see, smell or even think about food and not just when it enters our mouths. During the **'gastric phase'** the release of gastric juices and the churning movement is stimulated when food enters the stomach. Food remains in the stomach for up to three hours while chemical and mechanical digestion continues. The **'intestinal phase'** occurs when food enters the duodenum and activity in the stomach is inhibited. Secretion of intestinal juices is stimulated which also stimulates the release of pancreatic juice from the pancreas and bile from the gall bladder. Movement of food along the digestive tract is facilitated by a muscular action called **peristalsis**. This is the contraction and relaxation of muscles that line the oesophagus and intestines in a wave formation, and which squeeze food along the tubular structures.

Fact file

Peristalsis is analogous to squeezing and moving a blob of toothpaste from the end of the tube to the opening.

Theory into practice

Explain why some foods take longer to digest than others. What are the implications for body therapy?

Fact file

A carbohydrate-rich meal that is low in protein, such as tea and toast, will leave the stomach in about thirty minutes, while a varied, balanced meal will remain in the stomach for two and a half to three hours.

Chemical digestion:

Source	Secretion	Action
Mouth – saliva	Salivary amylase	Changes cooked starch into maltose and dextrin
Stomach – gastric juice	Pepsin, rennin, hydrochloric acid	Changes protein into peptides; coagulates milk protein into casein; stops action of amylase, kills bacteria, controls pylorus sphincter
Pancreas – pancreatic fluid	Lipase, trypsin, amylase	Changes lipids to fatty acid and glycerol; changes proteins to polypeptides; changes all starch to maltose and dextrin
Liver – bile	Bile	Emulsifies fats
Small intestine – intestinal fluid	Lipase, maltase, sucrase, lactase, peptidase	Changes lipids to fatty acids and glycerol; changes maltose to glucose; changes sucrose to glucose; changes lactose to glucose; changes polypeptides to amino acids

The final part of food's journey is elimination or **egestion**, which takes place when 'food' passes from the colon to the rectum. In fact, the material which enters the large intestine contains very little food at all since by then it has mostly been absorbed. The material entering the large intestine contains water, salt, indigestible cellulose and bacteria. Most of the water and salts are absorbed by the colon, which causes the bacteria to die, leaving only cellulose and dead bacteria that forms a paste. This paste becomes the **faeces**, which consists of a little water and a solid part made up of about 50 per cent dead bacteria and 50 per cent cellulose. The brown colour of faeces comes from the breakdown of old red blood cells.

Peristalsis occurs about three to four times a day in the colon, less frequently than in the small intestine, and this moves faeces from the colon to the rectum. The rectum becomes distended causing a reflex contraction of the muscles which expels the faeces via the anus. If defecation is delayed, more water is absorbed from the faeces which reduces the sensation of fullness but can, in time, cause constipation.

Assessment task 2.6

Outline the functions of the digestive system. (P)

Metabolism and energy

Metabolism is the collective term given to all physical and chemical changes that take place in cells and tissues to maintain growth and repair. **Catabolism** refers to all 'breaking-down' processes while **anabolism** refers to all 'building-up' processes. The functions of metabolism can be summarised as the provision of energy in the form of ATP and the exchange of carbon between molecules. Every process which uses energy, such as movement, respiration or circulation, is dependent on the functions of metabolism, as are the processes involved in digestion, which break down larger molecules into more usable substances.

We know that energy comes from food and is used by the body in the form of ATP. Nutrients are broken down in a catabolic process to provide energy and the exchange of carbon for synthetic purposes, i.e. to produce raw materials for tissues and cells. **Glycolysis** is the metabolic process of breaking down glucose, a carbohydrate, to produce pyruvic acid and ATP. Lipids are first broken down into fatty acids and then, during glycolysis, are broken down further to produce carbon dioxide, water and ATP. Amino acids, produced during the synthesis of proteins, can also be broken down further to produce energy.

The amount of ATP produced depends on the amount of food broken down, with carbohydrates and lipids being the greater sources of energy. Lipids produce approximately twice as much ATP per gram as carbohydrates and are therefore a better source of energy. However, lipids not broken down into ATP and used as a source of energy will be stored by the body as fat. The term **basal metabolism** is used to describe the basic amount of energy the body requires to maintain homeostasis.

Energy requirements

The body's nutritional requirements are affected by growth, pregnancy, breast feeding, activity, illness, convalescence and old age. These factors aside, the energy requirements of adults aged between 18 and 50 years remain pretty constant. When growth stops in the late teens, the body requires less energy since it has less work to do. However, it is necessary to maintain a nutritionally balanced diet in order for the body to function healthily.

The energy value of foods is measured in calories (or, more accurately, kilocalories – kcal) and this is listed, along with nutritional advice, on many food stuffs. In general, a daily intake of 2000 to 2500 kilocalories is ideal, with men requiring slightly more calories than women do. We also need slightly more calories in the winter than in the summer in order to keep warm. Thus, craving a hot filling meal on a cold winter's evening is both natural and necessary!

The amount of calories an individual requires will vary depending on how active the person is. It is therefore important to maintain a balance between food intake and energy output: tipping the balance in either direction will lead to weight loss or gain.

Calorie counting is difficult and often laborious for most of us and so the best advice is to eat a balanced diet each day. If this advice is followed, body weight should remain stable and the body will have all the nutritional requirements it needs to function effectively.

Theory into practice

Why do men require more calories than women do? Explain the dietary considerations of pregnant or breast-feeding mothers. How could an active person, possibly a teenager, supplement their diet to meet their higher energy requirements?

Fact file

Balanced diet:

- five servings (half a cup) of fruit and vegetables
- fat intake should be less than 30% of calorie intake
- intake of saturated fats should be less than 10% of calorie intake
- complex carbohydrates (starch) should be chosen over refined forms (sugar)
- 0.8 grams of protein per kg of body weight
- less than 6 grams of salt.

Remember:

- Weight gain arises when food intake exceeds energy output.
- Weight loss arises when food intake is less than energy output.

Theory into practice

Look at the packets of some common food stuffs and make a table of nutritional and calorific values.

Cellular respiration

All living matter is made up of single units called cells. Bacteria are the smallest, unicellular structures while humans are made up of millions of cells, each with different structures and functions. Cells have a number of common characteristics and one of these is the ability to perform activity. Even microscopic organic structures are capable of a particular form of activity. In order for activity to take place, structures require energy. Just as a car cannot perform without fuel, the body cannot function unless it is fuelled by food, particularly carbohydrates and lipids.

The combustion of fuel takes place in the presence of oxygen; in physiology, this is sometimes described as the **oxidation** of food. We acquire oxygen from the air we breathe while some aqueous plants and animals take in oxygen from water. The amount of oxygen required by the body depends on the amount of activity taking place. During sleep we require very little oxygen, but during vigorous exercise much more oxygen is needed so that combustion of food can take place, to provide the energy required to maintain the activity. As well as providing the body with energy, another function of fuel is to provide heat. The body works in such a way that it uses most of its food to provide energy and less of it to provide heat, keeping body temperature constant at around 37.5°C.

Food is thus the fuel that supplies energy and maintains body temperature but the process of combustion also produces waste materials in the form of carbon dioxide and water. All living structures take in nutrients and oxygen and give off carbon dioxide and water, and this is what we mean by the term *cellular respiration*.

Regulation of blood glucose

The typical blood glucose level is about 80–90 mg per 100 ml of blood. Glucose is present in higher levels after meals, particularly but not necessarily meals rich in carbohydrates. This is known as the **absorptive state**, when blood glucose levels rise to a maximum of 140 mg per 100 ml of blood. If glucose were transported immediately from the digestive system to other parts of the body, there would be a shortage of glucose between meals and blood sugar levels would fall dramatically. Glucose that is not immediately required for energy is converted into glycogen and triacylglycerols (fat) and stored in the liver, skeletal muscle and adipose tissue. Blood glucose levels typically return to normal within two and a half hours after eating, even though digestion can continue for longer.

During the **post-absorptive state**, when glucose is not entering the bloodstream from the digestive system, it is obtained from supplies built up in the liver, adipose tissue and skeletal muscle during the absorptive state, and also from the catabolism of proteins. The use of glucose is reduced to maintain stores and fatty acids are instead metabolised to provide energy. The pancreas also plays an important role in the regulation of blood glucose (see pages 40–4, functions of the endocrine system). Alpha cells secrete the hormone **glucagon** in response to a *fall* in blood glucose levels, and this stimulates the conversion of glycogen to glucose. Beta cells secrete the hormone **insulin** in response to a *rise* in blood glucose levels, stimulating the conversion of glucose to glycogen for storage.

A deficiency in insulin results in high levels of blood glucose known as **hyperglycaemia**, characteristic of the condition **diabetes mellitus**. As levels of blood glucose rise, the kidneys pass

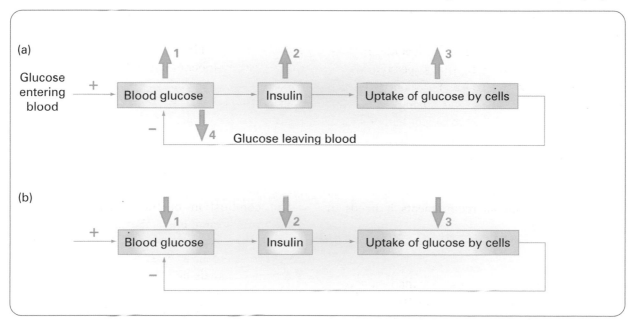

Insulin and blood glucose negative feedback system.

(a) **When glucose levels in the blood rise (1), so the level of insulin rises (2) and rate at which glucose is taken up by other cells also rises (3). This lowers the concentration of blood glucose (4).**

(b) **When glucose levels in the blood fall (1), so levels of insulin fall (2) and the amount of uptake of glucose by other cells is reduced (3). This reduces the rate at which blood glucose levels decline.**

Secretions of the pancreas:

alpha cells > hormone glucagon in response to
fall in blood glucose = glycogen > glucose
beta cells > hormone insulin in response to
rise in blood glucose = glucose > glycogen

greater amounts of urine which attracts more fluid and so produces more urine. Typical symptoms of untreated diabetes are a constant feeling of thirst and frequently passing large quantities of urine. If left untreated this can lead to dehydration, damage to the metabolism and even death. The diet for a diabetic should be the same as the recommended balanced diet for all adults: regular meals based on starchy foods which contain less sugar and fats. People suffering from diabetes might require more snack foods in their diet and should make sure that these are of nutritional value. Bananas are a rich source of the minerals potassium and magnesium which help maintain blood glucose levels.

Structure of the cardiovascular system

The cardiovascular system consists of a fluid – the blood; a pump – the heart; and a network of blood vessels, arteries, veins and capillaries. We will look at the structure of these in turn.

Blood

Blood is a thick, alkaline fluid which appears bright red in the arteries and dark red in the veins, depending on the presence of more or less oxygen respectively. It makes up about 8 per cent of our body weight, so the average volume of blood in an adult is between 5 and 6 litres. Blood contains about 55 per cent fluid in the form of **plasma** and about 45 per cent solid in the form of blood cells.

'Super foods' which are thought to affect the body:

Health concern	Food source
To boost collagen production and so maintain the firmness of skin	Blueberries
To prevent constipation	Peppers, which are rich in fibre, and water, to keep things moving
To delay the signs of ageing skin and help prevent wrinkles	Brazil nuts, which contain the antioxidant mineral selenium
To beat insomnia	Bananas, which help stabilise blood glucose levels: if levels are too low you can get overtired which makes it difficult to fall asleep
To banish the feeling of pre-menstrual bloatedness	Parsley, a natural diuretic which stimulates the kidneys to produce more urine
To fight off colds and flu	Salmon, which is rich in the fatty acid omega 3 necessary for the functioning of the immune system
To prevent brittle nails	Muesli, which is rich in vitamins B,C and E, needed to produce keratin
To give your hair a healthy, glossy sheen	Garlic
To prevent spots and aid healing	Kiwi fruit, which contains double the amount of vitamin C than found in oranges
To help prevent cancer	Processed tomatoes, which contain the antioxidant lycopene

Composition of plasma:

Components	Function
Water = 90% of total volume	Renews cellular fluid
Minerals: chlorides, phosphates, carbonates	Maintains pH of blood at 7.4; maintains electrolyte balance for correct functioning of body tissues
Proteins: albumin, globulin, fibrinogen, heparin	Make blood viscous (sticky) which controls its flow and maintains blood pressure
Nutrients: glucose, amino acids, fatty acids, glycerol, vitamins	Required for energy, heat and raw materials
Gases: oxygen, carbon dioxide, nitrogen	Required for/ produced by cellular respiration
Waste products: urea, uric acid, creatinine	By-products of metabolism
Antibodies and antitoxins	Protect against infection and neutralise some toxins which may enter the body
Hormones	See endocrine system (pages 39–44)
Enzymes	Produce chemical reactions in other substances

Blood cells:

Type of cell	Structure	Function
Erythrocytes (red blood cells)	Produced in red bone marrow of spongy bone. Minute biconcave discs, about 5 million per cubic mm of blood. Contain the protein **haemoglobin** which attracts oxygen to form oxyhaemoglobin, which is bright red in colour.	Carry oxygen to the tissues from the lungs and carry carbon dioxide away from the tissues to to the lungs.
Leucocytes (white blood cells)	Larger than red blood cells and less numerous. Three types: 75% granulocytes which can pass from blood stream to site of infection; 20% lymphocytes made in the lymph nodes; 5% monocytes.	Concerned with immunity. Granulocytes/phagocytes: ingest bacteria and cell debris (**phagocytosis**); lymphocytes: produce antibodies; monocytes: phagocytosis.
Thrombocytes (platelets)	Made in the bone marrow and are even smaller than red blood cells.	Concerned with clotting of the blood (haemostasis), which has three stages: narrowing of lumen in blood vessels; formation of platelet plug; clotting and retraction of fibrin.

Explain the function of each of the three stages of haemostasis. (Look also at wound healing in Unit 6: Dermatology and microbiology, pages 105–6.)

Structure of the heart

The heart is a hollow, muscular, cone-shaped organ located between the lungs and behind the sternum, slightly to the left side of the body. It measures about 12cm in length, 9cm in width and 6cm in depth. The heart is divided longitudinally and the two halves do not communicate. It consists of four chambers: the smaller, upper chambers, called the left and right **atriu** (singular: atrium) and the two lower chambers, called left and right **ventricles**. The heart also contains four main valves, which are mechanisms to prevent blood from flowing in the wrong direction.

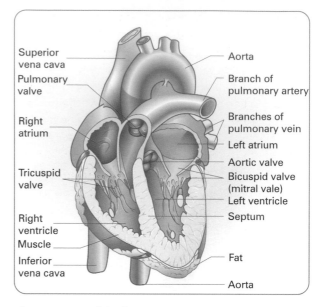

The structure of the heart.

A summary of the structure and function of the heart:

Structure	Location	Function
Left atrium/ right atrium	Upper chambers	Receives blood flowing towards the heart from the veins
Left ventricle/ right ventricle	Lower chambers	Directs blood away from the heart through the arteries
Right atrio-ventricular valve (tricuspid)	Between right atrium and right ventricle	Prevents backflow of blood into the right atrium during contraction of the right ventricle
Left atrio-ventricular valve (bicuspid)	Between left atrium and left ventricle	Prevents backflow of blood into the left atrium during contraction of the left ventricle
Aortic valve	Between the aorta and the left ventricle	Prevents backflow of blood into the left ventricle
Pulmonary valve	Between the pulmonary vein and the right ventricle	Prevents backflow of blood into the right ventricle

Structure of the blood vessels

Blood vessels are the tubes which form a network around the body for the transport of blood. When the ventricles of the heart contract, blood is pumped around the body via vessels called **arteries**, which branch into smaller vessels called **arterioles** and then even smaller vessels called **capillaries**. Because capillaries are small, superficial and carry blood at low pressure, the slightest external pressure forces blood out of them.

Capillaries form the link between arterioles and other tiny vessels called **venules**, which collect the

Press down on your fingernail and notice the change in colour from pink to white as blood is forced out of the superficial capillaries.

blood from the capillaries. Venules then unite to form **veins**, which carry blood on its journey back towards the heart. Arteries are thicker than veins and have larger lumen. With one exception, they carry oxygenated blood away from the heart. Veins carry deoxygenated blood towards the heart, with one exception: pulmonary vein. Unlike arteries, veins contain valves that prevent the backflow of blood. The largest artery in the body is the **aorta** which carries oxygenated blood from the left ventricle to all parts of the body (except the lungs). The largest veins in the body are the superior and inferior vena cavae. The **superior vena cava** carries deoxygenated blood from the upper parts of the body to the right atrium, and the **inferior vena cava** carries deoxygenated blood from the lower parts of the body to the right atrium.

Structure of arteries and veins

Arteries:
- carry blood away from the heart
- carry oxygenated blood (except pulmonary artery)
- have thicker muscular walls
- have no valves
- the blood flow is rapid
- the blood pressure is higher
- tend to lie deeper in the body.

Veins:
- carry blood towards the heart
- carry deoxygenated blood (except pulmonary vein)
- have thinner muscular walls
- have valves
- the blood flow is slower
- the blood pressure is lower
- tend to be more superficial in the body.

Functions of the cardiovascular system

The cardiovascular system has many functions. These include:

- transport nutrients to the tissues
- transport oxygen to the tissues in oxyhaemoglobin
- transport water to the tissue
- transport waste products to the organs of excretion
- transport hormones and enzymes
- leucocytes and antibodies help fight infection
- provide the raw materials from which glands produce secretions
- transport heat and regulate body temperature
- clotting mechanism prevents haemorrhage.

Pulse

As blood is pumped from the left ventricle into the aorta, the aorta is already full of blood and so it becomes distended in order to accept more. The left ventricle contracts which causes vibrations along the arteries due, initially, to the expansion of the aorta. The expansion and contraction of the aorta thus causes a wave of similar movements throughout the arterial network, and this is known as the pulse.

The pulse can be felt wherever an artery can be gently compressed against a bone. Pulse rate varies according to age, activity, emotion, gender, temperature and medication, and is measured as an indicator of the condition of the heart.

Theory into practice

Measure your own pulse 'at rest' and again after a period of brisk activity. Try to compare the pulse rates of people who differ according to the factors listed above.

Blood pressure

Blood pressure refers to the pressure exerted by blood onto the walls of the blood vessels. It is greatest in the large arteries leaving the heart, falls slightly in the arterioles, and is hardly apparent in the capillaries. Blood pressure is even lower in the veins, and in those veins entering the heart there is negative pressure, or suction, caused by the relaxation of the heart's chambers.

Blood pressure fluctuates with each pumping action of the heart. It is highest when the ventricle contracts, forcing blood from the heart, and lowest when the ventricle relaxes. The maximum value is called **systolic pressure** and the lowest value is called **diastolic pressure**. Blood pressure is measured by the weight of a column of mercury (Hg) the pressure can support, calculated in millimetres. Normal arteriole pressure is 110–120 mm Hg systolic pressure and 65–75 mm Hg diastolic pressure. The apparatus used for measuring blood pressure is called a **sphygmomanometer**.

High blood pressure, known as **hypertension**, occurs when blood is forced through the arteries at abnormally high pressure, which can damage the artery walls. At the site of damage, blood clots can form which can detach and travel along the bloodstream. If these clots then become detached in other parts of the body, they can obstruct the blood supply causing a stroke or heart attack. Low blood pressure, known as hypotension, describes systolic pressure lower than 110 mm Hg. It can occur after shock, haemorrhage or heart failure, and is dangerous because it results in an insufficient blood supply to the vital organs.

Assessment task 2.7

Outline the functions of the cardiovascular system. (P)

Assessment task 2.8

Explain in detail the interdependence of the digestive and cardiovascular systems. (D)

Structure and functions of the lymphatic system

The lymphatic system consists of lymphatic capillaries, vessels, nodes, ducts and the spleen. The capillaries and vessels form a network around the body which act as tunnels for the transportation of lymph fluid, in the same way that blood vessels provide a network for the transport of blood.

Lymphatic circulation
As blood travels through the capillaries in the body's tissues, fluid oozes out through the porous walls to form tissue or **interstitial fluid**. Interstitial fluid circulates through the tissues transporting nutrients and oxygen to the cells and carrying waste back into the blood. Excess fluid which does not return to the blood is called **lymph** and is collected and returned to the blood by the lymphatic system. Lymph travels from the **lymphatic capillaries** to the larger

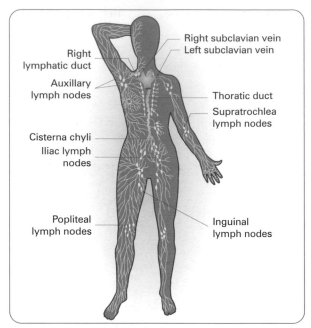

The structure of the lymphatic system.

lymphatic vessels. Along its journey it passes through **lymphatic nodes**, which are situated in areas of the body where there is a greater risk of infection. At these points the lymph is filtered and cleaned and **lymphocytes** are produced, which are antibodies that help to prevent infection. Having passed through at least one lymph node, lymph fluid travels into **lymphatic ducts**. The ducts pass lymph back into the blood circulation where it becomes part of blood, so that the cycle can begin once again.

Spleen
The spleen is a large nodule of lymphoid tissue located high at the back of the abdomen, to the left side and behind the stomach. It contains two types of cells: the first are similar to the lymphocytes of the blood and lymph nodes and produce leucocytes (white blood cells). The second type of cells are phagocytic and these engulf worn out erythrocytes (red blood cells) and destroy them. The spleen is nonessential to life and can be removed if it becomes unhealthy. Little else is known about the spleen, although it is believed to have a role in fighting infection because it becomes enlarged in certain diseases which infect the blood, such as malaria and typhoid.

A summary of the structures and functions of the lymphatic system:

Feature	Structure	Function
Lymph	Straw-coloured fluid	Carries more waste than nutrients
Lymphatic capillaries	One cell thick, hair like structures which combine to form lymphatic vessels	Transport lymph from the tissues
Lymphatic vessels	Larger and thicker than capillaries; contain valves which prevent backflow of lymph	Transport lymph through one or more lymphatic nodes
Lymphatic nodes	Vary in size from a pin head to an almond	Filter lymph to remove bacteria so can become swollen and tender if infection is present; produce some antibodies
Lymphatic ducts	Larger thoracic duct is about 45cm long, has valves and is located at the back of the abdomen; smaller right lymphatic duct is about 1cm long and is formed by the joining of the vessels from the head, thorax and right limb	Collect lymph and return it to the bloodstream Thoracic duct: receives lymph from vessels in the abdomen and lower limbs and empties into the left subclavian vein Right lymphatic duct: empties into the right subclavian vein
Spleen	Large nodular structure made up of lymphoid tissue	Produces lymphocytes, destroys worn out erythrocytes, assists in fighting infection

Structure and function of the respiratory system

The respiratory system consists of two parts: the structures leading to the lungs – nose, pharynx, larynx and trachea; and the structures within the lungs – bronchii, bronchioles, alveoli and capillary networks.

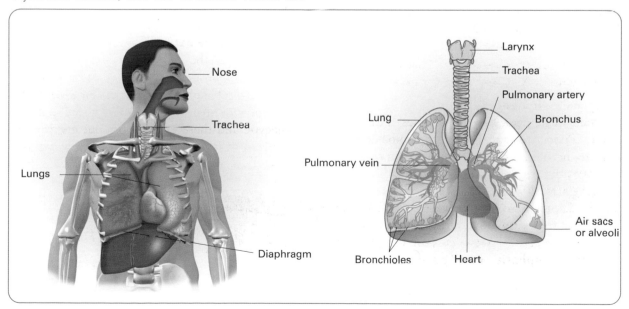

The respiratory system.

Breathing

Breathing consists of two parts: breathing in, or **inspiration**; and breathing out, or **expiration**. As we breathe air in, the chest expands to increase the depth of the thoracic cavity. The diaphragm is flattened and lowered, while the external intercostal muscles lift the ribs up and out. The lungs expand to fill the increased area and fill with air. During normal or 'quiet' breathing, expiration is passive; the intercostals muscles are relaxed and the diaphragm is dome shaped. Forced expiration causes the intercostals muscles to contract and lower the ribs. During deep breathing, or if the airways become blocked, accessory muscles assist the main muscles of respiration. The capacity of the thoracic cavity is increased by the sternocleidomastoid, which raises the sternum, while serratus anterior and pectoralis major pull the ribs outwards. During forced expiration, latissumus dorsi and the anterior abdominals help to compress the thoracic cavity.

Fact file

Chief muscles of respiration:
diaphragm and external intercostals.
Accessory muscles of respiration:
sternocleidomastoid, serratus anterior, latissimus dorsi, pectoralis major, anterior abdominals.

Theory into practice

Remind yourself of the locations, origins and insertions of the main and accessory muscles of respiration.

Gaseous exchange

Air is breathed in through the nose and travels along the respiratory tract to the lungs, unless the nasal cavities becomes blocked – in which case it is necessary to breathe in through the mouth. Inspired air travels in through the anterior nares (nostrils) and out through the posterior nares, via the pharynx, larynx and trachea. Next it enters the structures of the lungs: the bronchii which branch into small bronchioles, which then branch into even smaller alveoli. The alveoli are surrounded by a network of capillaries and it is here that gaseous exchange takes place between air in the alveoli and blood in the vessels. Deoxygenated blood enters the capillary network from the pulmonary artery, and oxygenated blood leaves the capillary network to enter the pulmonary veins on its journey around the body. Gaseous exchange in the lungs is called *external respiration* while in the tissues it is called *internal respiration*.

Gaseous exchange happens because of the scientific principle that gases diffuse from areas of high pressure to areas of low pressure. Oxygen in the alveoli is at a pressure of 100 mm Hg while that in the veins is at a pressure of 40 mm Hg. Therefore, oxygen diffuses from the alveoli into the blood to balance the pressure. Carbon dioxide in the blood is at a pressure of 46 mm Hg, so carbon dioxide diffuses out of the blood into the alveoli. Expired air therefore contains more carbon dioxide and less oxygen than inspired air; the nitrogen content remains unchanged.

A summary of the structures and functions of the respiratory system is given in the chart overleaf.

Fact file

Composition of inspired air:
▸▸ 79% nitrogen
▸▸ 21% oxygen
▸▸ 0.04% carbon dioxide
▸▸ traces of other gases
▸▸ water vapour.
Composition of expired air:
▸▸ 79% nitrogen
▸▸ 16% oxygen
▸▸ 4.5% carbon dioxide
▸▸ traces of other gases
▸▸ water vapour.

Assessment task 2.9

Outline the functions of the respiratory system. (P)

A summary of the structures and functions of the respiratory system:

	Structure	Function
Nose	Lined with ciliated mucus membranes which prevent the entry of foreign particles. Anterior nares (nostrils) lead in to the nose and posterior nares at the back lead out to the pharynx.	Vascular mucus membranes warm air as it passes through the nose; mucus moistens air and traps dust particles. Sense of smell is located in the highest part of the nasal cavity.
Pharynx	Leads from nasal cavity and is continuous with the oesophagus. Three sections: naso-pharynx (including the adenoids) behind the nose; oro-pharynx behind the mouth; and laryngeal pharynx behind the larynx.	Auditory tubes carry air from naso-pharynx to the middle ear. Oro-pharynx is part of the respiratory and digestive systems but cannot be used simultaneously, so breathing ceases momentarily during swallowing.
Larynx	Continuous with the oro-pharynx above and trachea below; consists of several cartilages including the epiglottis.	During swallowing the larynx shifts upwards and forwards so that the epiglottis blocks its opening.
Trachea	Below the larynx, extending down the front of the neck and into the thoracic region between the lungs. 12 cm long, consists of muscle, fibrous tissue and rings of cartilage.	Ciliated epithelium lining the trachea secrete mucus which combines with dust particles and is swept upwards away from the lungs by the cilia.
Bronchii	Two structures, one on either side, leading from the trachea to the lungs. Left bronchii is narrower to allow room for the heart. Similar structure to trachea.	Carry air from the trachea into the bronchioles.
Bronchioles	Bronchii divide progressively into smaller bronchii, the finest of which are the bronchioles which consist of muscular fibrous tissue.	Carry air from the bronchii towards the lungs.
Alveoli	Bronchioles branch to form minute tubes called alveoli.	Inhaled air reaches the alveoli via the respiratory tract.
Capillary networks	Network of blood vessels surrounding the alveoli.	Location of gaseous exchange between the air in the alveoli and the blood in the vessels.

Structure and function of the urinary system

Regulation of body fluids

About 60 per cent of our body weight is water. Certain systems work together to ensure that the water we take in and the water we lose are balanced, so that this value remains constant. Water is distributed around the body: about 70 per cent is inside the cells (**intracellular**) and 30 per cent is in the body fluids (**extracellular**). Of the extracellular water, about 15 to 20 per cent is in the interstitial spaces and about 10 to 15 per cent forms the fluid of the blood. You will know from your study of the systems so far that these volumes of water are separated by thin permeable cell or capillary walls, and that water constantly passes through from one area to another. Despite this, the volumes of water in different areas remain pretty constant.

In order to maintain these water levels in the body, water taken in must be in equal amounts to water lost. On average, we consume about 1.5 litres of water a day in drinks and about 1 litre a day in food, a total of about 2.5 litres. Water is lost from the body in similar amounts: about 400–500 ml by the lungs as water vapour; about 500–600 ml by the skin as sweat; about 1000–1500 ml by the kidneys as urine; and about 100–150 ml in the faeces.

Theory into practice

Explain how the volumes of water in our bodies are affected by hot weather and how water balance is maintained.

Electrolyte and pH balance

As well as maintaining volumes of water, the water must be of the correct composition. Water contains minute dissolved particles of salts, known as **electrolytes**. Electrolytes are charged ions: positively charged cations and negatively charged anions, which must be balanced.

Electrolyte distribution:

Ion	Symbol	Fluid
Chloride	Cl-	Plasma and interstitial fluid
Bicarbonate	HCO_3-	Plasma and interstitial fluid
Phosphate	PO_4-	Intracellular fluid
Sodium	Na+	Plasma and interstitial fluid
Potassium	K+	Intracellular fluid
Calcium	Ca+	Traces
Magnesium	Mg+	Traces

As well as maintaining certain levels of water and electrolytes, the body must maintain the pH of body fluids so that the various cell activities can take place. Body fluids are slightly alkaline with an average pH of 7.4. Venous blood is slightly less alkaline than arteriole blood because of the presence of carbon dioxide and other acids produced in the tissues. Interstitial and intracellular fluid is slightly more alkaline.

Alkalis and proteins neutralise acids produced during tissue activities. Acids, such as carbonates and chloride, neutralise alkalis so that the correct pH balance is maintained. If the body fluids become less alkaline than normal (i.e. more acidic), this can cause a condition called **acidosis** which can lead to coma and death. If the body fluids become more alkaline than normal, this can lead to a condition called **alkalosis**. Alkalosis can be caused by loss of acid from excessive vomiting, by retention of an alkali such as potassium as a result of renal failure, or by taking in high levels of alkaline salts such as sodium bicarbonate.

Theory into practice

Where else have you come across the conditions acidosis and alkalosis?

Urinary system

The urinary system consists of the kidneys, ureters, the bladder and the urethra. These structures play a key role in removing excess fluid from the body and in removing toxic waste materials in the form of urine.

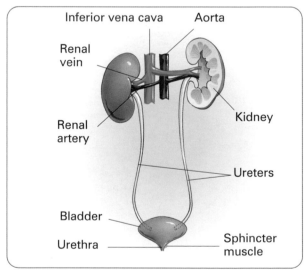

The structure of the urinary system.

The kidneys

The kidneys are two bean-shaped organs about 11 cm long, 6 cm wide and 3 cm thick. They are located at either side of the vertebral column in the posterior part of the abdomen, between the twelfth thoracic vertebra and the third lumbar vertebra. Each kidney is surrounded by a capsule of fibrous tissue and embedded in a bed of perirenal fat. The darker outer part of the kidney is the **cortex** and the paler inner section is the **medulla.**

The kidneys are made up of over a million minute twisted tubes called **nephrons.** Each nephron begins with a cup called the glomerular capsule into which leads a bunch of capillaries from the renal artery, called the **glomerulus**. The arteriole which brings blood to the glomerulus is the **afferent** vessel; that taking blood away is the slightly smaller **efferent** vessel. The nephron twists down into the medulla and back up to the cortex, and eventually empties into a straight tubule in the medulla. The efferent vessel divides to form a second set of capillaries where blood is collected by small veins, and these empty into the renal vein. In no other organ does blood pass through two sets of capillaries.

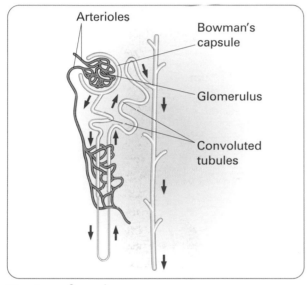

Structure of a nephron.

Theory into practice

You have come across the terms *afferent* and *efferent* before in this unit. Can you remember where?

Urine production

The function of the kidneys is to secrete and excrete urine which is produced by three processes: filtration under pressure, selective reabsorption and active secretion.

Filtration under pressure

The walls of the glomerulus are semi-permeable: they allow water and other small particles to pass through but not blood cells or protein. The blood in the glomerulus is under pressure so some of its constituents pass through into the glomerulus capsule. This fluid has a similar make up to plasma. It contains water, glucose, salts, fatty acids and urea, and is called the glomerular filtrate. In the presence of kidney disease, blood cells and proteins are also filtered.

Selective reabsorption

The cells surrounding the nephrons have the ability to absorb water, glucose and salts needed by the body. All of the glucose is absorbed and most of the water and salts, so that urine contains no glucose and only about 2 per cent urea. The acidity of urine varies according to the levels of salts, which helps to maintain the pH of blood at about 7.4.

Active secretion

The cells lining the nephrons have the ability to secrete some substances from the blood in the second capillary network.

Urine storage and release

Urine is stored in a reservoir called the bladder. The size, shape and position of the bladder varies according to how much urine it holds. The lower part is fixed about 3–4 cm behind the pubis symphysis, but as the bladder expands it moves upwards and forwards into the abdominal cavity. The bladder has the capacity to hold over 500 ml; however, this would cause great discomfort and usually we feel the desire to empty the bladder when it contains 250–300 ml of urine. The normal quantity of urine secreted in a 24-hour period is about 1.5 litres. This amount is increased by drinking lots of fluid and in cold weather, and is decreased by drinking less fluid and in warm weather. Urine is an acidic fluid consisting of 96 per cent water, 2 per cent urea, and 2 per cent uric acid and salts, although this composition is affected by certain illnesses.

Theory into practice

Try to find out the names of some medical conditions which can be detected by the composition of urine. You could collect leaflets and information from your doctor or a pharmacist.

Assessment task 2.10

Outline the function of the urinary system. (P)

A summary of the structure and function of the urinary system:

	Structure	Function
Kidneys	Bean-shaped organs located between 12th thoracic and 3rd lumbar vertebrae	Secretion and excretion of urine
Ureters	25–30 cm thick-walled tubes which undergo peristaltic contractions	Carry urine from kidneys to bladder
Bladder	Fixed opening behind pubis symphysis; location varies according to volume of urine	Reservoir for urine with a maximum capacity of 500 ml, though is usually emptied when it contains about 250–300 ml
Urethra	Tube extending from the bladder; 20 cm long in males, 4 cm in females	In males, functions as part of both reproductive and urinary systems

Assessment task 2.11

Explain in detail the interdependence of the digestive, cardiovascular, respiratory and urinary systems. (D)

Reproduction

The female reproductive system consists of ovaries, uterus, vagina and external genitalia. We shall also investigate the role, structure and function of the mammary glands in females, which are described as accessory organs of reproduction. The male reproductive system consists of the testis, epididymis, scrotum, sperm duct and penis. Both male and female reproductive systems serve to ensure the continuation of the species.

The female reproductive system:

	Structure	Function
Ovaries	Small glands the size and shape of almonds, located on either side of the uterus behind and below the uterine tubes.	Controlled by **follicle stimulating hormone (FSH)** and **lutenizing hormone (LH)**. Release ova at monthly intervals; secrete female hormones responsible for sexual development.
Uterus	Hollow, thick walled organ, 7.5 cm long, 5 cm across, 2.5 cm thick. Located between the rectum and the bladder at 90° to the vagina. Lined by the **endometrium**.	Receives fertilised ovum which grows to fill the uterus, then uterus grows with the foetus until birth. Placenta develops at the site of implantation to provide nourishment and oxygen to the developing foetus.
Vagina	Extends from uterus to labia, behind the bladder and urethra and in front of the rectum. The cervix enters the vagina at 90°.	Allows insertion of penis and deposit of seminal fluid during intercourse. Forms final part of birth canal during labour.
External genitalia	**Mons pubis**: pad of fat covered with skin and hair over the pubis symphysis; labia majora: two fleshy folds covered with skin and hair; **labia minora**: two smaller fleshy folds including the hood-like **prepuce**; **clitoris**: small, sensitive organ of erectile tissue; **vestibule**: cleft between labia minora.	Mons pubis and labia majora protect the internal structures; prepuce of the labia minora protects the clitoris; vestibule contains vaginal and urethral orifices which secrete lubricating fluid to moisten the vulva and assist penetration during sexual intercourse.

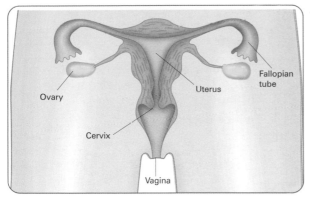

The female reproductive system.

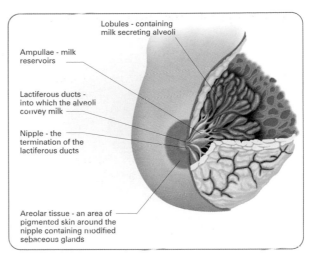

The structure of mammary glands.

Mammary glands

The female breasts or **mammary glands** are accessory organs to the female reproductive system. They consist of three types of tissue: glandular, fibrous and fatty. Each mammary gland consists of 15 to 20 lobes of glandular tissue, which in turn consists of several smaller lobes called lobules, which secrete milk during **lactation**. Small tubes, or ducts, leading away from the lobes and lobules are called **lactiferous ducts**. The ducts dilate at the centre of the mammary gland to form **lactiferous sinuses**, which are reservoirs for milk during lactation. Lactiferous sinuses form small ducts that open onto the surface of the nipple, lying at the centre of each mammary gland.

The mammary glands are supported and attached to the body by ligaments of fibrous tissue that are continuous with the pectoral muscles. Mammary glands do not contain muscle but can be maintained by exercising the supporting muscles of the chest wall. Breast tissue is almost entirely made up of fat, which covers the surface of the mammary gland and is present in between the structures. The amount of fatty tissue determines the size of the breasts, which can vary considerably between and within individuals. During puberty, an increase in adipose tissue stimulates the development of the mammary glands. The amount of adipose tissue decreases during menopause causing shrinkage of the mammary glands, which in turn become less full and more pendulous. An increased production of hormones during pregnancy stimulates further growth of the mammary glands and a change in the nipple, which becomes enlarged and darker in colour.

Theory into practice

Try to think of other conditions which alter the size and/or shape of the breasts.

Fact file

➤ Nipples and the surrounding areola are pink but become pigmented after the first pregnancy.

➤ A yellowy milk-like fluid called colostrum is secreted in small amounts during pregnancy and labour. True milk is not secreted until about day 3 after childbirth.

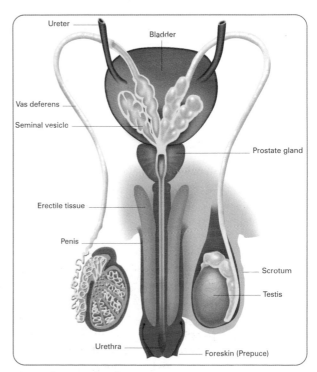

The male reproductive system.

The male reproductive system:

	Structure	Function
Testes	Reproductive glands which develop high in the abdomen but become suspended in the scrotum. Each testis contains 200–300 lobules, which contain three convulted tubes called **seminiferous tubules**.	Lining of seminiferous tubules develop into **spermatozoa**; interstitial cells in in connective tissue secrete **testosterone**.
Epididymis	Tightly coiled tubes attached to the back of the testes.	Seminiferous tubules open into epididymis, which leads to the deferent duct of the seminal vesicle.
Scrotum	Sac-like structure which hangs outside of the body.	Contains the testes.
Sperm duct	Formed by the deferent ducts and seminal vesicles, leading from the base of the prostrate to the urethra.	Passage for seminal fluid and sperm.
Penis	Tubular organ with plentiful supply of venous sinuses and a tip called the glans penis, covered with foreskin.	Becomes engorged with blood to cause an erection, which facilitates sexual intercourse.

Functions of the reproductive system

Fact file

> ▸ A **gamete** is a mature germ or sex cell that takes part in fertilisation, i.e. female ovum and male sperm.
> ▸ The term given to the production of gametes is **gametogenesis**.

Gametogenesis in males

A mature male is constantly producing sperm, although the production of an individual sperm takes about 64 days. Sperm production is most efficient at a temperature slightly lower than 37°C, which is why the testes are suspended outside of the body. Sperm production occurs in the seminiferous tubules and consists of three phases. During the 'mitotic phase', rapid cell division increases the number of cells. The second phase of 'meiotic division' reduces the number of chromosomes in each cell and provides individual combinations. The third phase of 'maturation and packaging' gets the chromosomes ready for transport from the body in the sperm, when 500 million or so sperm are released in a single ejaculation.

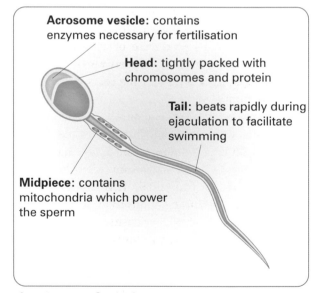

Acrosome vesicle: contains enzymes necessary for fertilisation

Head: tightly packed with chromosomes and protein

Tail: beats rapidly during ejaculation to facilitate swimming

Midpiece: contains mitochondria which power the sperm

The structure of a single sperm.

The production of sperm is controlled by hormones. Lutenizing hormone (LH) and follicle stimulating hormone (FSH) produced in the pituitary gland stimulate the testes to produce the male hormone testosterone. This is then converted to dihydrotestosterone (DHT) which stimulates the first phase of production, i.e. mitosis. FSH and LH also stimulate the production of DHT within the testes. Since sperm cannot live for more than a few days, local differences are maintained via levels of hormones in different areas, so that sperm production is staggered and a constant supply is maintained.

Gametogenesis in females

The female ova is one of the largest cells in the body, measuring about 0.1 mm in diameter. It contains a large amount of cytoplasm. This nourishes the growing embryo before the development of a placenta, which takes place two weeks after fertilisation. The production of cytoplasm uses up a lot of energy and raw materials and is subsidised by 'granulosa cells'. Egg production occurs in the ovaries and involves three phases. Mitosis and meiosis occur in a similar way to sperm production in males. The third 'growth' phase increases the amount of cytoplasm and occurs concurrently with the meiotic phase.

You might think that the production of a single ovum takes one month, i.e. the period of the menstrual cycle. In fact, it is a continual process which begins even before birth and continues until the menopause. When a female is born her ovaries contain more than two million partially produced ova, or **oocytes**; the total amount that she will ever produce. A few hundred of these survive until puberty but remain in a state of arrest. Following puberty a few are reactivated every day so there is a steady supply of oocytes and the release of a single egg each month.

The production of ova is controlled by hormones. During the first phase of maturation the follicle cells develop a sensitivity to FSH and LH, stimulating a further round of mitosis. The follicle cells also produce the female hormone oestrogen, which creates heightened sensitivity to LH. (Note that the oocyte itself is not sensitive to LH but the follicle cells are.) Sensitivity must continue to the final phase. During this final phase of maturation the follicle becomes a **corpus luteum** and secretes progesterone (instead of oestrogen) in preparation for a possible pregnancy. At the time of ovulation the oocyte is at the surface of the follicle. Increased fluid pressure within causes it to 'pop' and the ova is then ejected into the fallopian tube. If sperm are present in the fallopian tube, fertilisation can occur.

Assessment task 2.12

Outline the hormonal regulation of gametogenesis in the male and female. (D)

The menstrual cycle

The menstrual cycle describes the (approximately) 28-day reproductive cycle that occurs in females, although the length of the cycle varies between individuals. Day 1 refers to the first day of menstruation and day 14 is the day ovulation usually occurs. The menstrual cycle is controlled by the relative levels of the hormones oestrogen and progesterone, which determine whether an egg is released. When the levels of oestrogen reach a high level, secretion of FSH is retarded and secretion of LH is increased. Following ovulation, LH converts the ruptured follicle into the corpus luteum, which secretes progesterone and this continues the thickening of the endometrium. If the egg is not fertilised the corpus luteum degenerates, progesterone levels drop and the endometrium is shed as menstrual blood; the production of FSH is stimulated and the cycle begins once again. Menstruation usually begins between the ages of 12 and 15 years and continues until the menopause (about 50 years), with each period of menstruation lasting from 2–8 days. Menstruation also ceases during pregnancy.

Fact file

Common disorders of the menstrual cycle:

➤ **Amenorrhoea**: absence of menstruation which can be caused by a hormonal imbalance, psychological stress or anorexia nervosa.

➤ **Dismenorrhoea**: painful menstruation.

➤ **Endometriosis**: the endometrium attaches to other parts of the reproductive system, such as the ovary, uterus or fallopian tubes, causing pain and heavy bleeding during menstruation.

➤ **Pre-menstrual tension**: feelings of anxiety, depression, mood swings and irritability experienced by some women in the days prior to menstruation.

Theory into practice

Which, if any, of the conditions mentioned above would be a cause for concern during beauty therapy treatment? Why?

Fertilisation

Fertilisation describes the process of bringing together the male and female gametes in the fallopian tubes. Natural fertilisation occurs following sexual intercourse when the male penis deposits seminal fluid in the vagina.

> **Fact file**
>
> In vitro fertilisation (IVF) is the artificial process of fertilisation. This takes place in a laboratory before implanting the fertilised egg into the uterus.

Following ejaculation into the vagina, the sperm coagulate to prevent loss due to gravity. This only lasts a short time before it liquifies once again, but it is long enough for some sperm to have swum through the cervix and into the fallopian tubes. The sperm are helped by a number of physiological factors: the cervix, which is usually blocked by mucus, becomes more permeable during ovulation; cilia lining the entrance to the cervix waft the sperm through; sperm have a tendency to swim towards the fallopian tube containing the ovulated egg rather than the empty one, due to their response to chemical signals. Once the sperm reach the fallopian tubes they become activated and their life span is shortened considerably. The membrane surrounding the acrosome develops holes and releases an enzyme which destroys the follicle cells surrounding the egg. At this stage the membrane of one sperm fuses with that of the egg. Immediately the sperm stops swimming and the composition of the egg membrane adjusts to prevent any other sperm from entering it.

Pregnancy and birth

Normal pregnancy in humans lasts 40 weeks (which is nearer to ten months than nine) and involves a series of changes in the mother as well as in the developing foetus. These changes are far too complex to include in a short section such as this, or even a single chapter. Instead, an overview is provided for the purpose of interest and reference.

Before the seventh or eighth week of gestation, the foetus is a combination of cells – unrecognisable as a developing baby. Foetal growth occurs by an increase in the number of cells and is influenced by the health and nutrition of the mother as well as by the **placenta**, which is a rich supply of nourishment and oxygen after the second week. Foetal growth is not a linear process and the rate is slower towards the end of the pregnancy.

Foetal development from two to nine months follows these stages:

- ▶ 2 months: the embryo measures about 2–4 cm in length. The heart has divided into four chambers and the veins are visible.
- ▶ 3 months: the foetus is about 6–8 cm in length. The organs and muscles have begun rudimentary functioning.
- ▶ 4 months: the foetus is now covered with a layer of downy **lanugo** hair, has a clear heartbeat and may have even begun to kick!
- ▶ 5 months: a protective coating covers the skin. The foetus is about 20 cm in length and weighs about 450g.

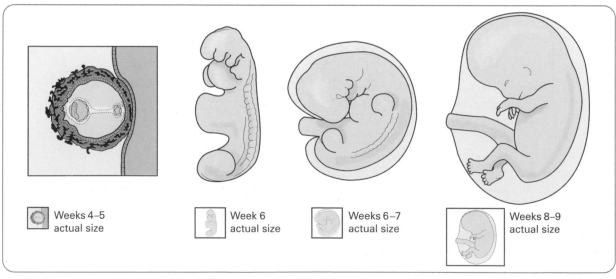

| Weeks 4–5 actual size | Week 6 actual size | Weeks 6–7 actual size | Weeks 8–9 actual size |

Weeks 0 to 8 of gestation.

- 6 months: the eyebrows and eyelids have developed. The respiratory system is functioning and the lungs are filled with amniotic fluid. The foetus has a developed sense of hearing.
- 7 months: the body is now well formed, even down to the fingernails. It measures about 30 cm in length and weighs about 1.1 kg.
- 8 months: the baby is now gaining about 225g each week as layers of adipose tissue develop, and will weigh about 1.8–2.2 kg by the end of the month. The head may have turned in preparation for birth.
- 9 months: the baby now weighs 2.7–3.6 kg and is preparing to be born. As he or she has increased so much in size, there is less room to manoeuvre and the mother will feel less movement.

Three stages of labour

There are several factors which can trigger labour, the main one being the baby itself. The baby's head must be engaged before normal labour can proceed; therefore babies are born when they are ready to be born! The placenta stops growing and its ability to supply nutrients declines, which prepares the foetus to become independent. The declining placenta stimulates the uterus to begin contracting. In addition, the stretching of the uterus over the enlarged foetus stimulates the pituitary gland to produce the hormone **oxytocin**, which also stimulates contractions. The foetal adrenal cortex grows late in pregnancy and produces large amounts of the hormone **cortisol**, which further encourages contractions of the uterus.

There are three stages of childbirth. Firstly, the plug of mucus blocking the opening of the cervix drops out and the cervix becomes dilated to a diameter of 10 cm, the approximate diameter of the baby's head. The contractions which open the cervix increase in strength and length over a period, which can last for more than 12 hours in a first labour. The second stage of labour usually lasts no more than an hour or two and involves pushing the baby out. Typically, the head comes first, then the baby twists to deliver one shoulder then the other, and finally the whole baby appears. The contractions of the uterus are sufficient in themselves but the urge to push is irresistible to most mothers.

The third stage of labour involves expelling the placenta, which will have become detached during the strong uterine contractions that forced the baby out. There is a risk of heavy bleeding at this stage and mothers are often injected with a drug to prevent this by constricting the blood vessels. The newborn baby must be kept warm as it has emerged from a temperature of 37°C to room temperature, which is about 20°C. The baby does not have to be fed immediately because stores of glycogen and fats have been built up during development in the uterus. However, the first meal should not be delayed too long as it also provides the opportunity for the mother and baby to bond.

Assessment task 2.13

Explain the hormonal regulation of the female reproductive system. (D)

Knowledge check

1 Explain the levels of biological organisation.
2 Describe the main structures of a cell.
3 Explain how structure and function of the nervous system are related.
4 Describe negative feedback.
5 Identify the main glands of the endocrine system.
6 Define homeostasis.
7 Identify the components of a balanced diet.
8 Describe food's journey from ingestion to egestion.
9 Describe catabolism and anabolism.
10 Draw a fully labelled diagram of the heart illustrating the direction of blood flow.
11 Define blood pressure.
12 Identify the chief muscles of respiration.
13 Describe the four main structures of the female reproductive system.
14 Describe the hormonal regulation of the menstrual cycle.
15 Define the three stages of normal labour.

Anatomy

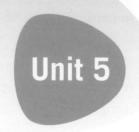

Unit 5

This unit introduces you to the anatomy or framework of the human body. It explores the structure, function and development of the human skeleton, including bones, joints and movement. You will also examine the muscles of the human body and their structure.

You will investigate the biological principles of support and movement by examining the co-ordinated actions of joints and muscle groups with an emphasis on posture and how it is maintained. The effects of the ageing process on bones, joints and muscles are also investigated.

As well as gaining a theoretical understanding of human anatomy, the concepts explored in this unit will enable you to assess human posture and movement practically, which is developed further in Unit 10: Body therapy. This chapter is closely linked to Unit 2: Human physiology.

In order to achieve Unit 5 in anatomy you must complete the following learning outcomes:

LEARNING OUTCOMES

1 Investigate the structure, functions and development of the the skeleton.

2 Relate the structure of joints to the movements they permit.

3 Explain muscle structure including the physiological basis of muscle fibre contraction.

4 Explore how the skeletal muscular system acts on the skeleton to maintain posture and produce body movement.

The skeleton

Functions of the skeleton

The human skeleton is a mobile, bony framework, consisting of approximately 206 bones. These establish its characteristic shape and differentiate humans from other animals. As well as providing shape, the skeleton has other important functions linked to its structure, which are summarised in the table overleaf and revisited throughout this unit.

Bones and bone tissue

The skeleton of a human embryo consists of a flexible tissue called **cartilage**, which is made of strong collagen and stretchy elastin fibres. Bone formation begins in the seventh week of development when cartilage is gradually replaced by hard bone tissue in a process called **ossification**. The bones of the head are not fully developed at birth, which allows the baby to mould to the birth canal during labour. Areas of incomplete ossification, such as the fontanelles in the skull and some small bones in the wrist, continue to develop through infancy.

Important functions of the skeleton:

Function	Summary
Support	Without a skeleton we would be a wobbly, floppy mass of cells and tissue, unable to stand, move or support ourselves.
Protection	The various parts of the skeleton protect the underlying structures, e.g. the cranium protects the brain and the thoracic cage protects the heart and lungs.
Attachment for skeletal muscles and leverage	Muscles attach to the bones of the skeleton and pull them into different positions, so that the bones act like levers. This allows many types of movement at joints.
Source of blood cells	Many bones are hollow and consist of spongy bone tissue which is filled with red marrow. Red marrow is the site for the production of blood cells in adults.
Store of calcium	Calcium makes bone hard and is used to maintain the compact tissue of bones. Its release into the bloodstream, initiated by **parathyroid hormone**, is required to maintain heart rate, respiration and muscle contraction.

Fact file

The skeleton grows quickly during infancy and adolescence. Children should take regular exercise to maintain healthy bones and joints but should refrain from using weights, which would put undue stress on the developing skeleton.

Nearly all cartilage is eventually replaced by hard bone tissue, although some remains on the joint surfaces of most bones in the form of **articular cartilage**. This is nourished by articular fluid and nutrients and is stimulated by activity.

It is therefore important that children are involved in regular physical activity to ensure good bone development and prevent thinning out of cartilage. Development of the skeleton continues until about the age of 25 years, by which time the final size and shape of the skeleton has been established. However, growth, destruction and repair of bone tissue, to maintain the strength and health of the skeletal system, continues throughout life.

Bone formation and growth

Bone tissue, unlike cartilage, is rigid and non-elastic. It consists of about 67 per cent calcium and 33 per cent organic matter, mainly collagen.

The process of bone formation is called ossification and depends on a delicate balance between the construction and destruction of bone tissue. This is maintained by specialist cells called

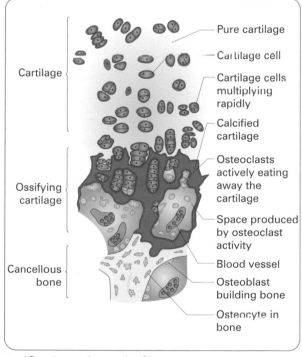

Ossification and growth of bone.

osteoblasts and **osteoclasts**. Osteoblasts make new bone tissue; they secrete collagen which forms a strong yet flexible framework. Mineral salts, especially calcium, are then deposited within this framework to provide hardness in a process called **calcification**. Osteoblasts become trapped in the framework of bone tissue and develop into osteocytes, which release further calcium ions that become part of the bone tissue. Osteoclasts contain **lysosomes**, which are enzymes that digest protein and also break down minerals in bone because of their acidic quality.

In this way the skeleton is maintained as osteoclasts destroy old bone tissue while osteoblasts construct new bone tissue. This process also allows bone tissue to act as a storage for calcium, which is required for the functioning of other areas of the body such as muscles, nerves and blood.

Theory into practice

Explain what you think might happen if osteoblasts became more active than osteoclasts, and vice versa.

Structure and classification of bone

There are two types of bone tissue – **compact** and **cancellous**. There are five types of bone: long,

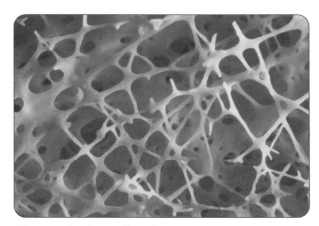

Micrograph of cancellous bone.

short, flat, sesamoid and irregular, which have structures suited to their function and position in the human body.

Type of bone tissue:

Type of bone tissue	Characteristic
Compact bone tissue	Hard, strong and relatively heavy. Forms the tough outer shell of most bones in the human skeleton.
Cancellous bone tissue	Spongy texture (also known as spongy bone tissue). Spaces in the tissue contain red bone marrow where blood cells are formed. Lightweight.

A summary of the structure of bone tissue:

Type of bone	Structure	Examples
Long	Consists of a shaft of compact bone tissue and two spongy extremities called epiphyses, made of cancellous bone tissue.	Femur (thigh) Humerus (upper arm)
Short	Short, irregular bones consisting of cancellous bone tissue surrounded by a thin layer of compact bone tissue. Lightweight.	Carpals (8 wrist bones) Tarsals (7 ankle bones)
Flat	Plate-like layers of compact and cancellous bone tissue make these bones strong yet lightweight.	Frontal (forehead)
Sesamoid	Oval-shaped bone located in tendons.	Patella (kneecap)
Irregular	Mass of cancellous bone tissue surrounded by a thin layer of compact bone tissue.	Vertebrae (spine)

Bone homeostasis

Homeostasis is the ability to maintain optimum conditions for health and development. In bones it is maintained by the balanced activities of osteoblasts and osteoclasts, which continually destroy and construct bone tissue.

Bone remodelling

Like other cells and tissues in the human body, bone tissue is continually being broken down and replaced in a process known as remodelling. This is achieved by a delicate balance of activity between osteoblasts and osteoclasts and is an example of homeostasis.

Responses to physical stress

The human body manages to protect itself from the external environment in a number of ways determined by structure. While the skeletal system provides protective cavities for the internal organs, it is protected from external physical knocks by the skin and underlying adipose tissue which acts to cushion any hard blows. If bones do fracture or break, osteoblast and osteoclast activity enables them to heal from within.

Membranes and ligaments also have a protective function against physical stress, an example of which is found in the lower leg. The interosseous membrane between the tibia and fibula distributes stress between the two bones when force is exerted on the talus during running or jumping. Between the vertebrae of the spinal column, collagen fibres and cartilage form intervertebral discs that act as shock absorbers, to protect against stress to the back bone. The joints and muscles of the body have specific ways of responding to physical stress, which are investigated in the following sections.

Bone injury and repair

The activities of osteoblasts and osteoclasts also play an important part in restructuring bone when it becomes injured. Bone tissue is able to heal itself in a process similar to that of skin healing (discussed in Unit 6, pages 105–6), which is an amplification of the normal process of cell renewal. The initial response to a break in the bone is pain, swelling, inflammation and localised heat, signalling an increased blood flow to the area. The fractured bone severs blood vessels in the area and, to prevent continued blood loss, a clot is formed known as a **fracture haematoma**.

Before a broken bone is set in plaster, the ends of the bones are aligned manually so that they can mend and remodel in place. Internally, osteoclasts remove cellular and bony debris and new blood vessels grow into the haematoma over a period of weeks. The haematoma changes into granulation tissue (as in skin healing) which contains a network of blood capillaries. Within about three weeks, fibroblasts and other cells produce a network of

A summary of bone tissue repair after injury:

Time scale	Physiological response	Physical response
Immediate	Bone fractures/breaks; severed blood vessels	Pain; internal and/or external bleeding
Within hours	Fracture haematoma; increased blood flow to area	Prevents further blood loss; heat, swelling, inflammation; manual realignment, set in plaster
Within weeks	Growth of new blood vessels, increased activity of osteoclasts	Removes cellular and bony debris
Up to three weeks	Haematoma becomes granulation tissue; increased activity of fibroblasts	Replaces damaged blood vessels; network of collagen and cartilage forms fibrous callus
Three to four months	Increased activity of osteoblasts Increased activity of osteoclasts	Builds pad of spongy bone tissue which is slowly replaced with compact bone tissue; trims away excess bony callus

collagen fibres and fibrous cartilage, which forms pads of tissue called calluses. In a process lasting three to four months, osteoblasts produce spongy bone throughout this pad, which eventually develop into compact bone tissue. Osteoclasts trim away excess bone callus, giving the broken bone the same appearance as healthy bone – even under x-ray. However, some muscle wastage may be apparent at the site of injury due to lack of use when the bone is immobilised in a plaster cast.

Children's bones, which are not yet fully calcified, are still quite flexible and may break with a **greenstick fracture**. These are so called because the broken bone resembles a new, green, flexible piece of wood, with one side breaking and the other side bending. Bone healing occurs more quickly in young people and is retarded by age. This may be due to poor blood supply or a reduced capacity for repair, due to a general slowing down of the metabolism. Poor nutrition may also be a factor.

Assessment task 5.1

Explain the process of growth and repair of bones of the skeleton with reference to osteoblast and osteoclast activity. (M)

Homeostatic imbalances

Homeostatic imbalances occur either when bone tissue is destroyed faster than it is replaced or replaced faster than it is destroyed, due to an imbalance of osteoblasts or osteoclast activity. Too much osteoblast activity would result in more bone tissue being produced than could be removed, and bones would become thick and heavy. Furthermore, if lumps were formed on bones this could affect joint activity and movement. If, on the other hand, osteoclast activity was higher, too much bone tissue would be removed. The bones would then become thin, weak and brittle.

As the body ages, compact bone tissue is lost more quickly than it can be replaced. Cancellous bone tissue loses some of its internal structure due to the breakdown of collagen fibres and so there is a reduction in bone mass and the bones become weaker. One of the most common homeostatic imbalances is **osteoporosis**, which occurs when bone mass falls below a certain level and the bones become more prone to fractures and breaks. This is usually associated with age and tends to affect women more than men. This is because women tend to have a lower bone mass than men at maturity and so the further reduction in mass causes them more of a problem.

Assessment task 5.2

Through research, provide an explanation of common homeostatic disorders of the skeleton. (D)

Effects of ageing

One of the greatest influences on skeletal development in infancy is nutrition. Vitamin A influences osteoblast and osteoclast activity, which is needed to maintain a homeostatic balance, and Vitamin D is required to aid the absorption of calcium from the intestine. Vitamins C and B12 are also essential to bone growth. Age-associated changes in the digestive system can radically effect the condition of the skeleton. Less calcium is absorbed from the diet, which appears to affect post-menopausal women more so than men of the same age, adding to the tendency towards osteoporosis. Changes in the digestive system also affect the absorption of vitamin D and changes in the skin slow down the production of vitamin D activated by natural sunlight. As the function of vitamin D is to transport calcium from the digestive system to the bones, a deficiency means that new bone tissue is produced slower than existing tissue is destroyed.

During middle age and into old age, bones start to shrink and the skin can become saggy as it fits less snugly on the internal framework. Bones in the face diminish in the same way as bones in the body do, and this bone shrinkage is partly to blame for the lack of tautness that is noticeable in mature skins.

Hormone replacement therapy (HRT) is commonly prescribed to women to treat the effects of the menopause. Treatment with the hormone **oestrogen** has been found to have a positive effect on calcium metabolism, which in turn reduces loss of bone density and reduces the risk of osteoporosis. Additional advice to clients would be to maintain regular gentle exercise, such as walking, which prevents bone mass loss and encourages the production of vitamin D in the skin via natural sunlight. Also, the diet should contain adequate amounts of calcium, which the body needs to produce new bone tissue. The recommended daily calcium intake is about 700 mg, or the equivalent of one pint of skimmed milk.

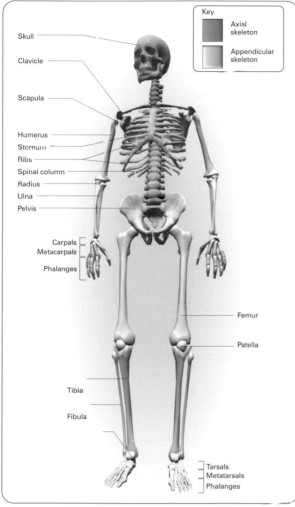

Theory into practice

Think about the appearance of the human body at different ages and explain the association with age-related changes in the skeletal system.

The skeleton

Key
Axial skeleton
Appendicular skeleton

Skull
Clavicle
Scapula
Humerus
Sternum
Ribs
Spinal column
Radius
Ulna
Pelvis
Carpals
Metacarpals
Phalanges
Femur
Patella
Tibia
Fibula
Tarsals
Metatarsals
Phalanges

The structure of the skeleton.

Axial and appendicular skeleton

The skeleton is divided into two parts: the axis or axial skeleton and its appendages, which are known as the appendicular skeleton. The axis of the body is made up of the 80 bones of the skull, ribcage and spinal column. The appendicular skeleton consists of 126 bones found in the upper and lower limbs, the pelvic girdle and the shoulder girdle.

Assessment task 5.3

Identify the bones of the axial and appendicular skeleton. (P)

Fact file

Axial skeleton:	Appendicular skeleton:
1 frontal	2 scapulae
2 parietal	2 clavicle
2 temporal	2 humerus
1 occipital	2 radius
1 ethmoid	2 ulna
1 sphenoid	16 carpals
2 lacrimal	10 metacarpals
4 nasal	28 phalanges
1 vomer	2 pelvic bones
1 maxilla	2 femur
1 mandible	2 patella
2 zygomatic	2 fibula
2 palatine	2 tibia
1 hyoid	14 tarsals
7 cervical vertabrae	10 metatarsals
12 thoracic vertabrae	28 phalanges
5 lumbar vertabrae	
5 fused bones of sacrum	
4 fused bones of coccyx	
24 (12 pairs) ribs	
1 sternum	
total = 80 bones	**total = 126 bones**

Relation of bone structure and function

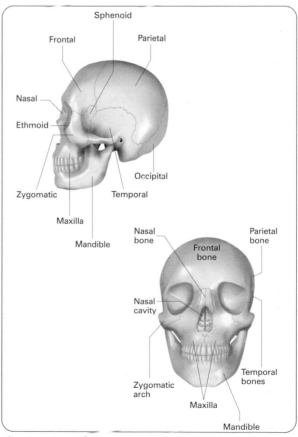

Sphenoid
Frontal
Parietal
Nasal
Ethmoid
Occipital
Zygomatic
Temporal
Maxilla
Mandible

Nasal bone
Parietal bone
Frontal bone
Nasal cavity
Zygomatic arch
Maxilla
Temporal bones
Mandible

The structure of the skull.

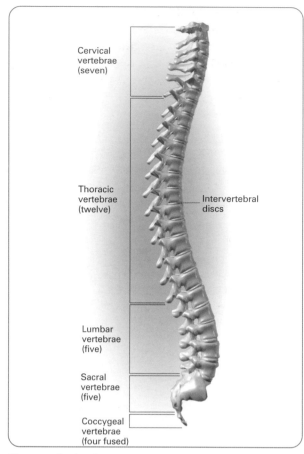

The vertebral column.

Relation of bone structure and function

The axial skeleton has a central position in the structure of the body and consists of the skull, vertebral column and thoracic cage. The skull has two parts: the cranium which forms the roof and back of the skull and contains the brain; and the face at the front of the skull which contains the eyes and teeth. The cranium forms a deep cavity to protect the brain and is constructed of flat bones which are strong yet lightweight. The facial bones are irregular and formed into peaks and furrows to protect the eyes, nasal cavities, teeth and tongue. The vertebral column consists of 33 individual bones, although some are fused together. Between each vertebra is a pad of fibrous tissue, called an intervertebral disc, which serves to act as a shock absorber against gravity and injury. Each vertebrae contains a hole in the centre and through this runs the spinal cord, which forms part of the **central nervous system** (CNS). The thoracic cage consists of 12 thoracic vertebrae, 12 pairs of ribs and one sternum. This cage protects the heart, lungs and major blood vessels, and is a point of attachment for the diaphragm and intercostal muscles which assist respiration.

The appendicular skeleton consists of the limbs, clavicle and scapulae. Together with muscles, the appendicular skeleton is responsible for voluntary movements. These can range from complex co-ordinations involving the whole body, such as walking and jumping, to small, specific movements such as writing or wriggling your toes.

Assessment task 5.4

Demonstrate a clear understanding of the relation between the structure of the skeleton and its function. (D)

Joints

A joint is formed where two bones meet. Without joints the skeleton would be static and movement would be limited. The most obvious joints in the human body are found at the knees and elbows, which allow movement of the upper and lower limbs. However, movement is also possible in the vertebral column, which enables us to twist and

Function of the axial skeleton:

Functions of skull	Functions of vertebral column	Functions of thoracic cage
Cranium protects the brain	Protects spinal cord	Protects lungs
Base of the frontal bone and zygomatic bones form the eye sockets	Provides attachment for ribs	Protects heart and major blood vessels
Mandible forms the lower jaw and aids mastication	Provides attachment for muscles	Provides attachment for diaphragm
Temporal bone protects the ear canal		Provides attachment for intercostal muscles

bend; in the hands and feet, enabling us to write, wave, pick things up, dance and walk; and in the thoracic cage, which enables respiration. There are three groups of joints – fibrous, cartilaginous and synovial – and these permit different types of movement; some allow no movement at all.

Types of joints

Fibrous

A fibrous joint occurs where two bones dovetail together, as in the cranium or where the roots of the teeth attach to the mandible and maxilla. The structures are separated by a thin band of fibrous tissue called a **suture**. These joints do not usually permit movement of any kind.

Cartilaginous

A cartilaginous joint occurs where two bones are connected by a pad of fibrous cartilage and ligaments which do not form a complete capsule around the joint. The most obvious examples are the joints between the vertebrae, which allow limited movement. The articulation between the pubic bones of the pelvis is another example of a cartilaginous joint.

Synovial joints

A synovial joint occurs where two or more bones are joined together by articular cartilage contained in a joint capsule, allowing free movement. Examples of free moving synovial joints are the joint at the knee between the femur and lower leg, the joint at the hip between the pelvis and the femur, and the joint at the elbow between the humerus and lower arm. Of these, the knee is the largest and most complex example.

In the knee joint, the femur, tibia and fibula are held together by **ligaments**, which are bundles of collagen fibres. The ends of the bones are covered

with **articular cartilage**, which allows the bones to move against each other without causing too much friction, and the joint is stabilised by pads of cartilage called **menisci**. The area around the bones contains pads of connective tissue called **bursae**, which contain **synovial fluid**, a sticky, nutritious liquid that enables free movement and also nourishes the cartilage cells. The main function of the bursae is to reduce friction as parts glide against each other. It is inevitable that, as the joint moves, some tissue is worn away; this is removed by **phagocytic** cells which are also contained in synovial fluid.

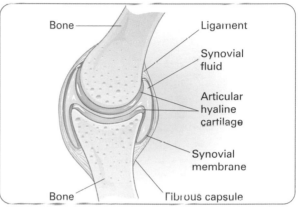

The structure of a synovial joint.

Assessment task 5.5

Explain the relationship between the structure and function of the hip, knee and ankle joints. (D)

Movements at synovial joints

Just from knowing your own body, you know that different areas are capable of different movements and you can probably work out why. The size and structure of bones, the type and size of joint, and the tone and structure of muscle, all play a part in movement.

The three types of joint:

	Characteristics	Range of movement	Example
▸▸ **Fibrous joints**	2 bones dovetail, separated by a suture	None	Between bones of skull
▸▸ **Cartilaginous joints**	2 bones connected by cartilage	Limited	Between vertebrae
▸▸ **Synovial joints**	2 or more bones covered with articular cartilage and contained within a joint capsule	Free movement limited by different articulating surfaces	Knee, elbow, hip, ankle, wrist

Joint movement:

Illustration	Anatomical term	Description
	Flexion	Reduces angle between two bones
	Extension	Increases angle between two bones
	Abduction	Moving away from mid-line of the body
	Adduction	Moving towards mid-line of the body
	Circumduction	Moving an extremity around in a circle
	Rotation	Turning on an axis
	Supination	Outward rotation
	Pronation	Inward rotation

Joint movement (cont.):

Illustration	Anatomical term	Description
	Inversion	Turning inwards
	Eversion	Turning outwards
	Elevation	Raising body part
	Depression	Lowering body part

You can train your body to be more flexible and you can facilitate movement through massage and passive exercise, but there remain limitations to the movements possible at different joints. Synovial joints are freely moving joints, although movements are limited by the shape of the articulating surfaces and the ligaments that hold the bones together. There are three types of movement possible at synovial joints. Angular movements include flexion and extension, abduction and adduction; rotary movements include rotation and circumduction; gliding movements describe movement where one part slides on another.

As body therapists you must be able to describe movements for the purpose of making accurate records, prescribing exercise and monitoring client progress. We therefore use anatomical terms to describe movements precisely.

Theory into practice

Anatomy is best learnt by experience. Put each of the movements described into practice, either with a friend or using your own body, and try to become familiar with the terms.

Types of synovial joint:

Type of synovial joint	Movement	Location	Movement range
Gliding	Multiaxial	Clavicle/scapula	Small, versatile
Hinge	In one plane only	Phalanges	Flexion, extension
Pivot	Around two axes	Radius and ulna	Pronation, supination
Ball and Socket	Around three axes	Pelvis/femur	Flexion, extension, adduction, abduction, pronation, supination
Condyloid	Around two axis	Carpals	Adduction, abduction, flexion, extension

Assessment task 5.6

Demonstrate a clear understanding of factors affecting movements in joints. (D)

Assessment task 5.7

Demonstrate a clear understanding of the movements possible in several joints during exercise. (D)

Homeostatic disorders of joints

Joints undergo a lot of wear and tear during a life time and it is common for older clients to complain of stiff, swollen or aching joints. However, it is difficult to separate age-associated changes from mechanical strain or injury. The repetitive actions of joints arising from occupation, sporting activities or strain caused by poor posture can certainly influence the stability of joints as we age. Cold weather and inactivity during sleep cause the body's circulatory system to slow down, and this can lead to a build up of fluid in the joints, resulting in swelling or discomfort.

A further age-associated problem is the loss of water from cartilage. Think again about the intervertebral discs. These 'cushions' contain water which is squeezed out by the pressure of gravity over time, making them less flexible and causing difficulties with lifting and bearing heavy weight. As the discs lose water they become flatter, which also explains why our height diminishes with age.

Fact file

Many joint disorders are reported to be worse in the morning or when the weather is harsh, i.e. cold and damp.

Theory into practice

Measure yourself when you get up first thing in the morning and again just before you go to bed at night. Explain the discrepancy between these two measurements based on what you have learnt in this section.

During a body consultation a female client aged 60 years complains of aches and pains in her knees and lower legs. You also notice swelling around the ankles. Think about the best way to proceed with the consultation, the treatment you would provide and the home care advice you would offer.

Inflammatory and degenerative conditions

Rheumatism is the term given to a variety of disorders of the joints and related tissues which are accompanied by pain, swelling and limited mobility. Rheumatic disorders are the main cause of disability in the UK, with an estimated 24 million sufferers.

Rheumatology is the study of disorders of the joints, tendons, ligaments and muscles.

Arthritis is inflammation of one or more joints which is characterised by pain, swelling and restricted movement. In some forms of arthritis the articular cartilage breaks down, causing painful friction between bones. Rheumatoid arthritis is a chronic, progressive condition that affects the elderly, particularly in the joints of their feet, ankles, fingers and wrists, and can cause immobility.

Spondylosis is a degenerative disease of the intervertebral discs of the spine which typically causes pain in the cervical and lumbar regions of the back.

Bursitis is an inflammation of the bursa, the small pads of tissue which reduce friction. The largest bursa is found in the knee and is known as the suprapatellar bursa. If the knee joint undergoes severe stress, the bursa produces more synovial fluid (water on the knee), which leads to swelling in an attempt to prevent further stress. The condition, colloquially known as 'housemaid's knee' is characterised by pain, swelling and restricted movement. The menisci which stabilise joints can suffer damage during exercise, causing the cartilage to tear. This is a common complaint of footballers who may have to undergo surgery to remove torn cartilage from the knee.

Tendinitis is inflammation of a tendon, usually caused by over-use, and is also known as **repetitive strain injury** (RSI). Tendinitis can also be the result of unaccustomed exertion or failing to warm up adequately before sport. The disorder known as 'tennis elbow' is an example of tendinitis caused by over-use of the arm; it causes the tendon at the elbow to become inflamed and painful.

A **sprain** is an injury to the ligament, cartilage or muscle in the locality of a joint which can occur

A summary of disorders of the joints:

Disorder	Description	Example
Arthritis	Inflammation of joints	Swollen, aching joints
Spondylosis	Degenerative disorder of intervertebral discs	Pain in cervical and lumbar region
Rheumatoid arthritis	Chronic, progressive disorder	Typically affects fingers, wrists, feet, ankles
Bursitis	Inflammation of bursae	Housemaid's knee
Torn cartilage	Damaged menisci	Footballing injuries to knee joint
Tendinitis	Inflammation of tendons	Caused by over use, e.g. tennis elbow or repetitive strain injury
Sprain	Over-stretched tendon, cartilage or muscle	Sporting injuries
Dislocation	Bones in joint become disconnected	Sudden or unnatural movements

when the joint is over-stretched or forced to exceed its range of movement. It is characterised by localised pain and swelling. Sudden or unnatural movements may cause the bones of a joint to become disconnected, causing damage to the ligaments and surrounding capsule. This injury is known as **dislocation** and can cause considerable discomfort.

Assessment task 5.8

Provide a clear description of two common disorders which could affect the wrist joint and two which could affect the knee joint. (M)

Muscle structure

There are three types of muscle tissue: cardiac muscle which forms the heart; smooth muscle which forms the internal organs; and skeletal muscle which is attached to bones. Cardiac and smooth muscle activity is involuntary and is responsible for functions such as heartbeat or the passage of food through the digestive system. Some skeletal activity, such as movement, is under conscious control. However, all types of muscle tissue share certain characteristics:

➤ muscle tissue is excitable (it responds to a stimulus)
➤ muscle tissue has the ability to contract (shorten)
➤ muscle tissue has the ability to stretch (lengthen)
➤ muscle tissue is elastic (it returns to its original shape after contraction or stretching).

This unit will examine skeletal muscle only.

Functions of skeletal muscle

Skeletal muscle:
➤ facilitates movement
➤ raises body temperature
➤ maintains posture
➤ assists venous return.

The most obvious function of skeletal muscle is to facilitate movement at joints and thereby increase or decrease the angle between two bones. Muscle is attached to bones via tendons at the point of **origin** and the point of **insertion**. When a muscle contracts, the origin remains fixed while the insertion moves towards it, thus reducing the angle of the joint. For example, sitting up from a lying down position shortens the angle between the trunk and the thighs as the abdominal muscles contract or shorten.

Theory into practice

Flex your arm so that the biceps muscle contracts. Decide where the origin and insertion of that muscle might be. Now extend your arm. Locate the muscle responsible for that action and again suggest possible points of origin and insertion.

As well as enabling movement, skeletal muscle is responsible for maintaining posture, which is achieved by the same concept of contraction. Under normal, resting circumstances the muscles are in a state of partial contraction known as **muscle tone**. If our muscles were completely relaxed all the time, our bodies would not be able to hold themselves upright; the weight of our bones and organs, particularly the skull and brain, would pull us over. Not surprisingly, the muscles with the greatest tonicity in humans are found in the neck and back. Postural muscles do not require conscious effort to carry out their function, although they can be affected by bad habits and improved through training.

Theory into practice

Explain, in anatomical terms, why the muscles of the neck and back have the greatest tonicity.

Another involuntary action of skeletal muscle is shivering. When the body feels cold, either because of external temperature or due to illness, muscle tone is triggered and the muscle contracts and relaxes very quickly to produce a shiver. This shivering action produces heat which is absorbed into the bloodstream and transported around the body to increase its temperature. Skeletal muscle also plays a part in returning blood from the body to the heart, known as venous return. This is achieved by the 'milking action' of skeletal muscle surrounding the blood vessels.

Blood is prevented from flowing backwards (away from the heart) by valves which open and close as the muscle contracts. Inactivity for long periods, perhaps due to illness, can halt this milking action. In addition, people who stand for long periods at a time, perhaps because of their jobs, may have weak valves in their blood vessels. This causes the blood to flow back down and accumulate in the vessels, thereby stretching them. These stretched blood vessels, characterised by enlarged, bumpy blood vessels close to the skin's surface, are called **varicose veins**. Because blood has a central pump – the heart – the milking action of skeletal muscle assists but is not wholly responsible for venous return. The lymphatic system does not have such a pump and so the milking action of skeletal muscle plays an important function in the movement of lymphatic fluid around the body.

Structure of skeletal muscle

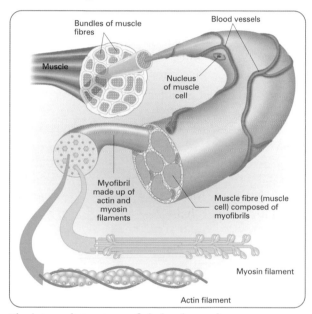

The internal structure of skeletal muscle.

Gross structure

> **Fact file**
>
> **Composition of muscle:**
> ▸▸ 75% water
> ▸▸ 20% actin and myosin
> ▸▸ 5% mineral salts, glycogen and fat.

Muscle tissue consists of large striated (striped) cells which are elongated and highly specialised. They are bound together, either in bundles or sheets, by connective tissue called **fascia**. This connective tissue is similar to the outer layer of a joint capsule and contains collagen and elastin

fibres which give muscle its strength and elastic properties. Its main purpose is to provide a surface for other muscles to slide against and it also gives the muscle its shape. The outer membrane of the muscle cell is a combination of plasma and sugar; this also contains collagen that links it to the surrounding fascia. Running the length of muscle cells are filaments of the proteins **actin** and **myosin**, which form **fibrils** or 'little fibres'. It is these fibrils of protein that give muscle its characteristic striped appearance. Within the bundles of muscle fibres there is also a rich supply of blood vessels and nerve attachments.

> **Assessment task 5.9**
>
> Explain fully, with the aid of illustrations, the gross anatomy of skeletal muscle. (M)

Cellular structure

A muscle cell is also called a muscle fibre because muscle fibres are unicellular. Microscopic examination of a muscle cell shows many muscle fibrils lying in regular alignment. The fibrils are composed of even smaller fibres called **myofilaments**, which are chains of protein molecules. Myofilaments of actin are thinner and more transparent than the thicker, darker bands of myosin, and this is why muscle tissue appears to be striated.

> **Assessment task 5.10**
>
> Illustrate and explain the structure of a muscle fibre. (D)

Contraction of skeletal muscle

Skeletal muscle is known as striped or striated muscle because of its appearance under a microscope. The stripes are formed by fibres of the proteins actin and myosin. Myosin filaments have projections which allow them to move along actin filaments when the muscle is excited by a stimulus. The filaments do not change in length but slide past each other; hence the term **sliding filament theory** of contraction. This can be illustrated using the simple analogy of a pack of cards. Imagine splitting the pack in two, one half representing actin and the other representing myosin. Then, reassemble the pack by flicking through the two halves so that the cards from each half of the pack are interwoven. The cards stay the same length but the width is lessened as they slide past each other to form one pile. In a similar fashion, sliding together shortens muscle and produces the state of contraction, while sliding apart lengthens muscle and produces the state of relaxation.

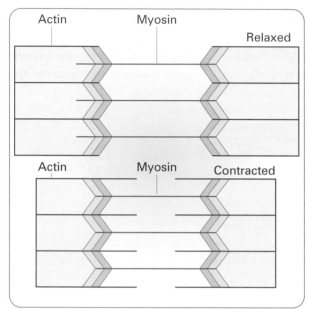

The sliding filament theory of muscle contraction.

Assessment task 5.11

Illustrate and fully explain the sliding filament theory of fibre contraction and the relationship between muscle fibre structure and function. (D)

Development of muscle tension

Activity is triggered by the occurrence of an action potential within an individual muscle fibre. Each individual action potential causes a small contraction known as a **twitch**. When a muscle fibre is activated, a mechanical force is generated within it. Therefore, the more muscle fibres that are triggered, the greater the force generated by the muscle. When the frequency of action potentials increases, twitches merge together in what is called **tetanus** (see below).

Fact file

Tetanus here describes the natural state of muscle tension and should be differentiated from the pathological condition of tetanus (known as lockjaw).

Thus, when a muscle contracts as a result of action potentials in the fibre, a force is generated which causes the filaments of actin and myosin to slide past each other in accordance with what is known as the sliding filament theory of contraction.

Muscle tone

Skeletal muscle is responsible for different types of contraction during dynamic or static activity. If the origin and insertion move closer together, the muscle is shortened or contracted and is said to be working **concentrically**. If the muscle tries to halt a movement during exertion it is said to be working **eccentrically**. The muscle attempts to contract but is extended by external forces which force the origin and insertion apart. If the muscle has to contract to prevent movement it is said to be working **statically**. Concentric and eccentric contractions are also known as **isotonic** contractions. Static muscle work is known as **isometric**, the term *isometric* means 'equal measures', as in a muscle working in equal measures with an external force to prevent movement. Isometric exercises are used to increase muscle strength by increasing tension without causing contraction, usually by pushing against a solid, immovable force. Isometric and isotonic contractions can be illustrated by considering the different types of muscle work involved in doing pull-ups on a high bar (see below).

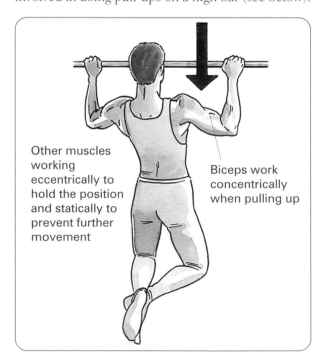

Other muscles working eccentrically to hold the position and statically to prevent further movement

Biceps work concentrically when pulling up

Pull ups - eccentric, concentric and static muscle work.

Energy for contraction

In order to work, muscles require an energy supply which is obtained from digested food. Carbohydrates are broken down into simple sugars called glucose, and if this energy is not immediately required it is stored in the muscles and the liver as **glycogen**. Muscle glycogen is a source of heat and energy which, when oxidised, produces a compound called **adenosine triphosphate** (ATP), which is also rich in energy. When a muscle is required to contract, energy is released from ATP and transformed into **adenosine diphosphate** (ADP).

Oxidation of glycogen also produces a by-product, pyruvic acid, which is broken down to produce energy, carbon dioxide and water. If sufficient oxygen is available, which it usually is during activity, this process produces more ATP and more energy. The process of using oxygen to produce energy, carbon dioxide and water is known as **aerobic respiration**. If insufficient oxygen is available, pyurvic acid is converted to **lactic acid** which builds up in the muscle and causes **muscle fatigue** in a process known as **anaerobic** respiration.

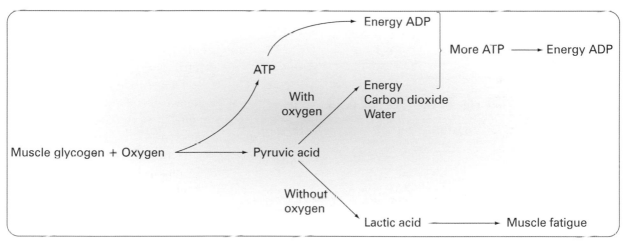

Aerobic respiration during muscle work.

The skeletomuscular system

Attachment of muscles to the skeleton

Skeletal muscles may be attached to bone, cartilage, ligaments or skin via **tendons** and **aponeuroses**. Tendons have the appearance of cords and consist of fibrous collagen tissues, while aponeuroses are a thin sheet of fibres that attach flat muscles, as in the abdomen. The most well-known tendon is the Achilles, which connects the calf muscles to the heel. Fibrous tissue also forms a protective and supportive sheath of connective tissue around muscles known as **fascia**, which contain a rich supply of blood and nerve fibres. Where muscles attach to each other the fibres of one interlace with the fibres of the other. In the muscles of the abdominal wall, the fibres of the aponeuroses interlace forming the linea alba, the shallow groove which leads from the umbilicus to the sternum.

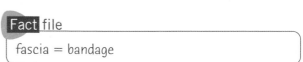

Fact file

fascia = bandage

Origins, insertions and actions

Chief muscles of the face and head

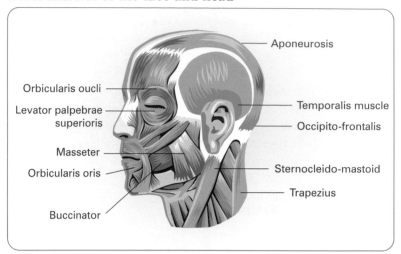

- Aponeurosis
- Orbicularis oucli
- Levator palpebrae superioris
- Temporalis muscle
- Occipito-frontalis
- Masseter
- Orbicularis oris
- Sternocleido-mastoid
- Trapezius
- Buccinator

Muscles of facial expression and mastication.

A summary of the muscles of the face and head:

Muscle	Origin	Insertion	Action
Frontalis	Epicranial aponeurosis	Behind eyebrow	Raises eyebrows, wrinkles forehead
Orbicularis oculi	Medial rim of orbit	Forms sphincter around eye area	Closes eyelid
Levator palpebrae	Back of orbit	Upper lid	Opens eyelid
Orbicularis oris	Sphincter muscle	Around mouth	Closes mouth
Buccinator	Maxilla and mandible	Angle of mouth	Compresses cheeks, aids mastication
Risorius	Maxilla and mandible	Angle of mouth	Retracts mouth
Elevators	Maxillae	Angle of mouth	Smiley expression
Depressors	Mandible	Angle of mouth	Sad expression
Nasal muscles	Maxillae	Nose	Compress and dilate the nostrils
Masseter	Zygomatic arch	Mandible	Raises lower jaw, aids mastication
Temporalis	Temples	Mandible	Raises, retracts lower jaw, aids mastication
Platysma	Fascia over pectorals and deltoid	Mandible, lower face	Draws down lip and jaw in yawning, wrinkles neck
Sternocleidomastoid	Sternum and clavicle	Mastoid process	Flexion of neck

Chief muscles of the arm and shoulder

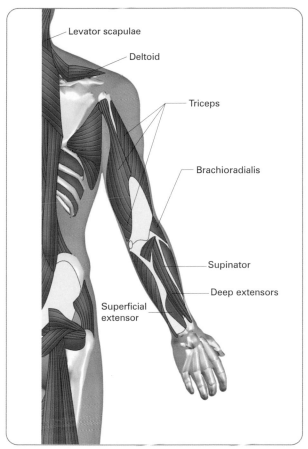

Muscles of the arm and shoulder: posterior view.

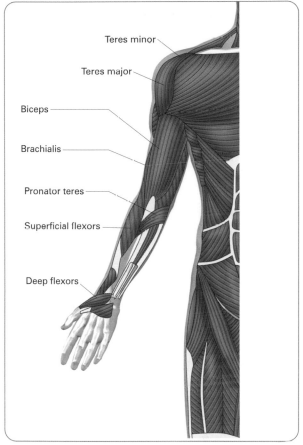

Muscles of the arm and shoulder: anterior view.

A summary of the muscles of the arm and shoulder:

Muscle	Origin	Insertion	Action
Biceps	Scapula	Tuberosity of radius	Flexion at elbow, supination of forearm
Brachialis	Shaft of humerus	Tuberosity of ulna	Flexion at elbow
Triceps	Scapula and humerus	Olecranon of ulna	Extension at elbow
Deltoid	Clavicle, spine of scapula	Tuberosity of humerus	Abduction of shoulder
Teres major	Inferior angle of scapula	Bicipital groove of humerus	Adducts arm, rotates inwards and back
Teres minor	Axillary border of scapula	Greater tuberosity of humerus	Rotates arm outwards
Levator scapulae	Upper four cervical vertebrae	Vertebral border of scapulae	Elevate shoulder, rotate scapula
Supinator	Lateral aspect of humerus	Lateral surface of radius	Supinates forearm
Pronator teres	Medial aspect of humerus and ulna	Middle of shaft of radius	Pronates forearm and hand

Muscle	Origin	Insertion	Action
Superficial extensors	Lateral aspect of humerus	Metacarpals and phalanges	Extension of wrist and fingers
Deep extensors	Ulna and radius	Phalanges of thumb and forefinger	Extension of thumb and forefinger
Superficial flexors	Medial aspect of humerus	Metacarpals, palmar aponeurosis, phalanges	Flexion of wrist and fingers
Deep flexors	Ulna and radius	Phalanges	Flexion of thumb and forefinger

Chief muscles of the leg and hip

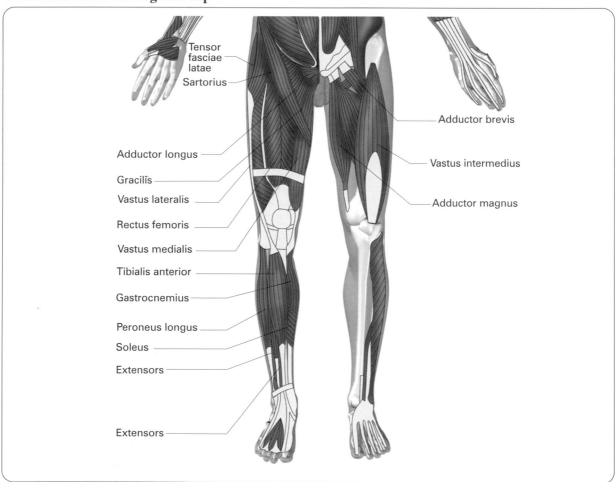

Muscles of the leg and hip: anterior view.
(A posterior view of the muscles of the leg and hip is shown on page 96.)

A summary of the muscles of the leg and hip:

Muscle	Origin	Insertion	Action
Quadriceps femoris: rectus femoris, vastus lateralis, vastus intermedius, vastus medialis	Anterior inferior iliac spine, greater trochanter, shaft of femur	Through patella and ligament to tubercle of tibia	Together: extension of knee; rectus femoris: flexion of hip
Adductors	Pubis and ischium	Linea aspera	Adduction, lateral rotation of femur
Tensor fascia lata	Outer surface of iliac crest	Iliotibial tract	Abduction of thigh and hip, extension of knee, medial rotation of femur
Sartorius	Anterior superior iliac spine	Medial condyle of tibia	Flexion and abduction of hip, flexion of knee, lateral rotation of femur
Tibialis anterior	Upper tibia	Intermediate cuneform and 1st metatarsal	Dorsiflexion and supination of ankle, inversion
Tibialis posterior	Posterior of fibula and tibia	Navicular	Plantarflexion and supination, inversion
Gastrocnemius	Lateral and medial condyles of femur	Through Achilles on heel	Flexion of knee, plantarflexion of ankle
Soleus (beneath gastrocnemius)	Head of fibula	Through Achilles to heel	Plantarflexion
Popliteus	Lateral condyle of femur	Shaft of tibia	Flexion of knee, medial rotation of tibia
Adductors: brevis, longus, magnus	Pubic bone	Linea aspera	Adduction at hip, rotation out (adductor brevis) and inward rotation (adductor magnus)
Iliopsoas: iliacus, psoas major	Lumbar vertebrae and surface of ilium	Lesser trochanter	Outward rotation of leg, lateral bending of spine
Gracilis	Pubis, ischium	Below medial condyle of tibia	Adduction and medial rotation of femur, flexion of knee
Gluteus maximus	Posterior pelvis, sacrum, coccyx	Outer aspect of femur	Adducts hip, outward rotation of thigh, extension of knee
Hamstrings: biceps femoris, semitendonosis semimembranosis	Ischial tuberosity, back of femur	Tibia and fibula at either side of politeal	Extension of hip, flexion of knee, lateral rotation of femur when semi-flexed
Gluteus medius	Outer aspect of ilium	Greater trochanter	Abduction and rotation of hip
Gluteus minimus	Under and behind gluteus medius	Greater trochanter	Abduction and rotation of hip

Chief muscles of the chest and abdomen

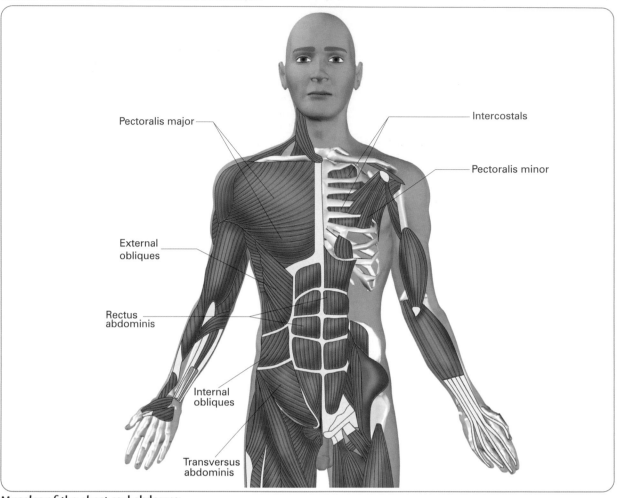

Muscles of the chest and abdomen.

A summary of the muscles of the chest and abdomen:

Muscle	Origin	Insertion	Action
Pectoralis major	Clavicle, sternum and costal cartilage	Lateral aspect of bicipital groove	Adduction, inward rotation of arm, supports mammary glands
Pectoralis minor (beneath pectoralis major)	Ribs 3–5	Coracoid process	Depression of scapula
Serratus anterior	Ribs 1–9	Inner aspect of scapula	Stabilises shoulder, forward rotation of scapula
Diaphragm	Tip of sternum, lower ribs, first three lumbar vertebrae	Central aponeurosis of abdominal wall	Flattens to create more room in thorax during inhalation
Intercostals	Lower borders of ribs	Upper border of rib below	Pulls ribs up and out during inhalation, maintains shape of thorax

A summary of the muscles of the chest and abdomen (cont.):

Muscle	Origin	Insertion	Action
Rectus abdominus	Pubis	5th–7th costal cartilages	Ventral flaxion of trunk
External obliques (form waist)	Lower 8 ribs	Iliac crest; linea alba through abdominal aponeurosis	Flex trunk ventrally, rotation of trunk
Internal obliques (form waist)	Inguinal ligament, iliac crest, lumbar fascia	Linea alba through abdominal aponeurosis	Flex trunk ventrally, rotation of trunk
Transversus	Inguinal ligament, iliac crest, lumbar fascia, lower 6 ribs	Linea alba through abdominal aponeurosis	Forced expiration, defecation, vomiting

Chief muscles of the back

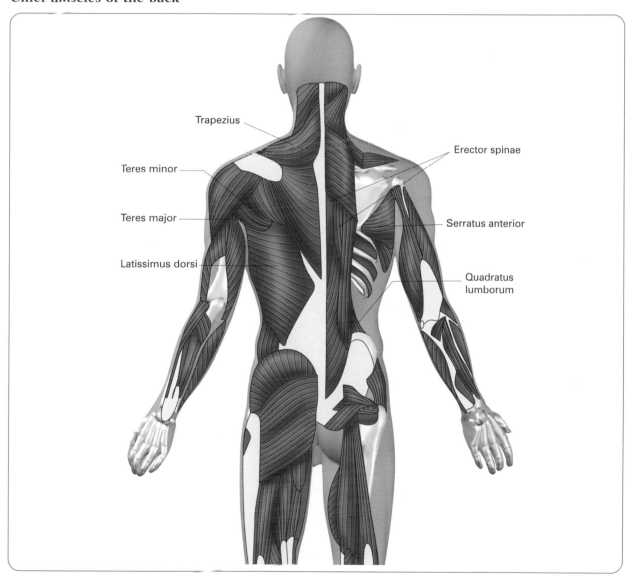

Muscles of the back.

A summary of the muscles of the back:

Muscle	Origin	Insertion	Action
Trapezius	Occipital bone, thoracic vertebrae	Clavicle, spine of scapula	Elevates and braces shoulder, rotates scapula
Erector spinae	Sacrum, iliac crest, ribs, lower vertebrae	Ribs, vertebrae, mastoid process	Extension of spine, lateral flexion of trunk, pulls head back, erect posture
Latissumus dorsi	Lower 6 thoracic vertebrae, lumbar vertebrae, iliac crest	Bicipital groove of humerus	Adduction of arm at shoulder, depression of shoulder
Quadratus lumborum	Iliac crest	12th rib, upper lumbar vertebrae	Extension and lateral flexion of trunk, steadies 12th rib

Shapes of muscles

Muscles of the body have different shapes and sizes which serve their position and function.

Characteristics of muscle types:

Type of muscle	Example	Characteristics
Biceps	Biceps at front of humerus; biceps femoris at back of femur	Two-headed muscle with great strength, responsible for powerful actions such as flexion and supination
Triceps	Triceps at back of upper arm	Three-headed muscle; antagonist to biceps, extends elbow and shoulder
Quadriceps	Quadriceps femoris at front of thigh	Four-headed muscle, actually consisting of four separate muscles which extend the thigh
Segmented	Rectus abdominus	Straight, abdominal muscle; supports posture
Serrated	Serratus anterior and posterior of the trunk	Provides stability and movement of the ribs to aid respiration

Direction of muscle fibres

Muscle fibres run in different directions according to their position in the body and the movements they control. They run from the origin, which remains in a fixed position, to the insertion, which moves towards or away from the point of origin during movement. For example, the biceps muscle at the front of the upper arm originates from the scapula and inserts on the radius so that the fibres run horizontally *down* the arm. When the muscle contracts, the fibres shorten to flex the arm at the elbow. The external obliques of the abdominal wall have origins in the lower ribs and insertions on the linea alba and iliac crest. The fibres run *around* the waist so that contraction of these muscles produces rotation of the trunk. Direction of muscle fibres can be observed in the diagrams and illustrated by the movements which each muscle performs.

Introduction to levers

During skeletal movement, bones act as levers. The joint acts as the balance part of the lever or **fulcrum**, and the part being moved is known as the **load**. Muscles provide the **effort**. Levers are classified according to the relationship between fulcrum, load and effort.

First class levers

The fulcrum is in a central position with effort and load on either side. Effort must therefore equal load, and movement of load results in movement of effort in the opposite direction. The head is an illustration of a first class lever, with the spine acting as fulcrum, the weight of the face as the load and the effort supplied by the muscles of the neck. To maintain an upright position the effort is minimal because the head is balanced centrally on the spine. Any movement of the effort results in movement of the load in the opposite direction. So, when the head is tilted forwards, the load in front of the fulcrum increases and greater effort is required from the neck muscles to hold it in position or pull it upright.

Second class levers

The load is in a central position with fulcrum and effort on either side. Movement of load results in movement of effort in the same direction. An illustration of second class levers is standing on tiptoe.

The fulcrum is the ball of the foot, the load is body weight and the effort is supplied by the calf muscles. As the centre of gravity shifts, increasing the load, so the effort is also increased. The effort is less than the load but the distance it moves is greater than the movement of the load.

Third class lever

Effort is in a central position with fulcrum and load on either side. Movement of effort results in movement of load in the same direction. Effort is always greater than load but any distance moved is less than movement of the load. Third class levers facilitate large movements with very little contraction of muscle and are the most common type of lever in the human body. One illustration of a third class lever is movement of the arm. The fulcrum is the elbow joint, effort is provided by the flexor muscles of the upper arm (biceps) which attach to the forearm, and the load is the weight of the forearm and hand. Flexion of the arm at the elbow results in movement of the load, i.e. hand and forearm, towards the effort, and movement of the effort in the same direction, i.e. contraction of the biceps.

Theory into practice

The concept of first, second and third class levers is quite difficult to grasp at first. Try to find a strategy for differentiating between (and remembering) the different types of levers. You could try anagrams, rhymes or mnemonics – whatever works for you!

A summary of levers:

Type of lever	1st class levers	2nd class levers	3rd class levers
Relative position	Effort – fulcrum – load	Fulcrum – load – effort	Fulcrum – effort – load
Direction of movement	Effort & load move in opposite directions	Effort & load move in same direction	Effort & load move in same direction
Relationship between effort and load	Central fulcrum: effort = load; fulcrum near effort: effort > load; movement: effort < load	Effort = load; movement: effort < load	Effort > load; movement: effort > load
Illustration	Effort = neck muscles fulcrum = spine load = weight of face	Fulcrum = ball of foot load = body weight effort = calf muscles	Fulcrum = elbow joint effort = biceps load = forearm & hand

Maintenance of posture and production of movement

Interaction of muscles and muscle groups:

Agonists	Antagonists	Synergists	Fixators
Muscles that contract to cause bending of a limb or the trunk	Muscles that work *against* each other so that contraction of one produces relaxation of the other	A muscle that works in conjunction with another muscle to produce the same movement	Muscles that maintain joints in a fixed position and produce limited movement
Flexors	Flexors and extensors	Hamstring group	Postural muscles
Triceps	Biceps and triceps	Gastrocnemius and soleus	Erector spinae

Maintenance of posture and anti-gravity muscles

Posture is an important part of our appearance and can convey a great deal about our clients. Healthy people with a positive outlook tend to have good posture whatever their age, although some changes associated with age can affect posture. Bone shrinkage and flattened cartilage reduces height but slouching reduces height further. Lifestyle influences posture: sedentary workers might have a tendency to round their shoulders; people who stand all day, such as teachers or hairdressers, might favour one leg over the other leg, which throws their posture off balance; a parent might carry a child on one hip or the shopping in one heavy bag. A tall individual who is self-conscious might develop a stoop, and people who are worried or stressed might develop a hunch – as if they really are carrying the weight of the world upon their shoulders.

It is important to maintain a steady body weight that is appropriate for your height, since any extra weight carried on the abdomen or buttocks puts a strain on the back. This is a common complaint in the later stages of pregnancy. Keeping fit and active maintains the strength of the muscles responsible for good posture at any age, while long periods of

A summary of postural muscles:

Postural muscle	Location	Action
Erector spinae	Either side of spine	Maintains upright position of the head and erect spine
Trapezius	Triangular muscle in region of scapula	Pulls the head upright
Rectus abdominus	Abdominal wall	Supports trunk, acts as an antagonist to the muscles of the back
Gluteals (esp. gluteus maximus)	Buttocks and hip	Tenses thigh, maintains upright posture of the trunk
Tensor fascia lata	Outer part of thigh	Tenses outer thigh, maintains posture when standing or walking
Tibialis anterior/ posterior, flexors/ extensors of toes	Lower limb	Maintains postural balance when standing, anti-gravity muscles

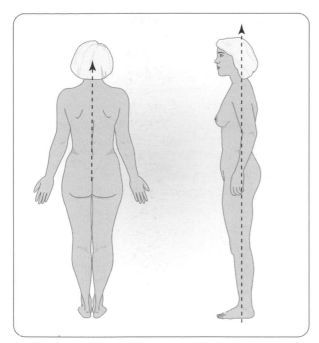

Posterior and lateral views of good posture.

remind them that good posture can take years off your appearance. The chief muscles responsible for maintaining posture are those of the neck, trunk and hip.

If posture is good you should be able to draw an imaginary line down the side of the body from the lobe of the ear and through the centre of the shoulder, the middle of the pelvis and the knee, finishing at the ankle bone. From a posterior view, the vertebral column should run in a straight line down the back. With the feet positioned at 'five to one', the knees and ankles should touch and there should be three gaps between the legs: between the top of the thighs, directly below the knees and below the calf. Posture and common postural defects are discussed further in the section on figure analysis in Unit 10: Body therapy, (pages 223–31).

Common postural imbalances

Poor posture can be caused by poorly trained postural muscles, wear and tear, lifting uneven weights and standing or sitting with weight unevenly distributed, i.e. on one leg. Carrying heavy weights or sustaining strain over long periods of time can cause the intervertebral discs to become flattened

inactivity causes them to weaken. It is important to advise clients to stretch out muscles and rotate joints to keep them working effectively, and to

A summary of postural imbalances:

Postural imbalances	Position	Conditions to note
Head and neck	Lateral view Posterior view	Forward tilt due to rounded shoulders Flexion to one side due to tension
Shoulders	Lateral view Posterior view	Rounded shoulders may be due to a heavy bust, self-consciousness, habitual or work-related poor posture Uneven due to carrying heavy weights
Pelvis	Lateral view Posterior view	Anterior tilt (common during pregnancy) or posterior tilt Uneven with uneven distribution of adipose; poor posture or spinal deformity such as scoliosis*
Abdomen	Lateral view	Protrusion may be due to muscle weakness (can it be sucked in?)
Spine	Lateral view Posterior view	Exaggerated thoracic curve (kyphosis*); Exaggerated lumbar curve (lordosis*) Winged scapula, lateral curvature (scoliosis*)
Legs	Lateral view Posterior view	Forward or backward tilt Less than three gaps may be due to bow legs, knock knees or excess adipose tissue

* abnormal spinal curvatures (see overleaf)

as fluid is 'squashed' out. Muscles can also become tense, bones displaced or cartilage worn down, which in turn can put pressure on nerves. **Sciatica** is the name of a common disorder whereby the sciatic nerve is irritated causing pain in the lower back and leg. Many of the postural imbalances mentioned can cause back pain which can be released by hanging the back over the legs with bent hips. This reduces pressure on the discs and unloads the pressure on the back.

> ### Fact file
>
> The back muscles work harder in a (static) seated position than they do in an upright position, and sitting produces greater pressure on the intervertebral discs than standing.

Abnormal spinal curvatures

Scoliosis is a spinal deformity which causes a lateral curvature of the spine. It might take the form of a single 'C' shaped curve or have a primary curve in one direction with a compensatory curve in the opposite direction forming an 'S' shape. It can develop in people whose legs are of unequal length, after significant trauma or following a stroke. **Lordosis** is a spinal deformity characterised by an exaggerated curvature in the lumbar region. This causes the abdomen and buttocks to protrude and the back to appear 'hollow'. It can be caused by obesity, hip deformities and is common during pregnancy. **Kyphosis** is a spinal deformity characterised by an exaggerated curvature in the thoracic region. This causes a hunch back or 'dowager's hump'. It can have a congenital cause but is more often the result of poor posture and weak back muscles.

> ### Fact file
>
> Remember…
> **SC**oliosis = '**S**' shaped or '**C**' shaped curvature of the spine.
> **L**ordosis = **L**umbar curve is exaggerated, hollow back.
> Kyp**H**osis = **H**ump backed, exaggerated thoracic curve.

Analysis of simple movements and exercises

Exercises for the back:

1   Lying face down, slowly raise the trunk. Load can be added to the lower back by stretching the opposite arm out in front of the body.

2   Lying face down, raise one leg at a time to train hamstrings, gluteals and lower back.

3   In standing position allow trunk to fall forwards by bending at knees and waist. Slowly roll up one vertebrae at a time to work the back muscles concentrically.

4   Lying on your side, raise the trunk laterally to strengthen quadratus lumborum.

Exercises for the abdomen:

1   Lying on your back with knees bent, use abdominal muscles to raise the trunk to a sitting position as if an apple were lodged between your chin and chest.

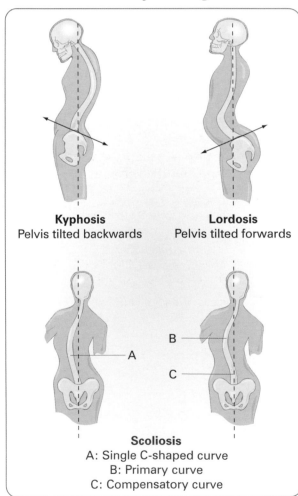

Kyphosis
Pelvis tilted backwards

Lordosis
Pelvis tilted forwards

Scoliosis
A: Single C-shaped curve
B: Primary curve
C: Compensatory curve

Kyphosis, lordosis and scoliosis.

2 Diagonal sit-ups raising the left shoulder to the right hip, working opposite external and internal obliques.

3 The load can be increased by straightening your arms down your sides, crossing your arms over your chest, adding weights, adjusting your legs so that your feet are flat against a wall at 90 degrees, or assuming a 'frog's leg' position with feet together and knees out.

Exercises for the chest, shoulders and arms:

1 With or without weights, raise the arms out to the side one at a time to strengthen the deltoids.

2 With or without weights and positioned on all fours, extend the shoulder backwards to strengthen the triceps.

3 With or without weights, flex the arm to strengthen the biceps.

4 Holding a parallel bar with or without weights, raise from chest to chin in a rowing action to strengthen the deltoids.

5 On hands and knees with a flat back, lower your body to the floor by bending the elbows out to the sides in a press-up, to strengthen the pectorals and deltoids.

Exercises for the legs and hips:

1 Squat with your back against a wall at 90 degrees to work the quadriceps statically.

2 Walk in long, exaggerated strides to work the quadriceps.

3 Lie on your back and pull one leg at a time towards your chest to work the hamstrings.

4 Place the balls of your feet on a low step so that they are higher than your heels. Alternate between this position and standing on tiptoes, to train the gastrocnemius and soleus.

5 Step up and down on a low platform to work all muscles of the leg and hip.

Assessment task 5.12

Devise a series of simple exercises suitable for toning 'thighs, bums and tums'. Locate the chief muscles involved in these exercises and identify their origins and insertions. (D)

Knowledge check

1 How many bones are there in the human skeleton?

2 Name the bones of the human skeleton.

3 Describe the process of calcification.

4 Describe the effects of ageing on bone tissue.

5 Explain how joint structure is related to function.

6 Identify and describe common homeostatic disorders of joints.

7 What are the main functions of skeletal muscle?

8 Explain the sliding filament theory of contraction.

9 Describe isometric and isotonic contractions.

10 What is aerobic respiration?

11 Define the following terms and give examples: agonists, antagonists, synergists, fixators.

12 Name the chief muscles of the leg.

13 Name the chief postural muscles.

14 Which muscles are responsible for raising the trunk to a sitting position?

15 Name the chief facial muscles.

A drawing to summarize the chief muscles of the human body is given overleaf.

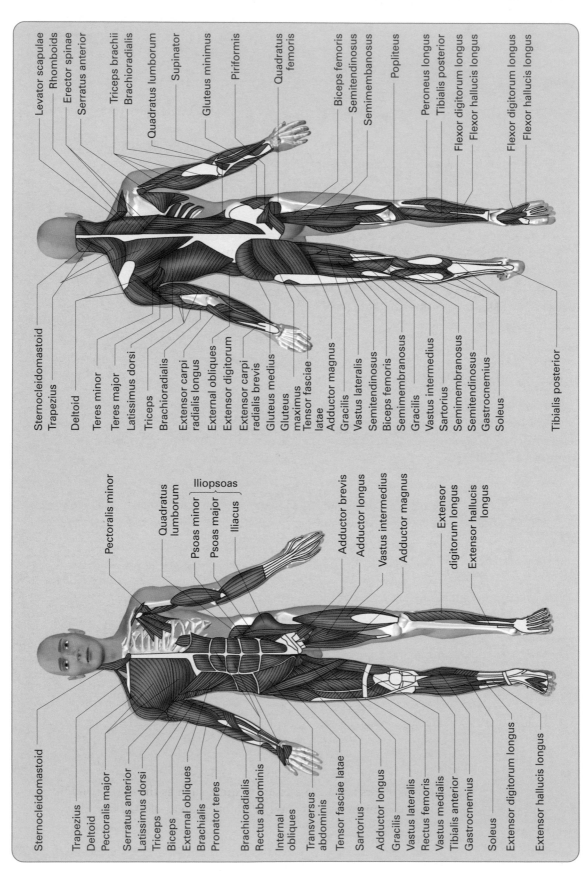

Chief muscles of the human body.

Labels (posterior view, top):
Levator scapulae, Rhomboids, Erector spinae, Serratus anterior, Triceps brachii, Brachioradialis, Quadratus lumborum, Supinator, Gluteus minimus, Piriformis, Quadratus femoris, Biceps femoris, Semitendinosus, Semimembranosus, Popliteus, Peroneus longus, Tibialis posterior, Flexor digitorum longus, Flexor hallucis longus, Flexor digitorum longus, Flexor hallucis longus

Sternocleidomastoid, Trapezius, Deltoid, Teres minor, Teres major, Latissimus dorsi, Triceps, Brachioradialis, Extensor carpi radialis longus, External obliques, Extensor digitorum, Extensor carpi radialis brevis, Gluteus medius, Gluteus maximus, Tensor fasciae latae, Adductor magnus, Gracilis, Vastus lateralis, Semitendinosus, Biceps femoris, Semimembranosus, Gracilis, Vastus intermedius, Sartorius, Semimembranosus, Semitendinosus, Gastrocnemius, Soleus, Tibialis posterior

Labels (anterior view, bottom):
Pectoralis minor, Quadratus lumborum, Iliopsoas, Psoas minor, Psoas major, Iliacus, Adductor brevis, Adductor longus, Vastus intermedius, Adductor magnus, Extensor digitorum longus, Extensor hallucis longus

Sternocleidomastoid, Trapezius, Deltoid, Pectoralis major, Serratus anterior, Latissimus dorsi, Triceps, Biceps, External obliques, Brachialis, Pronator teres, Brachioradialis, Rectus abdominis, Internal obliques, Transversus abdominis, Tensor fasciae latae, Sartorius, Adductor longus, Gracilis, Vastus lateralis, Rectus femoris, Vastus medialis, Tibialis anterior, Gastrocnemius, Soleus, Extensor digitorum longus, Extensor hallucis longus

Dermatology and microbiology

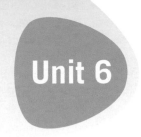

Unit 6

This unit introduces you to the biology of skin and its appendages. You will examine the structure and function of skin in some detail as well as exploring skin healing and the changes associated with ageing. You will also examine the structure and function of hair and nails and the changes associated with ageing.

In the second part of the unit you will explore common diseases and disorders that affect the skin, hair and nails. You will learn to recognise infectious and non-infectious conditions and to assess potential contra-indications to beauty therapy treatment.

The final part of the unit investigates **micro-organisms**, their transmission and effect on the body. You will learn how to minimise the risk of infection through procedures for health, safety and hygiene.

In order to achieve Unit 6 in Dermatology and microbiology you must complete the following learning outcomes:

Learning Outcomes

1 Explore the biology of skin, hair and nails through the lifespan.

2 Investigate the diseases and disorders of skin, hair and nails, and their contra-indications to treatment.

3 Describe the characteristics and transmission of micro-organisms which cause disease in humans.

4 Investigate the growth requirements of micro-organisms and relate these to the principles of personal and salon hygiene.

The biology of the skin

The human body is made up of 65 per cent water and the skin acts as a bag to keep the water inside. It also acts as a barrier in keeping other substances out, such as harmful bacteria, dirt and excess moisture. We are able to feel sensations, such as pain or heat, because of sensors in the skin that transmit messages to the brain about what is happening outside the body. Our skin also plays a major role in maintaining optimum body temperature and in protecting the body from harm.

The skin has many different surfaces. Some are smooth, such as the forehead or scalp, while others contain deep furrows, such as the palms of the hands. Some areas of skin, such as the face, are covered with fine, soft hairs. The head, groin and axilla are covered with much thicker, coarser hairs that serve a different function. Other parts of skin, such as the soles of the feet and palms of the hands, have no hair at all. Some areas of skin are thicker than others and have a coarse texture, such as the elbows and knees. Areas, such as the nose, might feel more oily than other areas of skin because of the larger number of oil-producing glands and the larger pore size. Some areas of the skin are much more sensitive to heat or pain than other areas are. Think about the sensation you feel when you step into a hot bath: the water temperature may seem comfortable when you dip in your hand but take the plunge and the skin of your thighs or abdomen might send a very different message to your brain.

Skin also comes in a variety of colours. We are aware of the variety of skin tones displayed by people of different nationalities and you will also be aware of the effect that sunshine has on different coloured skins. But have you ever noticed that areas of your own body can differ in colour from other areas? As well as the effect of sunlight and the **melanin** content, the colour of skin is also affected by the amount and condition of blood vessels and by the thickness of skin. Even the different areas of one person's face consist of a variety of skin colours and textures.

These are important considerations for beauty therapy treatments which involve the use of colour, such as the application of make up, eyebrow tints or nail enamelling. Skin colour, as well as texture, can also determine such factors as skin sensitivity, dehydration, allergy, illness and fatigue, and these will influence the analysis and diagnosis of clients for a variety of beauty therapy treatments.

In this part of the unit we will be looking, in some detail, at the structure of the bag we live in as well as investigating its main functions. Many people find the study of skin quite a difficult subject but most agree that it is fascinating. Before you start working through the section, take a closer look at your own skin and think about how different areas look and feel.

Functions of skin

The functions of skin can be neatly summarised in the acronym 'SHAPES':

▸ **S** – Sensation
▸ **H** – Heat regulation
▸ **A** – Absorption
▸ **P** – Protection
▸ **E** – Excretion
▸ **S** – Secretion

Sensation

The sense of touch is often considered the most important function of skin. We touch ourselves a countless number of times each day when we wash, dress, apply products, rub an aching limb or scratch away an itch. Touch is also an important way in which we communicate our feelings to others. A formal handshake, a hug of consolation, an affectionate kiss between a parent and child, hitting or punching and sensual stroking between romantic partners are all ways of touching which transmit varied messages between the transmitter and the receiver. Interestingly, studies have shown that the development of people who have been denied personal touch is severely retarded. Furthermore, touch is the basic technique of most, if not all, beauty and complementary therapy treatments; it is the underlying principle of what we refer to as manual or 'hands on' treatments.

In the same way that people transmit and receive messages through touch, the skin is involved in a communication process with the brain via sensory nerves that carry messages around the body. There are thousands of sensory nerve endings in the skin. These recognise sensations of pain, pressure, touch, heat and cold on the skin and carry messages about the sensations to the brain, which instigates a reaction. For example, if the finger is pricked with a pin, the sensory nerve endings in that area will recognise the skin damage and send a message to the brain. The brain will send a message back to the finger which is recognised as pain and instructs the finger to move. Of course, this all happens very quickly! Some messages do not travel as far as the brain, but instead produce automatic and immediate reflex actions in response to the stimulation of the nerve endings. Thus, the skin's function of sensation is a two-way process of receiving and transmitting information between the external world and the internal body systems.

Heat regulation

The skin plays an important role in helping to maintain the optimum body temperature for normal functioning. Normal body temperature, which is measured by a thermometer either under the tongue or in the axilla, is 36.8°Celsius, but it fluctuates slightly as a response to internal or external factors. However, extreme changes in body temperature can be dangerous, even fatal. As with sensation, temperature regulation is controlled via the brain, which stimulates specific nerve endings in the skin. Body temperature is regulated internally in two ways by sweating and vasodilation.

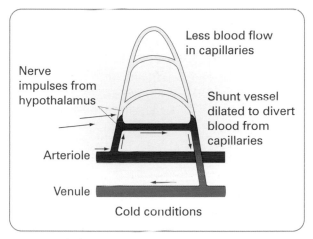
Body temperature is slightly higher at night than in the morning due to activity levels, and is higher in younger than older people as they tend to be more active.

Sweating

Sweat comprises water and waste products and the amount excreted varies according to changes in temperature. The body is producing small amounts of sweat all the time, which we are usually unaware of, and these serve to maintain the temperature of the body. When body temperature increases, more sweat is produced in an attempt to lower the body's internal temperature through the process of evaporation.

Fact file

Body temperature can increase as a response to external or internal factors, such as hot climate, vigorous activity, stress or illness.

Theory into practice

Think about what happens after a warm bath. If you don't dry your body but instead leave droplets of moisture on the skin, you will soon start to feel cold. This is due to the principle of evaporation. Body temperature is lowered as moisture evaporates from its surface, taking the heat with it and making you feel cool.

Vasodilation

The skin, like the entire body, contains a network of vessels which transport blood. The smallest and most superficial of these vessels are **capillaries**. Vasodilation of the capillaries causes them to expand, resulting in a larger superficial surface area. As more blood is brought closer to the surface of the skin it can cool down more quickly, thus cooling the body at the same time.

When the body feels cold the opposite happens. **Vasoconstriction** of the capillaries results in a smaller surface area and less blood volume close to the skin's surface, thus less heat is lost. Another change that occurs on the surface of the skin when the body feels cold is the appearance of 'goosebumps', which make the little hairs on the skin stand up on end. These hairs trap warm air close to the skin's surface, thereby providing insulation to help maintain the body's normal temperature.

Theory into practice

A good way to understand the effects of vasodilation and vasoconstriction is to think again about bathtime. If you screw up a wet towel and leave it lying on the bathroom floor, chances are that it will still be wet the following morning. If, on the other hand, you spread the towel out on a rail, thereby increasing the surface area, it will dry much faster. Moisture, and with it heat, evaporates more readily when the surface area is larger.

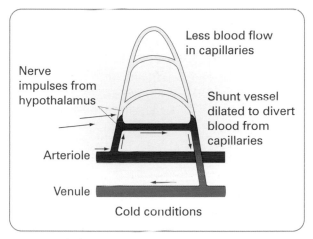

Vasoconstriction.

Theory into practice

When we feel too hot we might spread out our arms and legs and not want anyone to come too close. On the other hand, when we feel cold, we tend to fold our arms, scrunch ourselves into a ball or need a hug. Try to explain what effect these actions have on temperature regulation. Can you think what else you might do if you felt cold and the physiological effect these actions would have?

Absorption

One of the most important properties of the skin is its ability to repel moisture and bacteria and, on the whole, act as a waterproof seal. To this end, the skin has the ability to absorb only a small amount of oily substances. The outermost layer of the **epidermis**, the stratum corneum, acts as a barrier against water, although a tiny amount can be absorbed; oily substances can be absorbed via the hair follicles. Many molecules are simply too big to penetrate the skin. Manual massage and electrical current, which is applied in salon treatments such as galvanism or high frequency, aids absorption by dissolving larger molecules and thus assisting their passage through the layers of the skin.

The varying thicknesses of the stratum corneum affects the absorption of substances. Where it is thickest, on the soles of the feet, there is limited absorption. Where it is thinner, on the face and neck, absorption is greatest. Absorption is further assisted by manual or mechanical exfoliation which helps to remove the outer keritinised layers of the stratum corneum.

Protection

The skin serves to protect the body and its internal structures in a number of ways. Physical sensation alerts the sensory receptors to environmental factors that may cause damage, such as heat, cold and pain. Also, the skin is watertight; if it were not, the body would absorb the water it came into contact with whenever a person went swimming or took a shower; in addition, the water inside the body would escape. The stratum corneum, or horny layer, together with a layer of fatty tissue, provide this watertight seal. The fatty **adipose** tissue has a further protective quality; it cushions the body against knocks and blows, protecting the bones and internal organs from injury.

Ultraviolet light is a well documented enemy of the skin and exposure to it can cause severe, irreversible damage such as burning or skin cancer. When the skin is exposed to the sun, **melanocytes** are stimulated to produce increased levels of the colour pigment melanin. This darkens the outer layers of the epidermis and slows down penetration by ultraviolet rays to the deeper layers of the **dermis**. Melanin production protects the skin by blocking out some of the harmful effects of UV.

However, note that the alliance between the skin and natural sunlight also has a positive effect. Exposure to ultraviolet rays stimulates the production of vitamin D by the skin, which is necessary to promote healthy bone tissue. The skin requires protection from harmful **bacteria** and other disease forming micro-organisms. The stratum corneum blocks the invasion of foreign bodies while **sebum** has a mild antiseptic quality and can destroy some bacteria. Sweat and sebum combine to form the **acid mantle** which helps to prevent invasion by bacteria and fungi.

The acid mantle

If you think back to chemistry lessons you might remember learning about the pH scale. pH is short for 'percentage Hydrogen' and the pH value assigned to a substance tells us whether the substance is an acid or an alkaline. pH is measured on a scale of 1 to 14, where 1 is a strong acid, 7 is neutral and 14 is a strong alkali.

Fact file

```
--acid--      neutral    --alkaline--
 1  2  3  4  5  6  7  8  9  10 11 12 13 14
'neutral' pH = 7
'natural' pH of skin and hair = pH 4.5–5.5
```

You might have come across references to the pH scale in advertising, particularly for skin care where manufacturers might advertise that a product is pH neutral or pH 5.5. This may not mean very much to their customers who are neither chemists nor beauty specialists. The important distinction for you to make is that *neutral* and *natural* are not the same thing. The skin has the ability to balance acid and alkaline factors and maintain a pH of 4.5 to 5.5. This is what is known as the acid mantle.

The pH of differing products:

Substance	Nourishing products	Cleansing products
pH	Similar acidic pH to skin	Alkaline pH
Examples	Moisturisers, cuticle conditioners, massage mediums, nourishing masks, hair conditioners	Cleansers, exfoliators, cleansing masks, soap, shampoo
Precautions		Over-use can have a drying effect on skin, hair and/or nails

The acid mantle plays a part in the function of protection since it prevents the invasion of harmful microorganisms which could cause infection. Because of the alkaline content of cleansing products, over or incorrect use will have the effect of stripping the skin of its natural oils. As sebum has an anti-bacterial effect, the disturbance of the pH balance combined with the drying effect can leave skin prone to infection and irritation.

Theory into practice

Try to find out, or guess, the pH of some common substances such as washing detergent, cleaning preparations, toothpaste, perfume, bleach and foodstuffs. Think about their effect on skin and the implications for skin care.

Excretion

The skin eliminates waste products by excretion. The sweat glands excrete sweat which contains salt, urea and other impurities that would be hazardous to the body if not expelled. Excretion of sweat is minimal under normal circumstances.

Secretion

The skin secretes substances from specialised cells and glands which are beneficial to the health of the skin. For example, the sebaceous glands secrete sebum which is an oily substance made up of fatty acids and waxes. Sebum serves the purpose of nourishing the skin and hair and also plays a part in protecting against infection.

Theory into practice

Think about the difference between excretion and secretion. Try to think of other examples where excretion and secretion take place in the body.

Structure of skin

We have already discussed the main functions of the skin and mentioned some of its structures, such as sweat and sebaceous glands, blood vessels and nerves. The skin can be divided into three distinct layers. The outer layer is called the **epidermis** and beneath it is the **dermis**. These two layers are 'glued' together by the **basement membrane** and if they become separated, a blister is formed. Deepest of all is the subcutaneous or fatty layer which consists of adipose tissue.

Structure and biology of the epidermis

The epidermis consists of five layers called stratum corneum, stratum lucidum, stratum granulosum, stratum spinosum and stratum germinativum. The prefix 'stratum' means layer and the second part of the name refers to its structure or function.

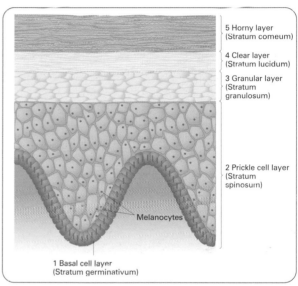

5 Horny layer (Stratum comeum)

4 Clear layer (Stratum lucidum)

3 Granular layer (Stratum granulosum)

2 Prickle cell layer (Stratum spinosum)

Melanocytes

1 Basal cell layer (Stratum germinativum)

The structure of epidermis.

1 Stratum germinativum

The deepest layer of the epidermis is the stratum germinativum, also known as the **basal cell layer** because of its position at the base of the epidermis. This layer consists of living 'parent' cells which reproduce by continually dividing to make new cells called **keratinocytes**. Keratinocytes produce the protein keratin, the main building blocks of skin, hair and nails.

2 Stratum spinosum

The stratum spinosum also consists of living cells which are plump and filled with fluid. This is also known as the **prickle cell** layer because of the way

Fact file

cyte = cell
melanocyte = cells that produce melanin
keratinocyte = cells that produce keratin

the cells look. They are shaped like spines or spikes, which allows them to attach to other cells.

3 Stratum granulosum

This granular layer contains living cells which are beginning to wear down. The cells are much flatter than those in the deeper layers and contain less fluid.

4 Stratum lucidum

Lucid means 'clear' and the stratum lucidum is a layer of dead, transparent cells. It is thickest on the soles of the feet and the palms of the hands which are subject to more wear and tear than other areas of the body. The thicker layer provides added protection.

5 Stratum corneum

The stratum corneum is a layer of cornified cells which forms the surface of the epidermis. It is the visible part of skin and the area where skin is shed. Here the cells are flattened, consist mainly of keratin and overlap to protect the skin from damage. The stratum corneum is sometimes called the horny layer because of the thickness of the, now dead, skin cells. Darker skins have a thicker stratum corneum than paler skins and therefore have greater protection from the damaging effects of ultraviolet light. The stratum corneum is thickest on the soles of the feet and thinner on the face, which affects the absorption of applied substances.

Keratinisation

Skin is continually making new cells in the stratum germinativum and shedding them from the stratum corneum in a process called **keratinisation**. The three lower layers of the epidermis contain living cells which are fed by the dermis, while in the two uppermost layers the cells start to die. A new cell is formed when a parent cell divides. It moves up through the layers and changes in shape and structure to become flatter and more horny. By the time the cell reaches the stratum corneum it is no more than a flat, empty shell, which is shed away. This natural shedding process is called **desquamation**. The process of keratinisation, which carries a new cell on its journey from the stratum germinativum to the stratum corneum, takes approximately 28 days. As a person ages, the process of keratinisation slows down. This explains why older people seem to keep a suntan for longer:

they hang on to their dying skin cells so that there is a build-up of old skin cells in the stratum corneum as they wait for new ones to push through. Beauty therapists use techniques to manually slough off dead skin cells, such as facial and body scrubs or electrotherapy such as **galvanism**, and these make the skin look brighter and fresher.

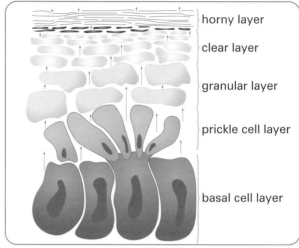

Keratinisation.

Theory into practice

Think about the structure and the functions of the skin. Explain why dark skins are at less risk from the effects of the sun. Explain why a suntan lasts for less time in a younger person than in an older person.

Structure and function of the dermis

The dermis contains much fewer cells than the epidermis and more connective tissue. The dermis is divided into two layers called the **papillary** layer and the **reticular** layer. In addition to these two main layers, the dermis contains a number of appendages such as sweat and sebaceous glands, hair follicles and nails.

Papillary layer

The papillary layer is the uppermost layer of the dermis. It is rich in nerves and blood supply which exist to feed the lower, living layers of the epidermis. Blood carries nutrients and oxygen to the cells and carries waste products away.

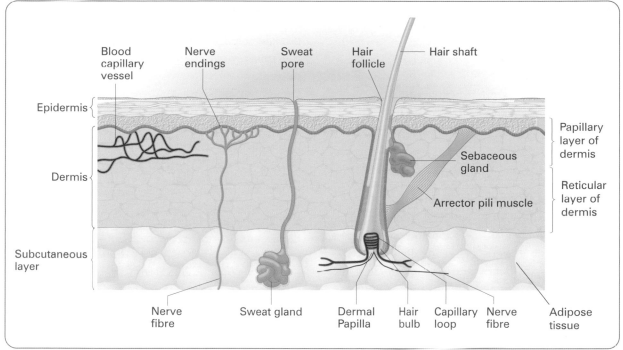

Cross-section of skin.

Reticular layer

The reticular layer is the deepest layer of the dermis and so the deepest of all the layers of the skin. It is made up of two types of protein fibres called collagen and elastin. These fibres are tangled together and form the connective tissue of the dermis, each with a separate structure and function.

Collagen fibres are thick strands of protein that provide skin with its structure and strength. Collagen fibres exist in bundles which run in different directions in different parts of the body.

Elastin is present in the dermis in tight bundles of fibres. These, along with collagen fibres, provide skin with its characteristic elasticity – the ability to stretch and return to its natural state. Renewal of elastin fibres slows down with age and the skin loses its elastic quality, appearing looser. A decline in the regeneration of collagen and elastin fibres of the dermis is the cause of lines, wrinkles and less pronounced facial contours that are characteristic of mature skins.

Fact file

If you pinch an area of skin you will see that it folds more easily one way than another. This is along a natural fold called a **cleavage line**. As a person ages, the collagen fibres gradually lose their strength and stretchability and the skin starts to sag into wrinkles along these cleavage lines.

Fact file

Collagen is a common ingredient in nourishing and anti-ageing products although some scientists argue that, due to the relatively large size of the collagen molecule, they cannot penetrate the stratum corneum. Recent developments in cosmetic surgery have seen an increase in the collagen injection, which is a way of overcoming this problem as the collagen is transported directly into the deeper layers of the skin.

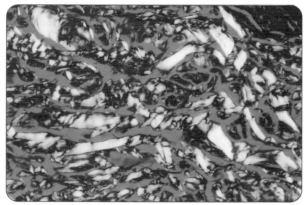

Collagen fibres seen under the microscope.

Gently pinch a piece of skin on the back of your hand and watch how long it takes to return to normal. Ask friends who are older and younger than you if you can try this on their hands (in the name of science!) and notice the difference. How would you explain this?

Epidermal derivatives

Sweat glands

There are two types of sweat gland – **eccrine** glands and **apocrine** glands. Eccrine glands are found all over the body but there is a greater concentration in the palms of the hands and the soles of the feet. They are constantly excreting small amounts of sweat, known as *insensible* perspiration, in order to maintain optimum body temperature. (*Sensible* perspiration is the term used to describe large amounts of sweat production.) *Apocrine* glands are attached to hair follicles under the arms, in the groin and around the nipples. They are the larger of the two glands and are activated when we are excited, stressed or anxious. Apocrine sweat also contains pheromones, which are the hormones thought to play a role in sexual attraction.

When sweat meets bacteria it causes an unpleasant smell known as body odour. Deodorants contain an antiseptic that decreases the activity of bacteria, while anti-perspirants contain an astringent which reduces the pore size, like in a toner, and thus less sweat reaches the surface of the skin. Both products commonly contain a perfume which masks body odour.

Sebaceous glands

Sebaceous glands secrete sebum, a natural oily substance, which moisturises the skin and helps to protect against infection due to its anti-bacterial quality. There are no sebaceous glands on the palms of the hands, the soles of the feet or the surface of the lips. Areas containing the most sebaceous glands are the scalp, the back and the chest. There are more sebaceous glands in a man's body than in a woman's body, and more in black skins than in white skins.

Factors affecting sweat production:

Factors which increase sweat production	Factors which decrease sweat production
Warm external climate or warm clothing	Temperatures lower than 36.8°C which result in vasoconstriction
Vigorous activity which increases muscle activity and body temperature	Limited activity which results in a lowering of body temperature
Hot, spicy foods and alcohol which can cause vasodilation of the capillaries	Removing certain foods from the diet which cause vasodilation
Skin colour – black skin contains more sweat glands	Skin colour – white skin contains less sweat glands
Certain illnesses or medical conditions are accompanied by a fever which results in a high temperature	Certain illnesses are characteristic of a decrease in sweat production, such as low blood pressure and diabetes
Hot flushes and sweating are characteristic of the menopause.	As the body ages, circulation becomes sluggish and the body has a tendency to feel cold
Certain forms of medication have side effects which increase body temperature	Reduction in sweating can help to prevent dehydration
Hormonal activity caused by an emotional response to fear or excitement, which causes vasodilation in all areas of the body	With age the sweat glands eventually become redundant due to inactivity

Structure and function of the subcutaneous layer

The subcutaneous layer separates the dermis from the muscles. The subcutaneous layer is therefore underneath the main layers of skin: the dermis and the epidermis. The function of the subcutaneous layer is as a storage area for fat. This layer of fat serves to protect the body against knocks and bangs by cushioning the blow. It protects the internal organs, the bones, the blood vessels and nerves. There is an abundance of nerves and blood vessels throughout the dermis and they are protected by fat cells.

| Fact | file |

sub = under and cutaneous = skin, so
subcutaneous = under the skin

The subcutaneous layer has another important function. Since fat is a poor conductor of heat, it insulates the body by preventing heat loss. The subcutaneous fat functions in the same way that draught insulation works in the home when it is fitted around doors and windows – it keeps the cold on one side and the heat on the other.

| Fact | file |

Women's bodies tend to look rounder than men's and this is because they have a fuller subcutaneous layer.

| Theory | into practice |

Illustrate how fat acts as an insulator by touching different areas of your body that contain more and less fat. Which areas feel warmer? Try this activity again the next time you exercise and notice the difference.

Know skin like the back of your hand!

Concentrate on a 2 cm square on the back of your hand and imagine that you could slice off a piece of skin just a few millimetres deep. There is no need to actually do this; imagining that you could is enough!

That small piece of skin on the back of your hand contains:

- 4 oil glands
- 12 metres of nerve fibre
- 8 metres of blood vessels
- 6 cold sensors
- 36 heat sensors
- 75 pressure sensors
- 9000 nerve endings
- 300 sweat glands
- 600 pain receptors
- 30 hair follicles.

Skin healing

The skin appears to have an amazing in-built ability to heal itself from external injury, but this healing process is, in reality, an amplification of the normal process of cell renewal which occurs constantly in the layers of the skin. The first reaction to skin damage is a rapid reflex action which removes it from the source of injury. Next, the nervous system responds to the collision by displaying a wound and then a series of wound responses on the way to regeneration of damaged skin. The physical signs of skin damage typically include inflammation, tenderness, redness and swelling, which illustrates increased blood flow to the area.

| Fact | file |

Healing means 'making whole' and involves the skin's capacity to repair itself in response to external trauma.

Skin's initial wound responses:

pressure = bruising
extreme temperature = burning
scratching = abrasion
cutting = bleeding

As soon as a blood vessel becomes damaged, blood flows rapidly to the area and **plasma** changes from its soluble form, **fibrinogen**, to an insoluble form, **fibrin**. These fibres of fibrin tangle together with other blood cells to form a clot which prevents further blood loss, and then dries out to form a scab. This all happens within a few hours of trauma, initiating further response. Platelets in the blood stimulate cellular activity in the epidermis, dermis

A summary of wound healing in skin:

Time scale	Physiological response	Physical response
Immediate reaction	Reflex action	Causes body to move away from source of injury
Immediate reaction	Nervous response	Appearance of a wound
Within hours	Increased blood flow to area	Localised inflammation
Within hours	Clotting mechanism becomes activated	Formation of a dry scab to prevent blood loss
Within hours	Increased cellular activity	Destruction of harmful bacteria
Within days	Dermal and epidermal cellular renewal	Fragile covering of new skin cells over wound
Within 3–4 weeks	Blood vessels contract	Hyper-pigmentation is reduced and skin colour returns to normal

and blood, and this stimulates the destruction of bacteria as well as the renewal of skin cells. Within a couple of days, the site of injury will have a thin covering of epithelium tissue which eventually grows into normal skin. At this stage the wound is particularly fragile and should be protected from further injury which can hinder the healing process.

During the final stage of healing, small blood vessels in the area contract and close as they are no longer required and the dark appearance of the wound gradually fades. The newly formed dermis reorganises itself into natural cleavage lines and the elastin fibres pack together. The epidermis is reformed and blends in with the mature tissue within 3 to 4 weeks. If the skin suffers a deep wound, damaging the dermal layers, there may be disturbances in the tissue and permanent scarring. A deeper wound can cause permanent damage to nerve fibres and hair follicles so that skin sensitivity becomes reduced.

Theory into practice

Think about the structure of skin and explain why some wounds bleed while others do not. Also, some areas may be insensitive to minor injury – why is that?

Changes associated with ageing

Professionals and non-professionals alike discuss 'ageing'; but what do we actually mean when we talk about the process of ageing? In this section, and the associated sections on hair and nails below and in Unit 5: Anatomy, you will explore what the ageing process involves physiologically, how it feels, and the effect it has on appearance and physical and psychological wellbeing. You will investigate age-related disorders and what, if anything, can be done to slow down the signs of ageing. Ageing is a personal, sensitive and sometimes controversial issue. People generally, and according to the media women in particular, do not enjoy ageing. It signals old age and age-associated ailments, and reminds us of our own mortality.

Biologists who specialise in the study of ageing suggest that old age begins at about 60 or 65 years, the age of retirement in the UK. The world population as a whole is ageing. In 1990 it was estimated that 1 per cent of people were over the age of 65 years and a further estimation suggests that by 2050 the number will have risen to 20 per cent. We are living thirty or forty years longer than our great-great-grandparents as a result of improved health and social care. However, it seems that we do not want to look our age, but want the age without the ageing. There are plenty of manufacturers who

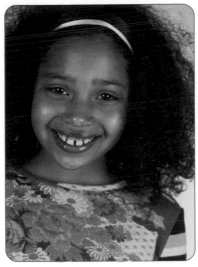
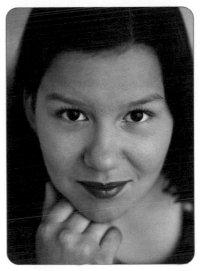
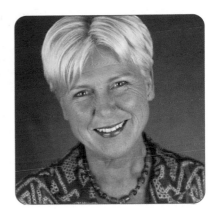

Our age is reflected in our face – but how accurate can estimations of age really be?

promise to help us, achieve that aim, thus ageing is big business.

Ageing is more than just numbers. There are enormous variances within peer groups on dimensions of health, ability and appearance. Internal and external characteristics combine to give very different images of ageing between individuals. Have you ever heard a person say something like, 'The stress of it all has aged me by ten years', or have you been surprised to hear that someone is much younger than his or her appearance suggests? These are some of the considerations to bear in mind as you proceed to think about age-related changes in the skin, hair, nails and bones.

In addition to universal age-related changes, there are other factors that influence the ageing process in skin and which should be considered by beauty therapists in consultation with clients.

The skin starts its journey of change before we are even born and goes on changing well into maturity As well as physiological changes in the skin itself, different areas of the body have different age-associated characteristics according to their underlying structures. The body, as a whole, tends to 'sag' as connective tissue loses its firmness, which leads to the condition known colloquially as 'middle age spread'. Facial contours slacken as the renewal of collagen and elastin fibres slows down, and lines and wrinkles start to appear. These are more apparent in some individuals who display tension or frown lines, or have lines around the mouth caused by years of smoking. Circulatory activity also slows as the blood vessels thicken, slowing the supply of nutrients and the removal of waste. Areas of skin, such as the backs of the hands and the temples, become thinner and blood vessels may become visible in these areas.

Theory into practice

Think about people in your own family of different generations, or celebrities in the media. Describe their appearance in relation to their age peer group.

If you can, discuss with people of different ages their awareness of ageing and what ageing means to them.

Ageing skin:

Factors which affect skin ageing	Universal characteristics of skin ageing
Exposure to UV	Dehydration
Diet and nutrition	Dark circles around the eyes
Stress and the ability to cope with stress	Appearance of lines and wrinkles
Social habits	Loss of freshness and 'bloom'
Alcohol, smoking, drugs	Facial contours become looser
Illness and medication	Skin appears thinner
Hereditary factors	Pigmentation spots

The skin through the ages:

Puberty – adulthood	Adulthood – old age	Ageing skin
Increase in hormonal and sebaceous activity	From about the age of 20 years body systems are fully developed and functioning	Regeneration in granular and prickle cell layers of epidermis slows; melanin concentrated patches appear; sweat and sebaceous activity slows
Texture is smooth, fine and firm with no lines or puffiness; good colour and fresh appearance	Characteristics of skin type become established	Texture is dry and dehydrated with uneven pigmentation; skin thinning and wrinkle formation
May be prone to comedones, acne vulgaris and outbreaks of blemishes	Skin colour and radiance begins to alter; some loss of elasticity and appearance of puffiness; texture is coarser	Possible vascular conditions or acne rosacea and pigmentation disorders; loss of facial contours

There are genetic differences between male and female skin. Male skin usually has a coarser texture and a darker colour than female skin, as well as a greater propensity to sweating, although sebaceous activity is almost the same. During the menopause, however, there is a sharp decline in sebaceous activity in women which leads to the characteristic dry, dehydrated skin type of mature skins, although the slowing down of sebum production in men is much less apparent. Female skin tends to retain more fluid than male skin and the subcutaneous layer is thicker giving it a 'softer' appearance.

The biology of hair

Structure and growth of hair

Types of hair

Hair can be grouped into different types: lanugo, vellus and terminal. **Lanugo** hair is found on the foetus before birth and is usually lost by the seventh or eight month of pregnancy. **Vellus** hair is the short, fine and downy hair found on the face and body. It does not contain pigment and is usually less than 2cm long.

Terminal hair is stronger than vellus hair and grows on the head, arms, legs, bikini area and underarms. It is composed of three layers – the cuticle, medullar and cortex – and grows to different lengths in different parts of the body.

The **cuticle** is composed of a single layer of scale-like cells, which point towards the tip of the hair. These cells overlap like the tiles on a roof, thus

Assessment task 6.1

Using detailed description and illustrations, relate the structure of skin to its functions. (M)

preventing the passage of foreign objects into the follicle. This overlapping allows the cuticle of the follicle to interlock with the cuticle of the hair, so holding the hair in place. A thin layer of lipids (fatty substances) and carbohydrates surrounds the cuticle and may protect the hair from the effects of physical and chemical agents. There is no pigment in this layer. The function of the cuticle is to confine and protect the cortex as well as giving the hair its elasticity.

The **cortex** lies inside the cuticle and forms the bulk of the hair. It consists of elongated keratinised cells cemented together. Melanin granules contained within this layer give the hair its colour. A number of air spaces are contained within the cortex. In the living part of the hair these spaces are filled with fluid, which gradually dries out as the hair grows. These spaces are larger at the base of the hair, becoming smaller at the tip.

The **medulla**, when present, is found in the centre of the hair. It may be continuous or discontinuous and may vary within the same hair. The medulla is formed of loosely connected, keratinised cells. Air spaces in the medulla determine the sheen and colour tones of the hair due to the reflection of light.

The structure and growth cycle of hair

The structure of the hair in the follicle

Hairs are formed from sac-like indentations of the epidermis known as hair follicles. The hair structure consists of keratin, a hard, horny substance composed of a combination of hydrogen, oxygen, sulphur and nitrogen.

The shape of the follicle determines the shape of the hair, i.e. straight hairs grow from straight follicles whereas curly or wavy hairs grow from curved follicles. Hair which is kinked or frizzy grows from follicles which have become distorted at the base as a result of mechanical interference such as waxing or tweezing.

The terminal hair is composed of three sections: the shaft, the root and the bulb.

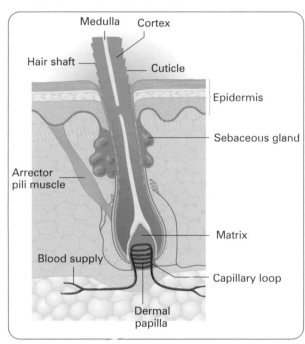

The structure of the hair in the follicle.

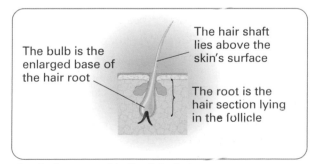

The shaft, root and bulb of the hair.

Dermal papilla

The **dermal papilla** is situated in the papillary layer of the dermis. It is connected to the resting follicle by a thin cord known as **the dermal cord**, which contains the hair germ cells. During anagen (active growth stage) the dermal cord grows down towards the dermal papilla. As the follicle grows in length so it grows in width until the bulb (which has formed at the tip of the dermal cord) engulfs the dermal papilla.

The dermal papilla is pear shaped in appearance and contains a rich vascular blood supply through capillary loops at the base. The blood supply from the dermal papilla provides nourishment to the follicle. At the widest part of the papilla an imaginary line divides the structure into two parts. The lower part contains undifferentiated cells that multiply rapidly. These cells are pushed up the papilla until they reach the critical level where they change, developing specific characteristics to form the hair.

During late catagen (transitional growth stage) the hair bulb separates from the dermal papilla and the hair starts to rise in the follicle. The follicle begins to collapse and shrink behind the rising hair. The dermal cord is reformed from undifferentiated cells.

The hair bulb

The hair bulb can be divided into two regions - upper and lower. In the lower bulb the cells are all the same; in the upper bulb they change in characteristics, differentiating into cells that produce the hair and the inner root sheath.

An imaginary line drawn across the widest part of the bulb would separate the two regions and is known as the *critical layer*. The *matrix*, also known as the germinal layer, lies below the critical level. This is the area where the cells actively reproduce by mitosis. The cells move up from the matrix into the upper bulb where they elongate vertically and increase in volume. As the cells move above the critical level into the keratogeneous zone, where keratinisation takes place, melanocytes, which produce melanin, give the hair pigment. Only a small amount of melanin is contained in the matrix, clearly showing the separation of the upper and lower bulb.

The upper bulb can be compared to the spinous layer of the epidermis. In both locations the indifferent epidermal cells become larger, acquire pigment, synthesise fibrous proteins, become reorientated and undergo the final stages of keratinisation. The keratogenous zone is located approximately half way up the follicle – this is where keritanisation takes place.

Inner/outer root sheath

The **inner root sheath (IRS)** holds the hair in the follicle by interlocking with the cuticle of the hair to the level of the sebaceous gland. The IRS is composed of three distinct layers:

1 The innermost layer is the cuticle, which interlocks with the cuticle of the hair.

2 Huxley's layer is the middle layer and is the thickest of the three layers.

3 Henley's layer is the outer layer and consists of a single layer of cells.

The inner root sheath originates from the base of the follicle, growing up in unison with the hair until it reaches the level of the sebaceous gland. The hair then continues to grow up, on its own, through the follicular (hair) canal.

The **outer root sheath** surrounds the inner root sheath and is continuous with the mitotic layer of the epidermis. At the level of the sebaceous gland, the cellular structure of this layer cannot be distinguished from that of the surface of the epidermis. Large amounts of water and glycogen are found in this layer, the highest concentration being found in the cells between the neck of the bulb and up to the level of the sebaceous glands. The thickness of the layer is uneven and, unlike the inner root sheath, it does not grow up in unison with the hair. The outer root sheath is the permanent source of the *hair germ cells* from which new follicles develop when stimulated by circulating hormones and enzymes. It is, therefore, important that these hairs are destroyed during treatment to prevent growth.

The bulge

The presence of the bulge has only become known as a possible source for follicle regeneration in recent years. It is the area where the arrector pili muscle is attached to the follicle. It is believed that the bulge is the storage area for hair follicle stem cells, which enable the follicle to regenerate if the dermal papilla is destroyed.

Moisture gradient

You will notice, as you gain practical experience, that the moisture content on the skin varies from one person to another, between different areas of the skin, and from one day to another. Moisture may be present at the surface of the skin; alternatively, the surface may be dry but the dermis may be moist. The moisture level in the skin and hair follicle is lower at the surface of the skin, and higher in the deeper layers of the dermis.

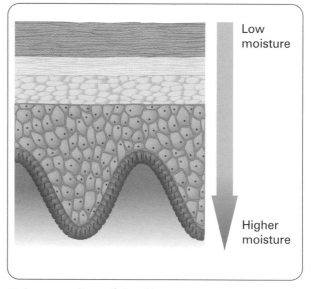
Low moisture

Higher moisture

Moisture gradient of the skin.

Sebaceous gland

Sebaceous glands are situated within the dermis, with their ducts opening into the hair follicle. Occasionally some ducts may open directly onto the skin's surface. They are absent from the palms of the hands and soles of the feet. Each gland is constructed of a single duct that ends in a cluster of secretory saccules, which are similar to a bunch of grapes.

These glands are highly sensitive to circulating androgens, which stimulate the growth of the gland and the production of sebum containing fatty acids, esters and other substances. Sebum production increases during puberty and decreases with age. Sebum is secreted onto the skin's surface via the hair follicle, its purpose being to keep the hair pliable and to lubricate the skin. Sebum is also responsible for making the skin waterproof and it plays a major role in the formation and maintenance of the 'acid mantle'.

Hair growth cycle

The hair and follicle goes through a continuous growth cycle, not dissimilar to the seasons of the year. Each phase passes smoothly into the next. In nature, winter is followed by spring, spring by summer and summer gradually and inevitably changes to autumn, and then back to winter. So it is with the hair growth cycle. Anagen can be compared to spring and summer, when the hair blossoms into growth and develops to its full potential; catagen, like autumn, is the transitional stage where hair growth slows down and comes to a stop, finally sliding into its resting or dormant stage (telogen). Then the process begins again.

Anagen

This is the active growth stage when the resting follicle begins to descend from its dormant position, just below the bulge and arrector pili muscle, down into the dermis, where it connects with the dermal papilla.

In the early stages of this phase the lower follicle is completely restructured. Hair germ cells contained within the dermal cord begin to multiply by mitosis (cell division). The dermal cord grows downwards into the dermis, at the same time growing in width, until the bulb, which has formed

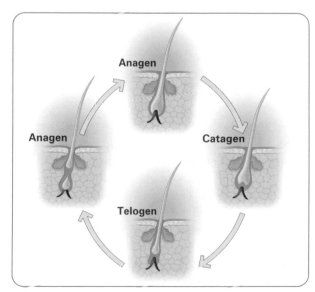

The different stages in the hair growth cycle.

at the tip of the dermal cord, encompasses the dermal papilla.

The new hair begins to form before the follicle has reached its full depth. Hair development occurs as a result of the cells in the *germinal matrix* (located in the lower bulb) becoming active. The undifferentiated cells develop different characteristics to form the hair and then the inner root sheath. The hair continues to form and grow upwards, eventually growing out through the follicle opening.

During late anagen, the pigment becomes lighter and thinner at the base of the hair shaft, melanin production stops and the melanocytes reabsorb their dendrites. Throughout the early and mid-anagen phases the follicle receives its nourishment from the dermal papilla. Research shows that the lower third of the *dermal sheath* is capable of supplying new cells for the regeneration of a *new dermal papilla*.

Catagen

Catagen is referred to as the transitional stage of the growth cycle (e.g. as late summer changes into autumn, late anagen changes into catagen). The follicle and hair stop growing, the *matrix* becomes detached from the dermal papilla and the bulb begins to shrink. The hair then starts to rise up the follicle, being held in place only by the cells of the inner root sheath. At this stage the nourishment is received from the follicle wall; water and glycogen are lost and the hair becomes drier. The epidermal cord is formed from undifferentiated cells as the follicle begins to shrink and collapse below the rising hair.

Telogen

This is the final phase of the growth cycle. The hair is dead with a brush-like end; it is dry, lacking in lustre and lifeless. It will either fall out naturally or be pushed out by the new hair that is developing when the anagen phase is repeated. Often there is no hair present in the follicle during the telogen or resting phase. However, in some instances this period of the growth cycle is very short and may occasionally be missed out altogether, with the follicle going straight from catagen into anagen. The telogen follicle is one-third of the length of a full anagen follicle.

The biology of nails

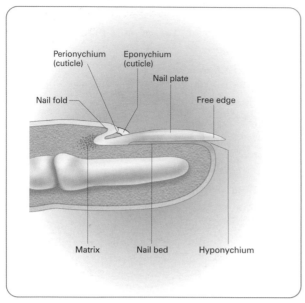

Cross section of nail in its nail bed.

Nails are tough, protective structures found at the end of the phalanges. The condition of nails, like that of skin and hair, reflects our general health and well-being. Healthy nails have a pinkish colour from the underlying nail bed and should be firm yet flexible, smooth and slightly curved with a natural sheen. This section will investigate the factors affecting nail growth and the structure of the nail in its nail bed.

Chemical composition of nails:

Carbon	51%
Oxygen	21%
Nitrogen	17%
Sulphur	5%
Hydrogen	6%
Oil	trace

Structure of the nail

The **nail plate** is a hard, protective structure constructed of layers of keratinised cells and forms the visible portion of the nail. The end portion of the nail plate extends over the tips of fingers or toes and is called the **free edge**. The majority of the nail plate rests on and is attached to the **nail bed**, which is the prickle cell layer of the epidermis. The nail bed is supplied by a great many blood vessels, which carry nutrients to the nail, and nerve endings which

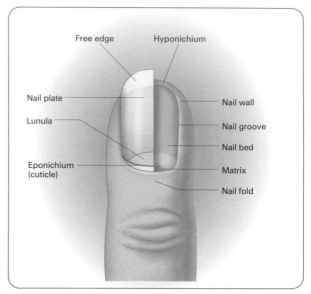

The structure of the nail.

serve as pain receptors if the nail receives trauma. The nail plate and nail bed have corresponding horizontal ridges, rather like corrugated cardboard, which ensure firm adhesion of one to the other. The **lunula** or 'half moon', at the base of the nail plate, is an area of incomplete keratinisation of the nail. It represents a bridge between the living matrix and the dead nail plate.

The **nail fold** or **mantle** is the fleshy part of skin at the first joint which protects the underlying **nail root** or **matrix**. Like any other root, this is the part of the nail that contains the 'parent cells' and is the site of cell division or mitosis. Cells push up the nail from the matrix, gradually dehydrating (in a similar process to keratinisation in skin). The nail plate actually consists of multiple layers of dead cells. External injury to the nail fold can result in damage to the matrix, which affects the growth of the nail and can result in permanent damage.

As the nail grows it forms a furrow between the nail wall and the nail plate called the **nail groove**. The **nail wall** slightly overlaps the nail groove to protect it from invasion of micro-organisms. Another structure which helps protect the nail is the **eponichium**. This is the fold of cuticle at the base of the nail which protects the matrix from invasion. A thickened portion of stratum corneum below the free edge, called the **hyponichium**, helps to protect the nail bed. This can become damaged by splinters under the nail. Both the hyponychium and eponichium can become damaged by the incorrect use of manicure equipment, resulting in infection.

Nail growth

The average rate of nail growth is about 0.5 cm per month, which means that a brand new nail can take up to six months to grow completely. Growth begins at the nail root, below the visible portion of nail, pushing the nail up onto its bed and extending past the tip of the fingers or toes. Nails grow faster in summer than winter due to more ultraviolet light and less dehydration from indoor pollutants, which cause nails to split. They grow faster on fingers than on toes, where they tend to be thicker, and in right-handed people they grow faster on the right hand. Nail growth in children is faster than in adults. The ageing process slows down nail growth but causes the nails to appear thicker. The reasons for these variations are the same: circulation.

Assessment task 6.2

Explain how the structure of nails determines growth. Describe the lifestyle and environmental factors which affect growth in nails and how these can be overcome. (D)

Diseases and disorders of the skin, hair and nails

Diseases and disorders of the skin

In order to carry out beauty therapy treatments without risk to yourself, your colleagues or your clients, you will need to recognise common diseases and disorders so that you can distinguish between treatable and non-treatable conditions.

Non-infectious disorders are those which vary from normal, healthy tissue but cannot be spread or made worse. Infectious diseases and disorders contra-indicate beauty therapy treatment and clients who show signs of these should be referred in the first instance to their GP.

Theory into practice

Explain the implications for beauty therapy treatment for each of the non-infectious skin conditions illustrated opposite and overleaf. What advice would you give to a client showing characteristics of each of these conditions?

Non-infectious skin conditions

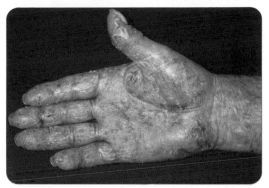

Dermatitis.

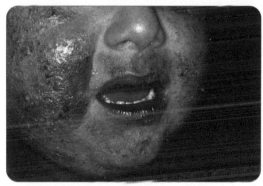

Eczema.

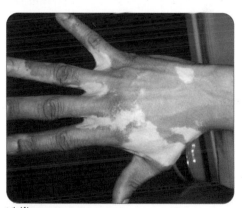

Vitiligo.

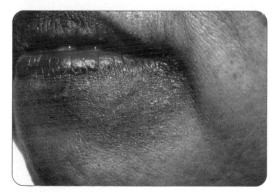

Chloasma.

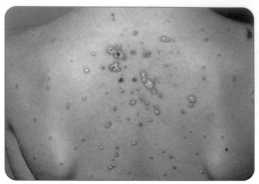
Psoriasis.

Skin cancer

Melanoma is a disease which affects tissues containing the colour pigment melanin, sometimes in the eye and more commonly in the skin. Professionals use the term **malignant** to describe a condition which is cancerous; the most dangerous form of skin cancer is therefore known as malignant melanoma. There are various types of skin cancer but for now we will use the term melanoma to refer to all skin cancers, although this is not strictly accurate.

Melanoma is on the increase amongst all populations and in all countries, with reported cases

Non-infectious skin conditions:

Condition	Cause	Appearance
Dermatitis	Usually an adverse reaction to an external irritant	Dry, flaky, itchy skin
Eczema	A sequence of inflammatory changes triggered by the skins intolerance to a sensitiser	Similar to dermatitis – dry, flaky, inflamed skin
Naevus (mole)	Usually congenital, may develop in puberty or increase with age	Flat, light to mid-brown in colour with smooth, even texture
Vitiligo	Under-production of melanin pigment	White patches; extra sensitivity, especially to UV light; more obvious in darker skins
Chloasma	Over-production of melanin, sometimes caused by sunburn or as a reaction to light sensitive ingredients or during pregnancy	Irregular patches of darker pigmentation, more obvious in paler skins
Psoriasis	Thought to be stress related	Reddened skin with silvery, scaly patches
Sebaceous cysts	Unknown cause	Nodular lesions with smooth, shiny surface situated in the dermis
Acne vulgaris	Hormonal changes typically during puberty, worsened by poor skin hygiene	Congested skin with comedones and pustules; can become inflamed
Milia	Build up of sebum	Small, white pearls beneath the skin
Acne rosacea	External or internal pollutants, more typical in mature clients	Red, couperose over nose and cheeks
Basal cell carcinoma	Usually over-exposure to UV; rare before puberty	Moles typically have a raised edge, are dark brown or black in colour
Melanoma	Usually over-exposure to UV light; rarely seen before puberty, can be benign or malignant	Moles usually dark in colour and irregular in shape; may be flat or nodular

rising by about 12 per cent each year. This increase is higher than for almost all other forms of cancer (except lung cancer in women) and illustrates that the number of melanoma patients worldwide is presently doubling every ten years. The Cancer Research Campaign, whose aim is to encourage public awareness and reduce cases, suggests that there are 40,000 new cases of skin cancer in the UK every year and of those about 2,000 individuals will die from the disease. There are more deaths in the UK due to malignant melanoma than there are in Australia, where public awareness of the dangers has been greater. Skin cancer can affect all areas of the body in all people and of all ages, but is rare before puberty. In the UK, melanoma is twice as common in women as it is in men and is most prevalent in the 15 to 34 age group. Almost 50 per cent of melanomas in women are seen on the lower leg, mostly between the ankle and knee, with some cases seen on the soles of the feet. In men, the most common site is the back. The face is the most common site of cancerous growths in adults over the age of 60 years.

Some skin growths are defined as pre-malignant and if left untreated have a tendency to become malignant. Pre-malignant growths must therefore be recognised and treated as soon as possible and early diagnosis is imperative. The term **benign** is used to describe a condition which is non-cancerous, is not likely to become malignant and does not pose a risk to health. A naevus is an example of a benign lesion. However harmless such a growth might be, an individual may choose to have a benign lesion removed for cosmetic reasons.

If malignant or pre-malignant conditions are identified and removed at an early stage, they are curable. It is only advanced melanomas which cannot be treated that are fatal, and it is therefore vital that health and beauty professionals learn how to detect the early signs of malignancy and pre-malignant growths, as well as how to eliminate anxiety by recognising benign pigmented lesions. To this end, they must properly educate their clients on methods of self-diagnosis and how to identify and eliminate the risk factors associated with skin cancer. As always, prevention is better than cure.

Ordinary moles

Moles are non-cancerous clusters of pigmented cells which are known as **benign melanocytic naevi**. Infants usually have few moles and most make their first appearance between the age of 8 and 20 years. Dermatologists are not clear as to the cause of moles, but note that children who have spent more time in the sun often have a larger number than individuals who have had less sun exposure. The average young adult in the UK will have between twenty and forty small brown marks on his or her skin which may be flat or slightly raised and are not painful. They are present all year round and do not fade in the winter as do freckles or **ephilides** (as they are known medically).

Many moles disappear without treatment and they decrease with age. In older adults they may be darker or more raised and some may have one or two

Analysing moles:

1 Size	A change in the size of an existing mole or a new mole which grows rapidly.
2 Shape	The appearance of a new mole which has an irregular shape or an existing mole which changes shape.
3 Colour	An existing mole which changes in colour, becomes darker or has an uneven pigmentation.
4 Diameter	The majority of benign naevi have a diameter at their widest part of 3–6 mm. New or existing moles with a largest diameter of 7 mm should be checked.
5 Inflammation	A benign lesion should not normally become inflamed; however, trauma or friction can sometimes cause redness.
6 Discharge	Benign moles should not bleed or ooze fluid, should not become sticky and should not have crusting. An early indication of melanoma is the reported sticking of clothes to existing lesions.
7 Sensation	Moles are painless and do not usually cause sensation of any kind. Early cause for concern is any form of mild itching.

hairs protruding from them. Medical advice is to leave moles alone unless their appearance changes, in which case medical attention should be sought. There is a well documented seven point checklist which assists in the analysis of pigmented naevi and which describes major and minor characteristics that require referral (see page 115). Please remember, however, that as beauty professionals we do not have the capacity to diagnose medical conditions and should never attempt to do so. Our job is to use discretion in alerting clients to conditions which should be checked by their doctor.

Risk factors associated with skin cancer

The main factor believed to cause skin cancer is exposure to ultraviolet light. Reported cases have risen in recent decades due to increased travel abroad and the prestige of sporting a deep suntan. With increased sun awareness it is hoped that the suntan will become less appealing and that people will choose to 'fake not bake'. The depletion of the ozone layer has also affected the amount of damaging rays which are reaching the earth, adding to the risk of skin cancer. Research suggests that fair-skinned people who expose themselves to the sun will burn in half the time today as they did in 1990 because the depleting ozone layer offers less protection against the sun's damaging rays.

Risk factors for sun damage:

Individual Risk Factors	Relative risk
Fair skin, does not tan, prone to burning	3
Fair hair colour	3
Previous sunburn	3
Previous melanoma	8
A large number of ordinary moles	20–30
Abnormal moles with no family history of melanoma	4–10
Abnormal moles with a family history of melanoma	100–400
Moles which change in shape, colour or texture	400

(From: Mackie, R.M. (1994) *Malignant Melanoma: A guide to early diagnosis:* University of Glasgow)

Individuals who emigrate to hot countries over the age of 15 years are less likely to suffer than those who emigrated earlier or those who were born there, which highlights the risk of childhood exposure. As well as the general causal effect of sun exposure, there are a number of personal risk factors to be considered.

More risk factors for skin cancer:

Pregnancy	Some individuals develop melanoma during pregnancy and they are at greater risk of melanoma in subsequent pregnancies. If melanoma develops in a non-pregnant individual there is no risk factor associated with pregnancy at a later time.
Contraceptive pill	Despite suggestions that the old, high-level oestrogen pill was a possible risk factor associated with skin cancer, continued studies show no evidence to suggest that the use of modern oral contraception is a risk factor.
Smoking	Smoking is not a risk factor for skin cancer.
History	Individuals who have had melanoma in the past are 10 per cent more likely to develop a second malignant growth on the same or another part of the body.

Medical diagnosis and treatment

Melanoma responds well to treatment and therefore early recognition, referral and removal can save lives. The most important consideration for treatment is the depth of the growth as this has implications for survival. Individuals with lesions less than 1.5 mm deep have a 93 per cent survival rate whereas for melanoma 3.5 mm deep or over this drops to 40 per cent. Doctors measure the depth of melanoma using a method called **Breslow thickness**, named after the pathologist who first recognised the importance of this measurement. The distance is measured between the granular layer of the epidermis and the deepest malignant cells. Growths are usually removed by a small operation under local anaesthetic.

Infectious skin conditions

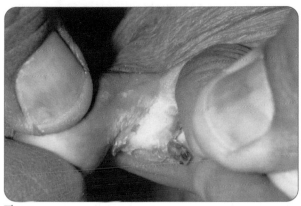

Tinea.

Theory into practice

For each of the infectious skin conditions described in the table below, demonstrate an understanding of the implications for beauty therapy treatment.

Some of the most common infectious skin conditions:

Condition	Cause	Appearance
Folliculitis	Bacterial infection of hair follicle; may be due to ingrowing hairs or poor skin hygiene	Inflammation, erythema, discomfort
Furuncle (boil)	Staphylococcal bacterial infection of hair follicle due to fatigue	Red, swollen, painful, pus-filled nodule, commonly found in axilla, neck, back of thighs
Carbuncle	Staphylococcal bacteria	Group of boils
Impetigo	Streptococcal and staphylococcal bacteria spread by dirty fingers	Weeping or dry crust on inflamed skin; commonly on facial areas
Wart	Virus	Raised, skin coloured; can be smooth or rough; vary in size
Plantar wart (verruca)	Virus	Painful, ingrowing wart on sole of foot
Herpes simplex (cold sore)	Virus; recurrent cold sores may be related to stress or illness	Usually on face or lips; tingling, red, raised; may weep
Herpes zoster (shingles)	Virus related to chicken-pox	Painful; erythema along nerve pathways; acute inflammation
Tinea (ringworm)	Superficial fungus	Typically red papules which resemble a ring
Scabies	Sarcoptes scabiei parasite or 'itch mite'	Itchy rash, commonly found in warm folds of skin between fingers, axilla and palms

Diseases and disorders of the hair

Some of the most common diseases and disorders of the hair:

Condition	Cause	Appearance
Alopecia	Age, illness, stress, self-harm	Loss of hair in defined areas
Tinea capitis (ringworm)	Superficial fungus	Round, scaly patches on the scalp; hair breakage near root
Dandruff	Dry scalp or irritation from chemicals or detergents	White scales which shed from scalp; sometimes have an oily texture
Pediculosis capitis (head lice)	Infectious parasitic infection	Lice lay nits which are small, round, white eggs that attach to clean hair
Endocrine disorders	Inherited or acquired disorders which cause hormonal imbalance	Male hair growth pattern in women

Diseases and disorders of the nails

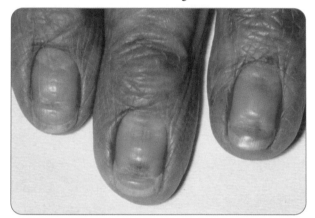

Beau's lines.

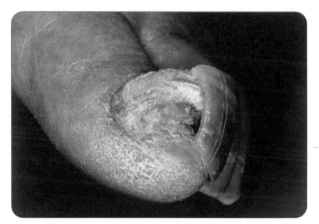

Paronychia.

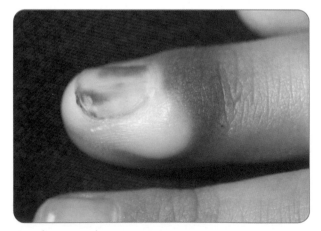

Onychocryptosis.

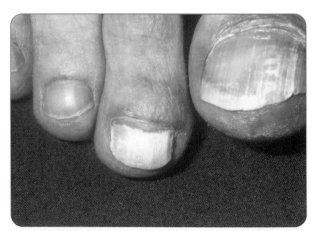

Tinea ungium.

Some of the most common diseases and disorders of the nails:

Condition	Cause	Appearance
Beau's lines	Serious illness which prohibits nail growth	Deep depression across all nails
Abnormal coloration	Illness, smoking, chemicals	Depends on cause; can be shades of blue or yellow
Onycholysis	Trauma, injury, illness	Separation of nail from its bed
Onycophagy	Acquired nervous habit	Chewed nail and cuticle, exposed hyponychium
Hangnail	Dehydrated cuticle, biting, injury	Cuticle in eponychium or nail groove splits
Onychocryptosis (ingrowing nails)	Ill-fitting shoes, incorrect cutting or filing	Nail grows into surrounding tissue, inflammation, bleeding
Pterygium	Poor circulation, injury, neglect	Thick overgrowth adhering to nail plate
Paronychia	Bacterial infection which enters broken cuticle	Inflammation around nail plate; painful, may weep
Tinea ungium/ onychomycosis (ringworm of nails)	Superficial fungus	Nails are brown, thickened and may shed
Onychogryphosis	Poor circulation, age	Thickening of nail, excessive ridges and curvature

Summary

Diseases and disorders of the skin, hair and nails have multiple causes. Some are infectious and others are not. Your job as a beauty therapist is to differentiate between treatable and non-treatable conditions and provide appropriate advice and recommendations. Those conditions described can be characterised according to the following causes:

▸▸ bacterial infection
▸▸ viral infection
▸▸ allergic reaction
▸▸ hereditary factors
▸▸ hormonal disorder
▸▸ fungal infection
▸▸ parasite
▸▸ pigmentation disorder
▸▸ stress
▸▸ cancer.

Theory into practice

Spend some time sorting the diseases and disorders of skin, hair and nails described in this section according to their cause. Think about the implications for treatment of each of these categories.

Assessment task 6.3

Complete the table below to categorise diseases and disorders of the skin, hair and nails according to viral, fungal and bacterial causes. (M)

	Viral	Fungal	Bacterial
Skin			
Hair			
Nails			

Characteristics and transmission of micro-organisms

Micro-organisms

A micro-organism is a minute living organism that can affect the body in a number of ways. If certain micro-organisms invade in sufficient quantities, or if the body has low resistance, they can cause illness and disease. The symptoms of disease are determined both by the type of micro-organism and the area of the body which is infected.

Bacteria

Bacteria are the simplest form of all living organisms and also the most abundant; biologists have identified almost 2000 different species. Bacteria reproduce rapidly by splitting so that a single bacterium can produce up to 16 million bacteria in just one day. Different bacteria survive in different environments ranging from sub-zero to near boiling temperatures. Some bacteria require oxygen to survive – **obligate** aerobes; others do not – **anaerobes**; and some bacteria can survive with or without oxygen – **facultative** anaerobes. Bacteria are decomposers that help break down organic matter but not all of them are harmful. So-called 'friendly bacteria' are non-**pathogenic**. They are present in the digestive system to help in the break down of certain vitamins. Bacteria are used in antibiotics and also in the production of foods such as cheese and yoghurt. Harmful bacteria are called pathogenic bacteria or pathogens, and these belong to a large group of bacteria known as *true bacteria*. They cause disease either by destroying the tissues of their host or by producing substances which are toxic to it. Pathogens reproduce rapidly in the right conditions.

Conditions required for the growth of pathogenic bacteria are:

» nutrients
» temperature 37°C – growth can occur within temperature danger zone: 8–37°C
» alkaline conditions
» moisture
» darkness
» some require oxygen, others do not.

Theory into practice

Study the conditions required for the growth of pathogenic bacteria listed above and explain the ways in which the body protects itself from the invasion of these harmful bacteria.

Structure

Bacteria are single cell organisms which consists of **cytoplasm** surrounded by a **cell membrane** and then a cell wall. The cytoplasm contains two types of nuclear matter: **DNA** containing fast growing chromosomes, and **RNA** which contains protein-

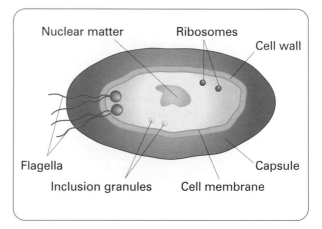

Structure of a bacterial cell.

The structure of different types of pathogenic bacteria:

Name	Structure	Disease
Bacilli	Straight, rod shaped	E.coli, tuberculosis, typhoid
Cocci	Spherical shaped	
Diplococci	Cocci formed into pairs	Pneumonia, gonorrhoea
Staphylococci	Cocci formed into clusters	Carbuncle, food poisoning
Streptococci	Cocci formed into chains	Impetigo, scarlet fever
Spirilli	Spiral rods	Cholera, syphilis

producing rybosomes as well as food reserves in **inclusion granules**. Some bacteria contain **flagella**, which are tadpole-like structures that enable movement. The cell wall is a combination of sugars and amino acids. Different types of pathogenic bacteria are classified by their shape: bacilli, cocci and spirilli (see table on page 120).

Protoctista

Protoctista are complex, single-celled organisms which usually reproduce asexually by mitosis (although some do reproduce sexually). Protozoa are a particular type of protoctista which are adapted to the environment in which they live and can be further divided into four groups differentiated by their method of movement. These are animal **flagellates**, **sarcodines**, **ciliates** and **sporozoans**.

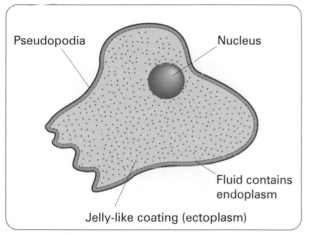

Structure of protozoa.

Structure of protoctista

Flagellates are the most simple forms of protozoa. They multiply by mitosis and generally have no outer wall. Some flagellates are parasitic, including the type that causes African sleeping sickness and another that survives in the digestive system of termites.

Sarcodines are amoeba-like organisms which survive in fresh and salt water. Those that live in the sea have snail-like shells made of calcium carbonate. The white cliffs of Dover and similar formations are the result of discarded chalky deposits from the shells of these micro-organisms. Some sarcodines are parasites, such as those which cause amoebic dysentery.

Ciliates are the most complex of protozoa. They contain cilia which enable them to stick together to form brush-like structures and they are capable of

'walking' or 'jumping'. Ciliates also contain a skin or cortex which includes the cell membrane. There are about 6000 types of ciliate which live in fresh or salt water, and most are non-parasitic.

The final class of protozoa, sporozoa, are parasitic. The best known of these is **plasmodium**, the type which transmits malaria back and forth between mosquitoes and humans. While male mosquitoes survive on nectar, the female requires blood for the development of her eggs and she acquires this by biting and drawing blood from humans. If the person she bites has malaria, the mosquito sucks up plasmodium with the blood which is stored in her salivary glands. The mosquito acts as a **carrier**, carrying the micro-organism to the next person she bites and injecting a droplet of saliva under the skin, thus infecting the victim with the sporozoa. These micro-organisms enter the liver where they sub-divide before being transported into the bloodstream at intervals of about 48–72 hours. This explains the episodes of chills and fever which are characteristic of malaria. If plasmodium is ingested by a mosquito at this stage, the cycle continues.

Fact file

Only certain types of mosquito – the female Anopheles – carry malaria. Before travelling abroad to high risk countries, you should seek advice from your GP about anti-malarial drugs. Seek immediate medical attention if you develop malarial symptoms or suffer an adverse reaction to mosquito bites while away from home or on your return from travelling.

Fungi

Fungi (singular: *fungus*) are larger than bacteria and can reproduce either sexually or asexually by forming spores. Some are so large that they are visible without the aid of a microscope, such as moulds and mildew. Like bacteria, fungi require nutrients, oxygen and a warm, dark, moist environment in order to survive. Some airborne spores are very small and can survive in the air for long periods and be carried great distances. Fungi live off host cells, digesting organic matter for nutrition. They grow rapidly, illustrated by the overnight appearance of a garden of mushrooms or toadstools. Along with bacteria, fungi are the chief decomposers of the world. Some fungi are parasites which live off host cells in plants or animals, including humans. They can attach to the skin or mucous membranes and cause disease. Other types of fungi live off dead organic matter. Some fungi are used in the production of Roquefort or Camembert cheeses and others are used in the manufacture of antibiotics which destroy bacteria, such as penicillin.

Structure of fungi

Some fungi are single celled, such as yeasts, while others are multicellular, such as moulds. Multicellular fungi contain a mass of filaments known collectively as **mycelium.** Spore producing fungi, such as mushrooms, consist of tightly packed filaments. Cellular structures, such as protoplasm, fungal nuclei and cytoplasm, flow freely within these filaments. The cell walls of fungi consist of a type of sugar unique to this species. Fungi Imperfecti is the class of fungi which cause disease. In humans, these include the following:

- tinea pedis (athlete's foot)
- tinea capitis (ringworm of the scalp)
- oral/genital thrush, caused by the fungus candida albicans
- tinea corporis (ringworm of the body)
- tinea ungium (ringworm of the nail).

Viruses

Viruses range in size but are larger than small bacteria and they cause a variety of illnesses. Cells infected by viruses must have a receptor for that particular virus; for example, the common cold is caused by a virus which attacks the mucus membranes of the respiratory tract, while chicken-pox is caused by a virus which attacks the skin cells. Viruses cannot reproduce. Like fungi they are parasites that live off host cells and cause them to make copies of the virus. While viruses can be more or less dangerous, some viral infections are potentially fatal, such as rabies, hepatitis and Human Immunodeficiency Virus (HIV). Some diseases such as cancer and multiple sclerosis are also thought to be viral in origin.

Structure of viruses

Viruses contain nuclear matter, either DNA or RNA, contained in a protein shell. DNA acts as a template so that the cells can produce more viral DNA, while RNA is responsible for enzymes and proteins. Viruses can digest and reuse the DNA and RNA of their host cells to produce more viral matter. The protein shell determines what type of host cell the virus will attack, for example, the skin or mucous membrane, and thus what type of disease it will cause.

Viruses are responsible for the following diseases and disorders:

- measles
- common cold
- warts
- herpes simplex (cold sore)
- chicken-pox
- rubella (German measles)
- influenza
- plantar warts (verruca)
- herpes zoster (shingles)
- polio.

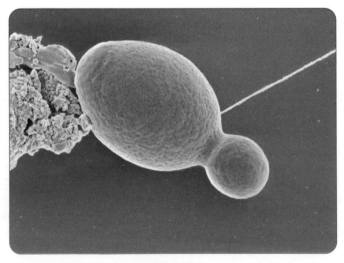

Thrush bacteria (Candida albicans).

Transmission of micro-organisms

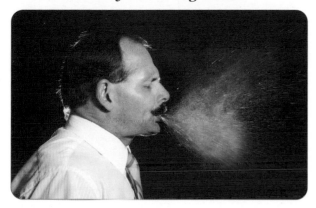

Airborne micro-organisms.

Micro-organisms can be transmitted (spread) in a number of ways, causing infection and cross-infection. Some illnesses are spread by the transmission of droplets in the air, such as the bacteria that causes whooping cough or the virus that causes influenza. Every precaution should be taken to avoid cross-infection of this kind in the workplace, ideally by staying at home until a full recovery from the illness has been made. Fungal spores can also be airborne, which results in the spread of moulds.

▸▸ **Practice point: Precautions**: If you have a cold wear a paper mask which covers your nose and mouth when working in close contact with clients. Always use a clean, disposable handkerchief to catch and contain droplets if you cough or sneeze, and wash your hands after each episode.

Other micro-organisms are spread in food, such as the bacteria salmonella which causes food poisoning or fungal moulds on rotting food, while others can be transmitted in contaminated water supplies or through poor sanitation.

▸▸ **Practice point:** Personal hygiene is of the utmost importance in beauty therapy and other professions which involve close contact with clients. When washing your hands use an antibacterial hand cleanser and thoroughly wash the fronts and backs, between the fingers and up the forearm. Always dry your hands thoroughly with disposable paper towels.

In the UK, we take certain things for granted such as clean running water, waste and sewage disposal and a reliable supply of uncontaminated food. Early in the twentieth century, however, things were very different, with a high proportion of infant mortality caused by diarrhoea as a result of contaminated water. In some third world countries poor sanitation, open sewers and contaminated drinking water are still the norm and cause much disease and fatality. Fleas, lice, mosquitoes and rats thrive in warm, damp conditions such as sewers, rubbish dumps and areas of poor sanitation, and are capable of transmitting disease between people or contaminating water supplies with their urine or faeces. The eradication in medical and public places of **vectors**, or disease carrying agents, has improved the health of the UK's population but remains a major concern for some developing countries. UK citizens travelling to certain countries can protect themselves by only drinking bottled water, being careful as to what they eat and being vaccinated against diseases such as hepatitis A, yellow fever and typhoid. Your GP can advise you of what precautions are necessary.

Some micro-organisms, such as those which cause hepatitis B, hepatitis C and HIV, are transmitted through body fluids. This might occur during sexual intercourse or the transfusion of contaminated blood. Medical and beauty professionals should take extra precautions when in contact with blood, tissue fluid and skin debris, and should seek information about a client's medical history during consultation. Disposable sterile needles should be used for epilation and disposable sterile micro-lances should be used for milia extraction. Care should be taken not to scratch yourself with used sharps and they should never be re-used. Clinical waste should be placed in sharps boxes for collection by the local authority and incineration.

▸▸ **Practice point:** You are more likely to come into contact with blood and tissue fluid during certain procedures such as bikini and underarm waxing, extraction and electrical epilation. Protect yourself and your clients by wearing disposable gloves for these treatments.

A number of micro-organisms are transmitted through direct contact with a carrier. Viral infections such as warts or herpes, bacterial infections such as impetigo, and fungal infections such as ringworm, are all transmitted in this way and are therefore contra-indications to all treatment. Some micro-organisms survive on inanimate objects such as tools, equipment and other surfaces, leading to cross-infection if the correct procedures for sterilisation are not followed. The bacterial nail disease paronychia can be transmitted on manicure tools; impetigo can be carried on facial cloths or sponges; and the fungus that causes ringworm can be transmitted on surfaces and floors. The HIV or hepatitis B viruses can be transmitted between clients on contaminated needles or tweezers.

Theory into practice

Think of a normal day in the working environment. Describe the many activities that would prompt you to wash your hands. Explain the other health and safety procedures that will help to protect yourself and others from cross-infection.

Growth requirements of micro-organisms

Historically, the main transmitters of disease causing micro-organisms were doctors and other medical professionals, and this recognition prompted immediate measures for prevention and control. Legislation was introduced regarding safe and hygienic practices in hospitals, which included sterilisation, disposal of waste, clean water supplies and the eradication of animal parasites which can act as vectors, such as fleas, lice and mosquitoes.

In 1796 Edward Jenner performed the first ever **vaccination**, the most effective method of control of viral infections. A vaccine is either a dead virus of the type that causes a particular disease or a closely-related but harmless virus. Vaccines are now used to immunise against a number of diseases but

A summary of disease causing micro-organisms and their methods of transmission:

Method of transmission	Micro-organism	Disease
Droplets in the air	Streptococcus bacteria, other airborne bacteria	Tuberculosis, whooping cough, scarlet fever
	Virus	Common cold, influenza
	Fungal spores	Cause moulds to spread
Ingestion	Staphylococcus bacteria, salmonella bacteria	Typhoid fever; food poisoning
Faeces, poor sanitation	E. coli bacteria	Food poisoning, typhoid fever
	Virus	Hepatitis A
Exchange of body fluids	Spirilli bacteria, diplococcus bacteria	Syphilis; gonorrhoea
	Virus	Hepatitis B, hepatitis C, HIV
Direct contact	Bacteria	Impetigo, carbuncle
	Virus	Wart, plantar wart, herpes simplex
	Fungus	Tinea – pedis, corporis, capitits, ungium
	Animal parasites	Scabies, head lice
Contaminated objects	Bacteria	Paronychia, impetigo
	Virus	Hepatitis B, HIV, plantar wart
	Fungus	Tinea – pedis, corporis, capitis, ungium
Vectors	Mosquito, rat	Malaria; typhoid fever

not all viruses can be controlled in this way. For example, there is still no cure for the common cold or influenza, the reason being that its structure changes so frequently that previously produced vaccines are unsuitable.

In 1929 another medical breakthrough took place when Alexander Flemming discovered the first **antibiotic** – penicillin. An antibiotic is, by definition, a chemical that is produced by a living organism and can inhibit the growth of micro-organisms. Penicillin inhibits bacterial growth by causing the cell walls to collapse. Today, antibiotics are produced synthetically and are used to treat a variety of illnesses. Medical intervention and the treatment of disease are the main reasons for the population explosion witnessed over the last century.

Assessment task 6.4

Give an example of one disease causing bacterium, one virus and one fungus. For each, explain clearly the structure, life cycle and means of transmission. (M)

Growth requirements of micro-organisms:

	Bacteria	Protoctista	Fungi	Virus
Water	✓ water supply	✓	✓ damp	✓
Nutrition	✓ parasite	Some are parasitic, some are non-parasitic	✓ parasite on live/dead host	✓ parasite
Temperature	37°C is ideal, refrigeration limits growth	Adapted to their environment	Flourishes in warm conditions	Flourishes in warm conditions
pH	Slightly alkaline			
Oxygen	✓ for aerobic respiration ✗ for anaerobic respiration	✓	✓ Although some survive for a short time without	

Health and safety

Handling techniques

The correct handling of goods and equipment, for their safety as well as your own, will become second nature to you before too long. The importance of good working posture cannot be emphasised enough, particularly when you are carrying out physically demanding treatments in body massage and body therapy; but good posture is just as important when performing seated treatments, such as facial therapy and nail treatments.

▸▸ Practice point: Good posture is when the body weight is distributed evenly between the head, shoulders, chest, abdomen, thighs and lower legs, and is over feet that are forward facing and slightly apart.

Many couches and stools are adjustable so that you can tailor them to your individual height. If you feel uncomfortable or are having to stretch or slouch, your body will become fatigued and you may cause yourself long-term injury which could affect both your career and your day-to-day activities.

As part of your job you may have to lift heavy boxes of stock or equipment and it is important to look after your back by doing this correctly. There are a number of disorders which can affect the muscular and skeletal systems if correct procedures are not adhered to, including postural defects, which are explored in Unit 10: Body therapy (pages 229–30), and repetitive strain injury (RSI). The **Manual Handling Operations Regulations Act (1992)** states the necessary measures to avoid these types of injury.

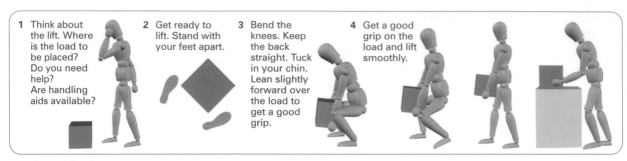

1. Think about the lift. Where is the load to be placed? Do you need help? Are handling aids available?

2. Get ready to lift. Stand with your feet apart.

3. Bend the knees. Keep the back straight. Tuck in your chin. Lean slightly forward over the load to get a good grip.

4. Get a good grip on the load and lift smoothly.

Watch your back!

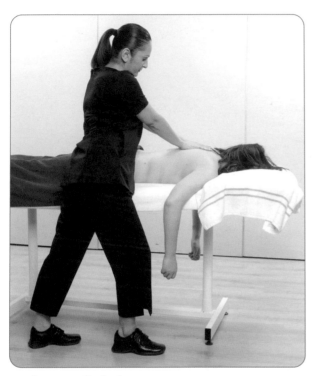

Good posture for body massage.

Sterilisation

Sterilisation is the method of completely destroying all living micro-organisms to prevent the spread of disease through cross-infection. Any piece of equipment or work surface which has been sterilised and is free from pathogenic micro-organisms is said to be **aseptic**. It is of paramount importance in the salon to ensure the safety of everyone who gives and/or receives treatment. There are different methods of sterilisation which are investigated in the Professional basics section (pages 12–13) and summarised at the end of this section (page 127). You must familiarise yourself with these procedures and the method most suitable for different tools and equipment.

Before sterilisation, you should thoroughly wash and dry all equipment to remove any barriers against sterilisation. Surgical spirit can be used on small items such as manicure tools, while other items such as vacuum suction, high frequency or mechanical massage attachments can be washed in hot soapy water. If tools or equipment become damaged, cracked or broken you must not use them as they might harbour bacteria in places which cannot be reached by sterilisation methods. Once sterilised equipment is exposed to the air it is no longer sterile, which is why all items should be sterilised both *before and after* use.

Correct clothing

Salon dress and personal hygiene is explored in the Professional basics section (pages 10–11). Your salon uniform should not be worn outside the working environment so that it remains in pristine condition and is not soiled by food, drink, pollution or smoke. Additional protective clothing may be worn for some treatments, such as a plastic apron for waxing, and some therapists choose to wear a tabard over their uniform which can be changed throughout the day as it becomes stained with products. Client clothing should be protected throughout the treatment with towels or tissues, and any clothing which has been removed should be stored safely away from products to avoid staining or damage.

Disposal of contaminated materials

Each work area should have its own lined bin with a lid that should be emptied at least once a day. This should only be used for salon waste, such as tissues, cotton wool, couch roll, etc., and not for food or other personal refuse. At the end of the session the liner should be removed, tied and placed in a large, sealed refuse sack for collection. The salon should have a separate bin for glass, either from breakages or product bottles. Glass items should be wrapped in sufficient quantities of paper towel or tissue before disposal. Clinical waste, which is contaminated with blood or other body fluids, must be disposed of separately to other waste in a yellow bin. Sharps boxes must be provided for the disposal of used epilation probes or micro-lances, which are then collected by the local health authority and disposed of by incineration.

A summary of sterilisation techniques:

Technique	Equipment	Method	Suitable for
Heat	▶▶ Glass bead	Glass beads at 190–300°C	Small metal items
	▶▶ Autoclave	Steam at 121–134°C	Metal and glass items
Disinfectant	▶▶ Alcohol	Does not kill micro-organisms, only reduces numbers	Sanitation only of metal and glass items
	▶▶ Quarternary ammonium		
UV radiation	▶▶ Cabinet	Method of sanitation only	Storage of sterile items such as brushes, sponges

1 Describe the main functions of the skin.

2 Explain how the skin helps to maintain body temperature.

3 What is the acid mantle?

4 Name and describe the layers of the epidermis.

5 Describe the skin's response to injury.

6 How does ageing effect the skin?

7 Describe the cycle of hair growth.

8 What external and internal factors affect the growth of hair and nails?

9 Name and describe the structures of the nail.

10 Describe the structure of a hair in its follicle.

11 Describe five non-infectious skin conditions.

12 Describe the seven point check list which is applied to moles.

13 Name and describe three viral, three bacterial and three fungal infections of the skin.

14 Describe three disorders of the hair with suggested causes.

15 Name and describe three treatable nail disorders and three which contra-indicate treatment.

16 Name three different types of bacteria.

17 How does the structure of a virus determine the type of disorder it may cause?

18 Describe the optimum conditions for the growth of micro-organisms.

19 Explain the importance of salon health and hygiene.

20 Describe additional hygiene procedures to ensure personal safety.

Organisational practices and procedures

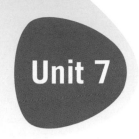

Unit 7

The success or failure of a business in many instances can be traced back to the management and organisational structure and procedures. Too often the salon owner has been too busy working *in* the business rather than *on* the business. Many salons have closed because their owners did not understand the importance and management of cash flow, or the necessity to produce accurate accounts for the Inland Revenue and records for Customs and Excise with regard to the quarterly VAT return.

This unit introduces you to the skills and knowledge you will require in order to set up and maintain key financial records, including PAYE, VAT, annual accounts and managing cash flow, both manually and with the aid of IT systems. You will be introduced to the merits of stock control, handling procedures and storage.

You will learn how IT systems can be utilised in the most efficient manner for financial records, appointment systems, keeping track of treatments and sales within the salon, stock control and recruitment.

You will also learn the steps to follow when recruiting the right employee for the needs of the organisation. These steps will cover recruitment procedures, interview techniques and induction procedures.

In order to achieve Unit 7 in Organisation practices and procedures you must complete the following learning outcomes:

LEARNING OUTCOMES

   1 Know and understand the financial records required to run a business.

   2 Describe and set up a stock control system.

      Have knowledge of COSHH regulations, storage of materials and safe practice.

   3 Evaluate the role of IT systems in the salon.

      Describe the different IT applications in the salon.

   4 Know the principles and procedures for recruitment and selection of staff.

Financial records and procedures

There are a number of financial records that must be kept in order to meet legal requirements. These include VAT, annual accounts and PAYE when employing staff.

VAT

VAT (Value Added Tax) is a tax on sales of goods and services. Virtually all the purchases made by the business will be subject to the addition of VAT. All sales and treatments made by the business will also be subject to VAT, and you must be familiar with the three rates in order to meet your obligations.

The three rates of VAT are:

- ▸ the standard rate of 17.5%
- ▸ the reduced rate of 5%, e.g. for water rates, electricity and gas (full details can be obtained from the Customs and Excise website: www.hmce.gov.uk)
- ▸ zero rated, e.g. for books and brochures, food, children's clothing (full details will be listed on the Customs and Excise website).

Certain services, such as banking, medical services, insurance and education, are exempt from VAT.

You must register your business with Customs and Excise for VAT when your turnover of supplied taxable sales and services exceeds £56,000 in the previous 12-month period, or if you anticipate reaching £56,000 in the next 30 days. To register you must contact the local VAT office; the contact number can be found in the telephone directory or by logging onto the Customs and Excise website.

When Customs and Excise have processed the registration you will be issued with a VAT registration number, which should be entered on all your invoices and stationery. You will also be assigned a 'tax period' and Customs and Excise will automatically send you a VAT return to coincide with this period. Businesses usually **account for VAT on a quarterly basis**.

You must keep accurate records giving full details of all invoices and cash receipts showing the net cost of purchases plus the VAT (input tax). You must also record all sales, such as retail products and treatments, keeping an accurate record of the net charge for the treatment plus the element for VAT (output tax).

VAT Returns and payments

The registered business must make a quarterly return to the Customs and Excise showing the amount of input tax on purchases and output tax on sales. You may submit your return and your payment by post or electronically via the Customs and Excise website. (You must still post your return form when you pay electronically.)

Your completed VAT return, together with the payment, is due one month after the end of your tax period. In other words, if your VAT quarter ends on 30 September, your payment and return should be received by Customs and Excise no later than 30 October. You will then need to adapt your daily accounting system to record all sales and purchases together with the relevant VAT.

The quarterly return should show the number of purchases and VAT paid out, and the number of sales together with the VAT received. The VAT paid by the business on purchases is deducted from the VAT received on sales. Where the Business receives more VAT than it has paid out, the difference must be paid to Customs and Excise.

As you will see from the example below, the business will pay VAT on purchases and charge VAT on its sales: the business will deduct the VAT paid on the purchase, e.g. £1.40 from the VAT received on the sale, e.g. £5.25. The business would then pay the difference of £3.85 to Customs and Excise.

PURCHASES (input tax)		SALES (output tax)	
Products for professional use	£5.00	Facial basic cost	£30.00
Tissues	£2.00		
Spatulas	£1.00		
	——		
Net cost:	£8.00		——
Add VAT @ 17.5%:	£1.40	Add VAT @ 17.5%:	£5.25
Cost to business:	£9.40	Cost to client:	£35.25

Flat rate scheme for small businesses

The flat rate scheme was introduced by the government in 2003 in order to offer small businesses, whose annual taxable turnover does not exceed £150,000, an alternative to the normal transaction basis of VAT accounting. The aim of the scheme is to simplify the way small businesses account for VAT so that they can save both time and money. In this system it is not necessary for you to record each and every transaction. Providing your business is eligible you will be able to calculate your VAT payment as a percentage of your total annual turnover. Full details of this scheme can be obtained from your local VAT office or the Customs and Excise website.

Fact file

Remember you will be penalised with a fine if you make a late VAT return either by forgetting to send the form or by sending payment late.

PAYE

Any business that employs staff must register as an employer with the local tax office. The tax office will issue the business with a reference number and send an Employers' Pack. This pack will contain the tables for tax deductions and National Insurance Contributions plus a CD with a set of forms. The tax year runs from 6 April to 5 April of the following year.

Employers are required to deduct tax and National Insurance contributions from their employees' earnings. These deductions, together with the employer's National Insurance contribution, should be paid over to the Inland Revenue through a PAYE payroll system.

What do you need to operate a PAYE payroll?

- Employer's tax reference.
- National Insurance and tax deduction tables.
- A National Insurance number for each employee.
- Employee's National Insurance number and tax code.
- P11 Deductions Working Sheet.
- Form P32: Employer's payment record.
- Employee's pay slip.

- P14: End of year summary for each employee.
- P35: Employer's annual return.

Operating the payroll

1 You will need to complete a P11 Deductions Working Sheet for each employee recording the following information: name; National Insurance number; tax and salary to date. This form must be updated every time the employee is paid.

New employees should hand a P45 form to their new employer. This will show a record of the employee's tax code, salary paid and tax deducted by his or her previous employer.

New employees who do *not* have a P45 should complete the form P46. This form will then be sent to the Inland Revenue who in turn will issue a Tax Code for the employee.

2 A payslip should be given to the employee on each pay day. This should include the following information:

- Gross salary, which is made up of basic pay, overtime, commission, and benefits such as medical insurance or company car; fixed deductions, i.e. tax and National Insurance Contributions.

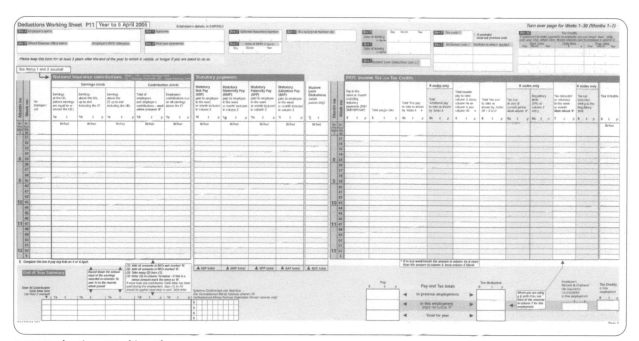

A P11 Deductions Working Sheet.

- Other deductions, i.e. those made to enforce a court order, e.g. child support (this is known as an 'attachment of earnings'); repayment of a student loan; or voluntary deductions such as a private pension scheme or stake holder pension, and private or medical insurance.
- Salary, tax deducted and National Insurance Contributions (NIC) paid in current tax year.
- Maternity pay, statutory sick pay.
- Net salary.

3 **Form P32: Employer's payment record**
   This form enables you to keep a detailed record of the total payments that you make to the Inland Revenue for each pay period, together with the date that the payment was made. The information kept on this sheet will help you to complete you employer's annual return accurately.

4 **Form P14: End of year summary**
   A P14 should be completed for each of your employees, listing all payments made to them and deductions from their salary during the year. The last page of the form is the **P60** Employee's certificate of PAYE, tax and National Insurance contributions.

5 **Form P35: Employer's annual return**
   The P35 shows the total Pay As You Earn (PAYE) deductions for all employees during the year. (Both the P14 and the P35 can be filed through the online PAYE services on the Inland Revenue website.)

Who is covered by PAYE and NIC?

- All employees whose earnings are above the PAYE threshold.
- Employees over the age of 16 years on all earnings over the NIC threshold.
- Employees over 65 years will be subject to PAYE but not NIC, providing they produce a certificate of age exemption.
- Casual and part-time workers – unless they work for you for less than one week in a pay period and less than the threshold amount during that time. You will be required to keep a record of payments you have made.
- Students – unless their earnings for the whole tax year will be less than the personal allowance, in which case they should complete Form P39(S).

Self-employed workers and sub-contractors

Self-employed workers and those sent a tax return by the Inland Revenue are required to fill in a self-assessment form listing all taxable income and gains received during the year and claiming any allowances.

Providing the form is returned to the tax office by 30 September following the end of the tax year on 5 April, the Inland Revenue will calculate the tax due. Individuals who wish to work out their own tax bill have until 31 January of the following year to submit their form. Fines or penalties will be imposed when forms are submitted after the deadline.

Income subject to tax deductions

This will include:

- basic pay
- commission and benefits
- statutory sick pay
- maternity pay
- statutory adoption pay.

Student Loans, Working Tax Credits and Statutory Sick Pay are also processed through the payroll. More information on these procedures can be obtained through the Inland Revenue website.

Payments to Inland Revenue

PAYE payments to the tax office should be correct and paid on time, which is within 14 days of each tax month or tax quarter.

Businesses whose combined National Insurance contributions and PAYE payments for all employees average more than £1,500 must make payments at the end of each tax month. Businesses with an average total of less than £1,500 may make payments once every three months.

The Inland Revenue will accept payment by one of a number of methods:

- BACS and CHAPS – direct electronic transfer
- cheque by post
- cheque or cash at a post office
- debit card over the Internet
- bank giro at your local branch office.

You will also need to complete a Payslip P30B (PDF). This form can be downloaded from the Inland Revenue website.

Annual Accounts

At the end of each trading year you will need to prepare a set of business trading accounts which will be used to determine the tax due to the Inland Revenue.

The way that tax is calculated will depend on the type of business, i.e. sole trader, partnership, limited company or public company. A set of accounts will consist of the following sheets:

1 Balance sheet

2 Profit and loss account

3 The budget (cash flow statement).

Balance sheet

The balance sheet provides the information concerning the assets and liabilities of the business at a particular point in time. Balance sheets are normally produced at the end of an accounting period. The balance sheet gives details of the assets that the business owns, i.e. equipment, money in the bank and the liabilities or the money that the business owes.

The balance sheet must always balance – in other words, the debits should equal the credits.

BALANCE SHEET AS AT 31 AUGUST 1999

	1999 £	1999 £	1998 £	1998 £
FIXED ASSETS		15,307		15,556
CURRENT ASSETS				
Stock	2,539		6,414	
Trade Debtors	-		180	
Sundry Debtors and Prepayments	708		-	
Cash at Bank and Building Society	13,154		-	
Cash in Hand	904		939	
	17,305		7,533	
CURRENT LIABILITIES				
Cash at Bank and Building Society	-		3,812	
Trade Creditors	3,641		11,584	
Sundry Creditors and Accruals	6,154		1,900	
Hire Purchase Creditors	2,795		2,681	
Bank Loan Account	10,095		-	
Loan Account 1	2,939		2,939	
P.A.Y.E and N.I.C.	1,296		3,142	
Value Added Tax	3,008		2,342	
	29,928		28,400	
NET CURRENT LIABILITIES		12,623		20,867
		£ 2,684		£ (5,311)
REPRESENTED BY:				
CAPITAL ACCOUNT				
Opening Capital		-		6,915
Net Profit for Year		26,625		237
		26,625		7,152
Opening Capital	5,311		-	
Drawings	18,630		12,463	
		23,941		12,463
		£ 2,684		£ (5,311)
Approved ————————				

A balance sheet.

Profit and loss

The profit and loss gives a clearly stated summary of the trading actions during the accounting year. It shows the financial health of the business and whether it is trading at a profit or a loss.

TRADING AND PROFIT AND LOSS ACCOUNT FOR THE YEAR ENDED 31 AUGUST 1999

	1999 £	1999 £	1998 £	1998 £
Sales		111,856		82,211
COST OF SALES				
Opening Stock	6,414		9,525	
Purchases	14,583		6,570	
Closing Stock	(2,539)		(6,414)	
		18,458		9,681
GROSS PROFIT		93,398		72,530
Sundry Income		3,330		934
Royalties Received		2,307		282
Rent Income		18,892		2,773
		117,927		76,519
LESS OVERHEADS				
Salaries and National Insurance	36,453		36,774	
Motor and Travelling	2,641		1,324	
Telephone Charges	796		719	
Printing, Stationery and Advertising	7,361		2,748	
Equipment Lease	6,659		1,753	
Sundry Expenses	2,432		1,290	
Heating and Lighting	867		1,646	
Repairs	1,217		500	
Cleaning	270		303	
Rent, Rates and Insurance	20,784		20,028	
Subscriptions	356		170	
Loan Interest	413		-	
Hire Purchase Interest	518		240	
Bank Commission and Interest	3,934		2,168	
Professional Fees	2,801		1,681	
Accountancy Charges	1,850		1,850	
Bad Debts	-		120	
Depreciation-Vehicles	396		528	
Depreciation-Improvements to Leasehold	4,996		1,393	
Depreciation-Fixtures and Equipment	1,194		1,047	
Profit/Loss on Sale of Assets	(4,836)		-	
		91,302		76,282
NET PROFIT FOR THE YEAR		£ 26,625		£ 237

A profit and loss account.

This information is obtained by deducting the expenses of the business from the income. The remaining sum will be the profit or loss.

Cash flow statement

It is vital to the health of any business that a sharp eye is kept on the movement of cash into and out of the business at any given time. For the business to trade at a profit it is necessary that more income (cash) is received than is spent.

The cash required to finance the business on a daily basis is known as working capital. This is used to purchase stock, such as retail products and consumables used during treatments, as well as to pay wages, telephone, rent, rates and VAT. When expenditure exceeds the monies received (income) the situation must be addressed immediately to determine the cause and rectify the problem. The situation may be resolved on a short-term basis by means of a cash injection provided by the proprietor, an overdraft or loan. However, the root cause of the shortage must be examined and a solution found.

Factors which affect cash flow could include:

- customers not paying for treatments or goods that they have received
- keeping too much stock on the premises

- treatments that have not been correctly priced to include an element for profit
- lack of staff due to illness or holidays
- spending more than the business can afford, i.e. expenditure is greater than income
- taking on a loan or overdraft facility that the business is not able to maintain.

Organisation requirements

The business will need to set up and maintain accurate financial records in order to be able to complete accurate VAT returns and annual accounts for the Inland Revenue.

Day books

These should be completed on a daily basis. The following information should be included:

- details of payments received from treatments, sales and other income
- method of payments, e.g. cheque, credit/debit payments or cash
- payments from petty cash for sundries, petrol, postage, stationery, etc.
- amount paid into bank and cash in hand/float or petty cash net of VAT
- VAT element.

Purchase Invoices File

Purchase invoices are issued by the supplier as a request for payment. Invoices will give details of:

the products/goods/services supplied; the cost net of VAT; the amount of VAT; the name and address and contact number of the supplier; the supplier's VAT registration number; the customer's name, address, account number, terms and due date for payment.

Purchase invoices should be filed in order and paid by the due date. For reference purposes it is helpful to record the date the invoice was received and the due date for payment. Enter the method of payment onto the invoice, e.g. cheque and cheque number, or when paying online enter the date and method of payment and the account from which the payment has been made.

Company credit card statements

A detailed record should be kept of all credit card payments made in connection with the business. Payments made for personal purchases should be identified by highlighting the relevant transaction on the monthly statement. Keep itemised receipts with the relevant credit card payment slips and file with the monthly statement for easier identification.

Cash receipt file

Cash receipts are given when a purchase is made for goods or services but an invoice is not issued, e.g. purchase of petrol, where the money is handed over at the time of purchase. A detailed record of cash purchases should be kept together with the reason

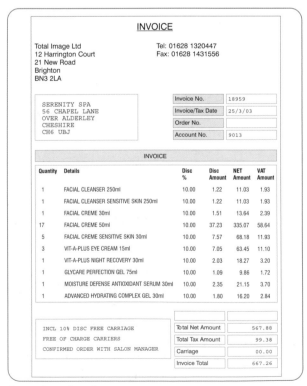

A purchase invoice.

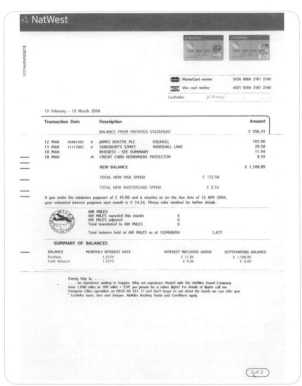

A credit card statement.

for the purchase, e.g. milk, stationery, postage, petrol, etc.

These receipts should also be filed in order and dated. It is often easier to keep the cash receipts with the day sheets, particularly if the money has been taken out of the till or from petty cash.

Bank statements

Your bank will send you a statement on a regular basis (usually monthly) showing all transactions that have occurred. These will include cheques that have been presented, direct debits, standing order payments, online payments, bank charges (and interest if applicable) as well as deposits into the account.

When your bank statement arrives you should reconcile it with your accounts. For this you will need your cheque book, paying-in book, purchase invoice file and record of all online transactions.

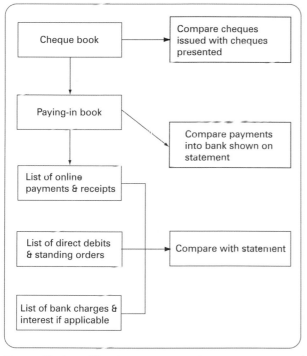

Reconciliation of bank statement and accounts.

The reconciliation is the process of agreeing account entries between the statement and the accounts. In the event that errors have been made by the bank you should notify your manager immediately.

Sales receipts

A number of clients may request a receipt when making payment. This should include the name and address of the business, their contact number, the VAT registration number, the amount received from the client and what the payment was for, e.g. products or treatment. The method of payment could also be included on the receipt, e.g. cash, credit card, cheque, etc.

Costing of treatments

One of the major mistakes made by small salon owners is that not enough thought is put into the costing of treatments. Too often a salon owner just under-cuts the competition without giving sufficient thought to the true cost of the treatment or making allowance for the profit margin that is essential to a healthy business.

▶ **Practice point:** Before finalising your treatment costs you must remember to include a margin for profit.

The following costs need to be considered when setting treatment fees:

▶▶ cost of materials
▶▶ cost of equipment (leasing, rental or depreciation element)
▶▶ cost of overheads (rent, rates, heating, lighting, etc.)
▶▶ therapist's salary
▶▶ advertising and promotional costs
▶▶ unique selling point
▶▶ demand
▶▶ time allocated for treatment room
▶▶ profit margin.

Theory into practice

List the costs that should be taken into consideration when setting the price list. Recommend a price for a full leg wax, taking the profit element into consideration. Give evidence of how you arrived at your decision.

Monitoring

Treatment fees and costs need to be monitored on a regular basis in order to retain the profit margin. Treatment fees should be revised on an annual basis. Before setting revised fees you will need to look at any changes that have occurred in the costs, e.g. suppliers of consumables increasing their prices, increases in business rates or salaries – in fact, all the elements that are taken into consideration as shown in the costing of treatments overleaf.

There are several areas that you will need to monitor in order to stay one step ahead of your competitors, as shown overleaf.

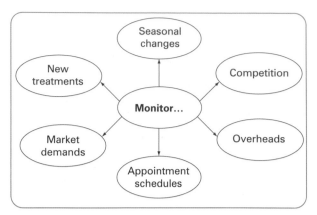

Monitoring these areas is essential to stay ahead of the competition.

Keep up to date with market trends by reading professional publications and attending trade conferences and exhibitions. It is important to be one step ahead of the competition without putting strain on the cash flow when introducing new treatments.

Look at the booking trends and analyse when the salon is quieter and when the busy times are; perhaps you could consider special promotions and offers which may only be booked during the quieter periods.

It is wise to keep an eye on your competitors and their pricing schedule, but beware of undercutting prices. Clients are often happy to pay a little more for the same treatment if: the standards are higher; the client feels that you genuinely have his or her welfare at heart; the surroundings are more relaxing.

In other words, you must have 'that something extra' compared to your competitors.

Budgeting

Every successful business has a business plan and budget that should be updated regularly. The minimum this should be done is annually, but you could update it more frequently if the need arises, e.g. when introducing a new treatment or new equipment, or if the cash flow is under pressure.

The budget or cash flow forecast takes a little time to prepare but is well worth the effort. You will need to take an educated guess as to the level of income that will be achieved from sales and treatments. You then need to list your running costs including fixed costs (those that have to be paid whether your premises are open or closed), e.g. rent and rates, followed by variable costs such as salaries, VAT element, heating, lighting, telephone, stationery, leasing/hire purchase cost, etc.

Work out what your overheads and costs are and when they are due for payment, e.g. telephone and rent are usually paid quarterly, whereas rates are often spread over 10 months; consumables may be paid as cash on delivery but some suppliers may allow 30 days for payment from the date of the invoice.

The example overleaf shows a basic cash flow forecast for six months trading (25 per cent of the trading year). The figures illustrated are fictitious but are intended to give you an idea of the information that should be included. The figures shown are not exhaustive.

The aim of the cash flow forecast is to list all your anticipated income as shown overleaf; you then need to list as accurately as possible all your expenditure – in other words every payment that you have to make in connection with the business. Hopefully your income will exceed your outgoings, which is essential if you are going to trade profitably.

Cash Flow forecast   Six month period

Income (List all sources of income)	January	February	March	April	May	June	Total
Treatments	11,500	11,000	12,500	13,000	14,500	15,000	77,500
Sales	1,900	1,500	2,350	2,600	2,800	3,000	14,150
Net VAT	13,400	12,500	14,850	15,600	17,300	18,000	91,650

Expenditure (list all items of expenditure you v which will include the some or all of the following)							
Salaries	2,680	2,500	3,000	3,200	3,460	3,600	18,440
Stock	1,340	1	1,250	1,560	17,300	1,800	23,251
Rent	2,500			2,500			5,000
Rates	295	295	295	295	295	295	1,770
Telephone	185			185			370
Advertising	500	500	500	500	500	500	3,000
Heat/light	95	95	95	95	95	95	570
							52,401

	Sales	91,650
minus	**Expenditure**	52,401
		39.249

Cash flow forecast.

Cash transaction procedures

Cash

There are a few clients who prefer to pay by cash. When taking cash, enter the amount onto the day sheet by the client's name, and although it is not essential it is often advisable to issue a receipt. The cash is then accounted for at the end of the trading day and paid into the bank.

Cheque payments

A number of clients prefer to pay by cheque. To process a cheque payment you should make sure that certain information is included on the cheque:

Fact file

> **Remember:**
> For your daily cash to balance you should deduct any cash payments made from the till from cash received.

- date in full
- figures and written amount match
- client's signature
- the name of the organisation to be paid
- cheque card guarantee number.

Credit and debit cards

Credit and debit cards are now the most popular method for payment. The card is swiped through the machine or inserted into the chip reader, and you enter the amount and follow the instructions on the screen. You then hand the top and bottom slip to the client for signing, making sure to check the signature against the signature on the card. Hand one copy to the client and the other copy should be placed in the till.

Organisational requirements

You will need to open an account with a bank. Before choosing which one, do your research and visit a number of banks. Arrange a meeting with the manager to discuss the facilities the bank will provide and the business terms, e.g. bank charges for handling cash, cheques, debits, standing orders and returned cheques, etc. In addition, discuss the interest rate on overdraft or loan facilities if applicable. Remember to take your business plan and budget with you.

You will need a paying in book to allow you to deposit cheques and cash received by the business as well as a cheque book. The type of account you open will depend on the needs of the business.

You could open a current account with a cheque book (many banks now pay a small amount of interest when the account is in credit) and this is the most popular account with smaller businesses.

You may require an overdraft facility. This will allow you to draw funds or issue cheques when you do not have the money in your account. The size of the facility will be agreed with the bank and you will be charged interest on the amount that the account is overdrawn. The facility is set for a period of time, after which the needs of the business will be reviewed with the manager. The balance of the overdraft will alter as funds are paid in and out of the account.

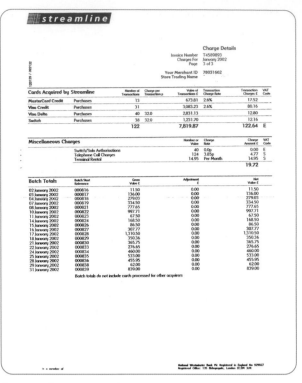

A streamline statement.

The business may require a loan for a specific purpose, e.g. to fund the purchase of new equipment or new premises, etc. A loan is a set amount that is agreed with the bank. It will be taken out for a set term, such as three or five years, and you may be required to provide some form of security. Repayments are normally paid monthly, which will be part payment of the original loan and part interest. A loan will incur interest at a set rate agreed in advance. When taking out a loan it is advisable to ensure that you will not be charged a penalty for early settlement of the loan. Payment protection insurance should also be considered in the event of your not being able to make repayments due to sickness.

Credit card payment facilities

The majority of clients pay for their treatments and products with credit cards or debit cards. You will find that it is a simple procedure to install this facility; to do so, you need to contact a bank such as Natwest Streamline, Lloyds Cardnet or Barclaycard. Discuss their terms and choose the one most suited to your business needs.

You will be provided with a machine that you connect to a telephone line. You are provided with a retailer's merchant number and payments go directly into your bank. You will be sent a monthly statement by the bank that supplies the facility detailing the payments that have been made (the total number of payments, the invoice for the rental charge and the bank's charge for processing the payments. The fees due to the provider will be taken from your current account by direct debit.

Safety and security

Security must be taken seriously when there are large amounts of cash on the premises. With regards to general security it is advisable to have an alarm system installed, preferably one that is connected to the police through the alarm company's system. Doors and windows must be securely locked when the premises are empty. In one salon a fire was started by vandals because a small window was left open overnight. The vandals had pushed lighted paper into the building through the open window, resulting in damage to the building and disruption to the business. Trading was affected and there was a subsequent loss of income whilst the building was out of use.

Clients generally pay by cheque or credit card. However, there are still some people who prefer to pay by cash. Extra care should be taken to keep cash as secure as possible.

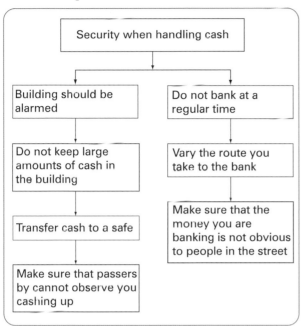

Security when handling cash.

Financial records should be kept in a locked fireproof metal filing cabinet, so that in the event of a fire valuable records are not lost.

Data that is stored on computer should be backed up daily. Two sets of back-up discs should be kept and it is advisable to keep one set in a different location. When backing up onto floppy disc the back-up discs should be renewed approximately every three months to reduce the risk of disc corruption.

Credit

Credit can refer to money due to a company or person for payment of goods or services received, or the time given for payment, e.g. 30 days from date of invoice. It may refer to a person's ability to pay, for example, a company will agree credit terms when opening a new account for a business, and individual and credit card companies set a credit limit when issuing cards.

A *creditor* is a person or company to whom the debt is owed.

A *credit note* may be issued when goods are returned to the retailer or supplier. The note will usually be to the value of the original cost of the goods and allows purchases to be made at a later date to the same value.

Refunds

A refund refers to the return of monies received for goods or services, e.g. if a client returns a product to the salon because it was faulty or the client experienced an allergic reaction and you therefore return or repay the original payment.

When the purchase has been made with a credit card, the refund should be made to the credit card. This is because the salon will have been charged a percentage of the original purchase payment by the bank that the business has the service contract with, such as Streamline, Barclaycard or Cardnet.

IT systems

Computers have made a powerful impact on businesses. The computer has become an essential tool in the battle to run a profitable and efficient salon and stay ahead of competitors. But before buying your first computer you need to decide what you will be using it for.

Do you want to keep your financial records electronically? (In the near future the Inland Revenue will require you to make your employer's annual return electronically.) Do you want to electronically analyse treatment trends, generate cash flow reports, produce mail-shots, book appointments, and keep track of stock, employees' attendance and treatment/sales records, etc.? Or perhaps you would find the online banking facility helpful? Your requirements will have an influence on the computer system you choose and the software that will be installed.

A computer and software package that has been chosen with your needs in mind can save you many hours of work by generating valuable information that takes much longer to produce by hand. The information can also be cross-linked to give a wider picture of the financial health of the business. Remember that whichever system or package you choose, you should not overlook the importance of IT training. Training courses are available from LearnDirect, technical colleges, IT training systems and the software supplier.

Financial software

Proprietary system

There are several software packages that are specifically designed for keeping accounts; these include Sage, Pegasus and Quicken. The complexity of the package you choose should depend on the size of your business, ranging from the sole trader through to large corporate companies. Some packages, such as Sage, will permit you to keep details of more than one company/business. When making a decision on which package to use, ask about the possibility of upgrading to a more comprehensive package as your company grows.

Operating the payroll electronically is a real timesaver. The time taken to input the initial information such as employees' details, names, addresses, National Insurance numbers, tax codes, basic salaries and commission structure is balanced by the speed with which you can generate the payroll at the end of the month. The system will keep a record of your National Insurance payments and PAYE, and generate the end of year returns. The software company will keep you up to date with the changes that occur with tax codes, PAYE and NIC tables. (Changes are dictated by the government of the day.)

Bespoke systems

You may decide that you would prefer to have a system custom built to match the specific needs of your business. There are a number of companies that provide salon management systems for hairdressing and beauty salons. The most well known include:

- Precision Business Software
- Premier Spa
- Chase Business Systems.

Contact numbers and website addresses are easily located in professional publications such as *Health and Beauty Salon*, *Guild News* and *Professional Beauty*. Beauty exhibitions are also a good place to look, ask questions and compare the pros and cons of different suppliers.

Fact file

Remember:
Do your research carefully before making your final decision on your choice of computer system and software.

Before deciding which company you are going to use, you need to determine the following points:

- Can the programme be integrated with other packages such as Microsoft® Word?
- Will the system live up to the claims made by the company?
- What training is provided and will it meet the salon needs? If additional training is required will there be a further charge and, if so, how much will it be?

- Are technical support and a help line provided? What is the cost of this service?
- Is the supplier willing to adapt the programme to meet your salon's specific needs?
- Will the supplier keep you up to date regarding upgrades?

Database/spreadsheets

A database is an organised set of information or data. It consists of the data and the tools needed for gaining access to the information. You can set up a very simple database consisting of your clients' names, addresses and contact numbers; or you can be more adventurous and set up a more complex database whereby you can enter the treatments your client has received, the retail products he or she has purchased, and the marketing information you have sent, etc. You might prefer to take the easier option and purchase a software package which has been specially written for use in beauty salons, such as Precision Business Solutions and Premier Spa.

An **electronic spreadsheet** such as Microsoft Excel® is used to organise, analyse and calculate data. You can use a spreadsheet for many purposes such as producing invoices, budget/cash flow forecasts, analysing salon takings, treatment trends and therapists' takings, or producing accounts, monthly, quarterly and annually.

Inventories

An inventory is a detailed list such as a comprehensive record of equipment, stock, stationery, etc. This should be updated regularly with a full inventory being taken at the end of your financial year.

Data protection

It is a legal requirement for the user to register with the Data Protection Registrar when records containing personal information relating to clients are kept on a computer. Only information of a professional nature should be recorded, together with appointments. Data must not be kept for longer than is necessary and should be updated regularly to ensure that the information held is accurate.

The law applies to all businesses and records held, no matter how small the business is. There are some exceptions to this rule, but failure to register is a criminal offence and can result in a fine of several thousand pounds.

Assessment task 7.2

Based on Assessment task 7.1, analyse the effects of correctly maintained records on the profitability of your business. With the aid of a spreadsheet, state the potential problems and discuss suitable solutions. (D)

Network systems

Management information systems

Larger businesses that own more than one salon, e.g. Regis, SAKS or a leisure group such as David Lloyd, need to be able to monitor as well as keep in touch with each establishment. The most efficient way of doing this is to set up a computer link to the head office.

Alternatively, computers can be linked together with a piece of software called PC Anywhere. This enables head office to download information from individual establishments. This information could be salon takings, stock movements, staffing levels, staff performance, new client's attendance and conversion to regular clients, the amount each client spends, frequency of visits, etc.

The information system enables you to gain the facts and figures that you need to manage the salon. You will be able to gather and analyse information such as treatment trends, sales trends, staff performance and attendance, cash flow, etc. This is a great help when you are updating your business plan and budget.

Internet

The Internet is a system that allows you to communicate with other computers worldwide. To connect to the Internet you need to register with a service provider such as AOL (America on Line) Microsoft Network (MSN), Virgin Net or Wanado.

The Internet allows you to: send mail electronically by email; access websites; transfer documents and files; and obtain files from electronic libraries.

Online banking

This facility enables you to access your bank account directly from your computer. The advantage of this is that you can: keep track of the account on a daily basis; pay invoices, standing orders and direct debits; and see the balance without having to telephone or go into the bank. To use this service you must register with the bank's online banking service. You will then be issued with an access code to which you add your own password.

Website

The addition of a website is becoming an excellent way to promote your business – the services you offer and the retail products you stock. To get the best results from a website it needs to be simple, eye catching and easy to read. You can have as few or many pages as you wish. There are many companies that specialise in website design. The fees for this vary but some help towards costs may be available through your local Business Link. A good website should be updated regularly – one way of doing this is to include regular salon newsletters, promotions and special offers.

Email

Electronic mail (email) can be a real asset, giving you the opportunity to send letters, correspondence, files and photographs/pictures quickly – provided that the recipient is also on email. However, there is every probability that you will receive a number of unsolicited emails from companies trying to sell you their services or goods. Unless you know the company you would be wise to delete these emails without opening them since viruses can be introduced onto computers via unsolicited emails.

To receive email, you will need an email address, which acts in a similar way to your postal address when you receive mail.

World Wide Web (www)

The Web is a software system running on the Internet which allows you to gain information. Via the Web you can gain access to electronic libraries for research purposes, access competitors' websites to keep abreast of their progress, research new treatments and products, or use it to shop online, e.g. Amazon is excellent for books or booking holidays.

Stock control and material handling

Stock control procedures

Stock rotation

You will need to rotate stock to ensure that it does not stay on the shelf or in the stock room until the quality of the product deteriorates or it reaches its expiry date. The most effective way of achieving this is to place new stock at the back of the shelf or storage area and bring the older stock to the front – in other words: first in, first out. This will ensure that the older stock is used before the new stock.

Stock levels

An efficient and profitable business needs to keep stock at a level that meets the needs of the business. When too much stock is kept on the premises (stock pile) valuable cash is tied up, thereby affecting cash flow. Conversely, a lack of retail products may mean that sales are lost and there is a loss of income for the business. When insufficient professional stock is kept it may not be possible to carry out the treatments to achieve the best result for the client. Monitoring stock levels carefully and efficiently therefore contributes to the health of your business. It is helpful to set a minimum and maximum stock level for each product that you use. This can be altered as demands dictate.

Stock orders

The most efficient method of maintaining stock levels is to order regularly and only what you need. Do not be tempted by special offers for retail unless you can be certain that you will be able to sell the items you have ordered. It is very easy to get carried away when it comes to buying Christmas stock and gift packs!

When placing an order you should refer to your minimum/maximum stock levels. Take a stock check to see what you need. Make a list of the order, the items you require, the product reference numbers and the wholesale cost. You should remember to record the date the order was placed, and the name and contact details of the supplier. Always include your own contact details and order reference.

There are a number ways in which you can generate an order, so choose the method that works best for you. The most efficient way of placing orders is by fax or email, but orders can also be placed by telephone. When ordering by telephone read the order clearly and slowly, then have the order read back to you to minimise the possibility of errors occurring. Orders can also be placed directly by post or with the company's sales representative when she or he visits the salon.

Fact file

Remember:
An efficient stock control system can result in retail products being sold before you are required to pay the invoice. This in turn helps your cash flow.

Stock records

Maintaining accurate stock records is a major contribution to the financial health and wellbeing of your business. It is helpful when producing the annual budget because you will be able to see the seasonal changes in certain areas, such as increased purchases of sun protection products and depilatory wax in the summer or Christmas gift lines during November and December.

Stock records are not difficult to produce, either manually or by computer. The information that you will need to record is:

▸ the supplier's name and address
▸ the product name and reference number
▸ the date of the opening order
▸ the minimum and maximum levels for each product
▸ the level of stock received in the opening order
▸ the date of stock checks and the level of stock on the premises
▸ the amount of stock that needs to be ordered to maintain stock levels.

Using a spreadsheet, design a simple stock control system. Evaluate the role of the stock control system in the salon.

Databases/spreadsheets

As we have seen, a database is an organised set of information or data. You can set up a very simple database for stock control, recording details of retail products, salon products, stock codes and prices, etc. You could also purchase a software package which has been specially written for use in beauty salons.

An electronic spreadsheet such as Microsoft® Excel is used to organise, analyse and calculate data. You can use a spreadsheet to keep track of the turnover of each product and to analyse the trends with a specific product or a complete range.

Handling procedures

Delivery

When your order is delivered to your salon you will be asked to sign a form to state that you have received the delivery in good condition. It is advisable to delete the words 'in good condition' and replace with 'not inspected'. A delivery note, listing the contents, should be enclosed with the order. Whenever possible ask for the delivery to be taken directly to the area where it will be unpacked.

The order should be opened and processed as soon as possible. Check the items against the delivery note as each item is unpacked. Price each item and put it onto the shelf or into the stock cupboard, making sure that new stock is placed behind the old stock.

Once the order has been unpacked and put away, compare the items on the delivery note against the original order. Details of the delivery should then be entered onto the stock records. Notify the supplier of any discrepancies in the order immediately.

Professional products are delivered in salon sizes that are normally larger than the retail size. It is good practice to decant this into smaller bottles and jars, which must be clearly and correctly labelled, and place in the treatment rooms. This helps to reduce waste and deterioration in the quality of the product.

Manual handling

The Manual Handling Operations Act 1992 comes under the umbrella of the Health and Safety at Work etc. Act 1974.

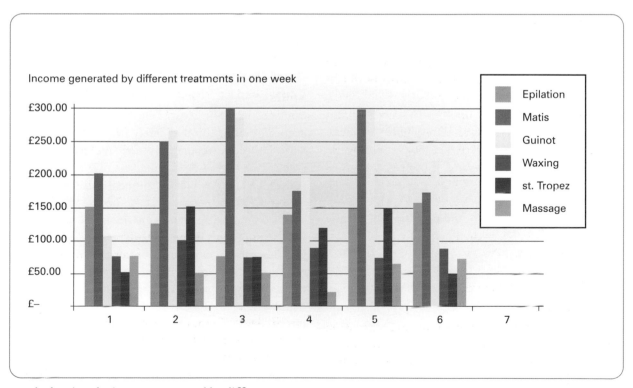

Graph showing the income generated by different treatments.

The purpose of the Act is to regulate the moving and lifting of heavy equipment or loads to ensure the health and safety of the individual carrying out the procedure. This Act implements a European Directive on the manual handling of loads, to prevent injuries such as sprains, strains, back injuries or cumulative damage which causes incapacity.

Orders of stock should be delivered to the area where they are to be unpacked. When a box or container is to be lifted from the floor onto a higher surface, then the correct lifting procedure (as illustrated on page 126) should be followed in order to reduce the risk of injury.

Large equipment should not be moved unnecessarily. Whenever possible, machinery or equipment should be moved on a trolley. Before moving or lifting a load, make sure that all obstacles have been removed and that all cables have been unplugged and tidied out of the way.

When removing an object from a shelf that is above shoulder level, care must be taken to avoid head injuries or a fall as a result of over-balancing.

Damaged goods/discrepancies

If there are any damaged items, you should make a note of these and record the damage against the delivery note. There are times when the delivered order does not match the order you placed. This could be due to the supplier being out of stock or an error on the part of the packer. You should contact the supplier immediately with details of the damage or discrepancies – certainly within 48 hours.

The supplier will normally replace damaged goods and may ask you to return the damaged items either by post or via their company representative. If it is not possible to replace the item you should receive a credit note for the item.

When an item is temporarily out of stock the supplier will often include a comment such as 'out of stock, item to follow' or 'out of stock, please re-order' on the delivery note.

> ## Assessment task 7.5
>
> Choose a suitable professional/retail skincare range. State the procedures to be followed from the initial order to the subsequent re-order. (M)

Deterioration

The business will lose money if stock is allowed to deteriorate or reach its expiry date. There are several ways to avoid deterioration or at least keep it to a minimum.

- Dummies should be used for window displays where strong sunlight over a period of time could cause the products to deteriorate.
- Stock should be stored in a cool dark stock room. Heat can result in the cosmetic ingredients separating, which will affect the consistency of the product since oils may become rancid. Sunlight will affect the colour of the product and the quality.
- Once products have reached their expiry date they begin to deteriorate. It is therefore advisable to reduce the price of products when they get close to the expiry date.
- Leaving tops off bottles and jars allows the air to get into the product. Some products will evaporate, others will change in consistency. A frequent cause of stock deterioration relating to nail polishes, base coats and top coats is a build-up of polish around the neck of the bottle. A few seconds taken to wipe round the top of bottles with cotton wool and enamel remover will prolong the shelf life considerably. Accumulated dry polish around bottle necks allows air to get into the polish which then thickens over a period of time. Thinning the polish out with nail polish remover affects the quality of the product (the polish will soon chip).

Spillage

Spillages must be cleared up immediately and also according to health and safety procedures, together with COSHH regulations and recommendations (see page 145–6). Spillages of a hazardous substance such as bleach, surgical spirit, warm wax or equipment cleaner must be dealt with as specified on the salon's risk assessment sheet.

When spillages occur on the floor and it would be possible for a person to slip or fall as a result, a chair or obstacle should be placed either over the area or immediately in front of it. A warning notice should be attached to the obstacle to prevent it being moved before the spillage has been attended to. The spillage should then be wiped up and the floor washed and dried thoroughly.

Where the spillage might have affected a client or member of staff, details should be recorded, e.g. the nature and substance concerned, the effect on the client – such as skin burn or wax on a client's clothing – and the action taken.

Disposal

Sharps (epilation needles, microlances, etc.) should be disposed of into the sharps bin immediately after use. When it is full, the sharps bin must be sealed and made ready for collection, after which it will be incinerated. There are different companies who will change sharps containers; these can be contacted through the Yellow Pages or your local environmental health office.

Each treatment room in the salon should contain a bin, lined with a plastic liner, for waste such as tissues, cotton wool, wax strips, spatulas and disposable gloves, etc. The bin should be emptied every day and the waste transferred to a waste bin kept outside the building. Arrangements should be made for external bins to be emptied on a regular basis; the local Environmental Health department will be able to give you advice on this.

Used or out-of-date chemicals must never be disposed of down the drain or placed where they can get into the wrong hands, e.g. be accessed by children. Refer to the manufacturer's safety data sheet or contact the manufacturer directly.

Fact file

> **Remember**:
> All salon waste must be disposed of safely and without causing damage to the environment or any individual. It is necessary for salons to comply with the Environmental Protection Act 1990.

Storage

Workplace Regulations

The workplace regulations apply to workplaces where persons are employed to work, but do not apply to workplaces used only by the self-employed. The Act requires employers to carry out a fire risk assessment to:

▸ identify hazards and people at risk
▸ remove or reduce the hazards
▸ manage the remaining risks to acceptable levels
▸ provide and maintain a means of escape, emergency lighting and fire safety signs
▸ provide and maintain fire fighting equipment, e.g. fire extinguishers.

Stock and consumables should be stored in a manner that takes into account both the Workplace Regulations and COSHH Regulations. The risk of fire should be minimised by storing all flammable liquids in a locked metal cupboard. Naked lights, such as matches and candles, should not be used where there is a possibility of paper and flammable products catching fire.

Fact file

> **Remember**:
> Aerosol cans have been known to explode when exposed to excessive heat. Aerosol cans should never be pierced or used when damaged.

COSHH regulations

These regulations cover the storing and use of products containing hazardous substances, for example, surgical spirit, glutaradehyde, chlorhexidine and bleach. These products should be stored in a locked metal cupboard with the correct signage attached.

The Regulations require that all products that contain substances known to be present as a hazard to health should be subject to a risk assessment, to consider safe use, first aid measures and details of

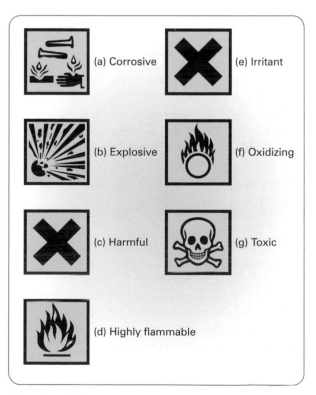

(a) Corrosive
(b) Explosive
(c) Harmful
(d) Highly flammable
(e) Irritant
(f) Oxidizing
(g) Toxic

Hazard symbols.

action to be taken in case of accidental exposure and disposal. All members of staff should be made aware of the risks of these substances and given the necessary training with regard to handling and use.

Safety and security

Risk assessments should be drawn up for all items of stock, both professional and retail. You should take COSHH regulations into consideration when writing the risk assessment.

▸ Stock should be stored in a cool environment away from direct light.
▸ Combustible or flammable substances should be stored in a locked metal cabinet.

▸ Retail stock should be kept in locked display cabinets rather than on open shelves. Products that disappear through clients or staff helping themselves is cash lost to the business. It is a sad fact that it is not uncommon for staff to help themselves to products, seeing it as a 'perk of the job' rather than theft!

Theory into practice

Write a risk assessment for surgical spirit, warm wax equipment cleaner and after-wax lotion. Evaluate the risks involved and compare the degree of risk between each product.

Assessment task 7.6

Identify potential problems associated with stock control and suggest logical solutions. Discuss the requirements of COSHH with regard to salon stock and demonstrate a clear understanding of how you would comply with these regulations. (D)

Recruitment and selection

Recruiting, appointing and employing staff can be one of the biggest headaches that an employer has to contend with. Getting the mix of employees right, so that they work together as a team and their skills are complementary to one another and to the benefit of the business, takes skill and careful organisation.

Recruitment

The aim when recruiting staff is to attract the best people for the job and appoint the person most suited to the position and the salon's needs. Appoint the wrong person and you will find that the clients will not be happy, morale of the other staff may be affected, and the business will suffer. In addition, repeated recruiting costs mount up.

The different stages involved in the recruitment process include the following:

▸ job analysis/design
▸ job description
▸ personnel specifications
▸ application form
▸ recruitment methods/advertisement
▸ shortlist
▸ interview
▸ appoint/job offer
▸ induction.

Job analysis/design

The first step in recruiting staff is to decide what the business needs are. Are you looking for one member of staff to add to an existing team or to replace someone who is leaving? Are you starting a new business and need to fill several vacancies? Is the position going to be full-time, part-time or perhaps job share? What hours need to be covered?

Is the person you appoint going to be employed by the business, freelance or self-employed?

What is the level of the work involved – manager, therapist, receptionist or administrator?

What skills will be required? Does the position require multi-skilled talents, e.g. beauty therapists, or a specialist such as an acupuncturist or osteopath?

Job description

When you have considered the questions above your next step is to write the job description.

Example of a job description:

Position	Manager, therapist, receptionist. Who the successful applicant will be working for and liaising with.
Description	Take over an existing client base. Build up or develop a new client base. Provide a range of treatments, e.g. Cathiodermie, body treatments, epilation, glycolic peels. Promote a range of retail products, e.g. MD Formulations, Matis, Guinot, Darphin. Stock control. Assist with marketing and promotional events, etc.
Working conditions	Salon environment and opening hours. Hours for position involved. Holiday entitlement, pension scheme. Benefits such as private health care or company car. Opportunities for continued professional development, e.g. additional training opportunities.

Theory into practice

Imagine that you own a busy salon with five treatment rooms, four beauty therapists and two part-time receptionists. The salon is open six days a week with three late evenings. The increase in business means that you need to recruit a full-time and part-time therapist. You offer a comprehensive range of treatments as well as three professional skin care ranges.

Develop a job description for both vacancies, then design the application form.

Personnel specifications

The next stage is to assess what qualifications, skills and experience you are looking for in your new employee(s). You should look at the applicant's qualifications, the date he or she qualified, post-qualifying experience and frequency of attending post-graduate courses. Membership of Professional Associations and attendance at beauty exhibitions and congresses indicate that the individual is interested in keeping up to date with trends within the industry. Are you looking for a multi-skilled member of staff who may have more than one role in the business?

Do you have a specific personality in mind, e.g. lively, sense of humour, good listener, interested in other people?

Recruitment methods/advertisement

There are different methods for recruiting staff. Each has their benefits and drawbacks. You need to be sure that you prospective employees will get to know about the vacancy.

Methods of recruiting staff:

Advertisement	You need to be confident that you are placing the advertisement where it will be read by prospective employees. This could be a professional publication, such as *Health & Beauty Salon* or *The Guild News*, or in the recruitment section of your local paper. This can be a costly but not necessarily effective method.
Job Centre	The local job centre will take details of your vacancy free of charge. It will post the details in the centre as well as nationally on its website.
Word of mouth	Networking or word of mouth is often the most effective way of finding the right person for your business. It is also the most cost effective
Internet	Professional associations, such as BABTAC and The Guild, have their own websites. They usually include a section for recruitment. The fees for advertising are very reasonable.

When you place an advertisement you must take care with the wording in order to:

a) put the message across effectively

b) ensure that you comply with employment legislation with regard to age, gender, race or disability.

You should monitor the response and attend to enquiries immediately they are received. When a request for an application form is made, details of the job description should be included.

Theory into practice

Design an advertisement for a full- and part-time therapist. You must take current legislation into consideration, e.g. regarding sex, age and racial discrimination. Research legislation using the Internet, the library or your local job centre.

Selection

Application forms/CVs

Each applicant should complete an application form and return it to you together with a written letter of application and their CV (Curriculum Vitae), which is usually typed or word processed.

The application form should give the name of the post, the salon's name and address, and request the following information:

▸▸ name, address and contact details of the applicant
▸▸ date of birth
▸▸ general education and achievements
▸▸ professional training and qualifications
▸▸ employment record
▸▸ post graduate qualifications/courses
▸▸ reasons for applying for the advertised position
▸▸ interests and hobbies
▸▸ present salary
▸▸ names and contact addresses of two or three referees
▸▸ closing date for return of the application forms.

Shortlisting

When you receive the letter of application, CV and completed application form, read it thoroughly. Look at the information given against the job description. If the applicant does not meet your needs then write immediately, but tactfully, with your decision. Keep letters of rejection short and sweet.

When the closing date has been reached:

▸▸ draw up your shortlist of candidates
▸▸ set a date for interviews, giving sufficient time for candidates to make arrangements to attend
▸▸ inform those individuals who are on the shortlist of the time, date and location of the interview
▸▸ give clear instructions as to what you want the candidates to bring with them on the day
▸▸ inform candidates if a trade test will form part of the interview and what the test will include.

Interview skills

Fact file

Remember that an interview is a nerve-wracking experience for the applicant.

The purpose of the interview is to provide an opportunity for the employer to meet all the suitable applicants and assess their strengths and weaknesses. First impressions are important for both sides.

Interviewing:

Interview	Features
Location	Easy access.
	Welcoming – not daunting, to encourage applicant to project his or her personality and suitability.
Aim	To appoint the person who matches the requirements of the vacancy.

Methods	▸▸ Visual observations:
	  - first impression
	  - dress
	  - shoes – clean?
	  - hands and nails – well manicured or bitten?
	▸▸ Make-up – often indicates type of personality.
	▸▸ Body language.
	▸▸ Handshake – firm or limp?
	▸▸ Confident/nervous/self-opinionated?

Interviewing (cont.):

Interview	Features

	▸ Questions:
	  – open ended, so requiring more than yes or no as an answer;
	  – test knowledge, skills and experience, particularly in relation to the treatments and retail products offered in your salon.
	▸ Evidence of continual professional development?
	▸ Short-term aims of applicant?
	▸ Long-term goals:
	  – reasons why the applicant feels that he or she is the best person for the job?
	  – reasons for applying to your salon?
	▸ Why does the applicant feel that you would benefit by appointing him or her to fill the vacancy?

Trade test – preferably on a senior member of staff who knows how the treatments should feel	Assess: ▸ efficiency and approach to preparation of work station and client ▸ communication skills ▸ treatment procedure ▸ completion of treatment ▸ sales opportunity.
Question the client on completion of the trade test	▸ How did the treatment feel? ▸ Was the client happy with the treatment? ▸ Would she book further appointments with the applicant? ▸ Ask for both positive and negative feedback.
Allow the applicant the opportunity to ask questions	Note the questions asked by the applicant, e.g. future development of the salon, opportunities for CPD, opportunities for promotion, etc.

When you are interviewing a number of applicants it is advisable to keep a list of questions and checklist for each interview with a scale of one to five for each area. Leave a space for general observations. This will help to refresh your memory and assist when comparing one applicant with another. Should you find that you are spoilt for choice, thus making a final decision difficult, then arrange for a second interview before making your final decision. It is very easy to appoint a new member of staff but not so easy to terminate his or her employment.

Appointing the wrong person (which is easy to do when you are short of staff or desperate to fill a vacancy) can be disruptive to the clients and other members of staff and, worst of all, detrimental to the health of the business.

Assessment task 7.7

Why is it important for an organisation to develop recruitment and selection procedures? Evaluate the benefits to the business. Look at and discuss different sources and methods of recruitment and selection. (M)

Assessment task 7.8

Identify potential problems associated with recruitment and selection of staff and suggest logical solutions. Gather evidence of alternative recruitment procedures. (D)

Letter of appointment

When the interviews are completed and you have made a decision you should take up references. (Telephone references should be confirmed in writing.) This reference should be kept with the personnel file. Subject to satisfactory references a letter of offer should be sent to the successful applicant to confirm:

1 the position offered

2 the starting date

3 the salary

4 any trial/probationary period (usually twelve weeks) that has been agreed for both parties.

Terms and conditions of employment can also be included at this stage.

Induction

▶ **Practice point:** Every new employee should be taken through an induction programme. This will help him or her to learn the organisation's procedures and housekeeping.

Benefits of induction

The benefits of a well conducted and organised induction programme are numerous. The new employee is given the opportunity to meet existing members of staff and gain knowledge of the salon's working procedures. The new employee will be shown around the premises and given information concerning the day-to-day running of the salon. She or he will be made aware of the salon policies regarding fire regulations and evacuation procedures.

The aim of the induction programme is to make the employees feel welcome, to familiarise them with salon procedures and to help them to settle in quickly and efficiently.

Induction procedures:

Welcome	Introductions to all members of staff. Tour of salon to familiarise new employee with salon layout, e.g. treatment rooms, stock room/storage area, reception, toilets, staff room, emergency exits.
Facilities	Staff room. General facilities, e.g. lights, heating, alarm system, access, telephone system, booking procedures.
Health and safety policies	First aid/accident book. Fire extinguishers – location and use. Evacuation procedures. COSHH sheets and procedures.
Internal systems	Reception procedures. Booking appointments. Cancellation policies. Telephone. Cashing up, petty cash, expenses. Record keeping. Filing.
Products and services	Product ranges. Treatments. Future development.
Training and CPD	Familiarisation with salon policy and procedures for treatments. Product knowledge of each professional and retail range.
Role/job information	Job title. Areas of responsibility and accountability. Contribution the role will bring to the salon. Who the employee reports to/is accountable to. Members of staff who will assist the individual in key areas. Working rosters/hours. Salon policies for sick leave, absence and annual leave.

Evaluation

When the induction programme has been completed, you should ask the new employee to complete an evaluation sheet. This should cover the benefits of the induction process as well as reference to any gaps in the procedure. This could also include room for the employee to suggest improvements to the induction programme.

1 Define the following terms:
   a PAYE
   b NIC
   c VAT.

2 Describe the procedure to be followed when registering a business for VAT.

3 What is the difference between PAYE and NIC?

4 List the forms that an employer needs to complete for the Inland Revenue.

5 State the information that should be included on an employee's salary slip.

6 What are 'annual accounts?' What information should be included in the annual accounts?

7 List the business records that should be kept in order to complete accurate reports and returns for:
   a Customs and Excise
   b the Inland Revenue.

8 Evaluate the benefits of computerised records in the business.

9 Define:
   a database
   b spreadsheet
   c website
   d electronic mail.

10 List the benefits of:
   a the Internet
   b the World Wide Web
   c online banking.

11 Define stock rotation.

12 Describe stock rotation.

13 Explain how you would maintain accurate stock records.

14 State the purpose of The Manual Handling Operations Act 1992.

15 How would you lift a box of stock?

16 List the conditions that cause stock to deteriorate.

17 Describe how 'sharps' should be disposed of.

18 Define COSHH.

19 Explain how a magnifying lamp can be a fire hazard.

20 List the stages involved in recruiting staff

21 State the different methods of recruiting staff.

22 What is a Curriculum Vitae?

23 State the purpose of an interview.

24 List the information that should be included in a 'letter of offer'.

25 Why should references be obtained before appointing a new member of staff?

References and bibliography for Unit 7: Organisational practices and procedures

Inland Revenue Publications – which can bedownloaded from the Inland Revenue website: *www.inlandrevenue.gov.uk*

H.M. Customs and Excise, *The VAT Guide* – which can bedownloaded from the Customs and Excise website: *www.hmce.gov.uk*

Basic skills in beauty therapy

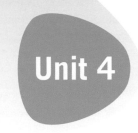

Unit 4

The purpose of this unit is to prepare you for commercial work in the beauty therapy salon and therefore a strong emphasis is placed on good practice, especially in relation to health, safety and hygiene. This unit introduces you to and develops your knowledge of the skills required to carry out some of the most popular beauty therapy treatments, including: treatment of hands, feet and nails; the temporary removal of facial and body hair; cosmetic eye treatments, such as eyelash tinting and eyebrow shaping; basic make-up and simple camouflage techniques.

As well as guiding the development of your practical skills, this unit will enable you to design suitable treatment programmes and provide homecare advice and retail recommendations to clients.

In order to achieve Unit 4 in Basic skills in beauty therapy you must complete the following learning outcomes:

Learning Outcomes

1 Investigate and apply treatments for the nails, hands and feet.
2 Explore and demonstrate the temporary removal of body and facial hair.
3 Investigate and apply eyebrow and eyelash treatments.
4 Explore and apply basic make-up and simple camouflage techniques.

Nails, hands and feet

Manicure and pedicure are popular salon treatments which can be performed on their own as part of a general grooming programme or as 'add-ons' to other services, such as facials or hairdressing. The manicure or pedicure can be extended to provide a luxury treatment or shortened to an express file and varnish. Nail technology is a specialist branch of beauty therapy that develops techniques in artificial nails and nail decoration. In this section, and other associated chapters, you will learn the practical skills and product knowledge associated with basic and special manicure and pedicure treatments for the purpose of maintaining healthy nails, hands and feet.

Pre-treatment preparation and procedure

Before the client arrives for a manicure or pedicure treatment you should ensure that the work area is prepared with the appropriate products, tools and equipment, and with due regard to health, safety and hygiene. Methods of sanitation and sterilisation are discussed in Section 1: Professional basics for beauty therapy (pages 12–13), and these should be referred to alongside the summary table overleaf.

As with all practical treatments, you should begin by carrying out a consultation to establish the client's needs and requirements. This will enable you to develop a good professional relationship as well as to design a suitable programme of treatment, after-care and retail recommendations.

There are many reasons or **indications** that a client might present for requesting this type of treatment, which include the following:

Indications for manicure:

» general grooming
» treatment of dry skin and nails
» post-acrylic
» to encourage nail growth
» special occasion
» as encouragement to stop nail biting.

Indications for pedicure:

» general grooming
» treatment for dry, cracked feet
» pre-holiday
» special occasion
» relaxation
» during pregnancy.

The indications for manicure and/or pedicure will also help you to design a treatment plan and make suitable home care and retail recommendations to your client. If the treatment is being performed for the maintenance of hands and nails it can be repeated as often as the client requires, usually about once a month. For the intensive treatment of a particular condition, such as dry skin and cuticles, a course of manicures closely spaced may be more beneficial, such as weekly treatments for four or five weeks or a monthly treatment using paraffin wax. The same is true for pedicure appointments, although most clients tend to have foot treatments more regularly during the summer months when their feet are on show. Well-applied nail enamel should last for a week on the fingernails and two weeks on the toenails, depending on the client's post-treatment activities.

As with all practical treatments, the techniques and products used as well as the effects of the treatment and any advice given should be recorded and kept on file for future reference (see Section 1, pages 8–10).

Advice and recommendations

You should be aware of and able to recognise common diseases and disorders of the nails, hands and feet, which are described in Unit 6: Dermatology and microbiology (pages 113–7) and are listed overleaf. It is important that you are able to differentiate between treatable and non-treatable conditions in order to ensure the safety of yourself and your clients.

Common concerns and their treatment:

Concern	Home care advice	Retail recommendations
Dry hands	Wear washing-up gloves; wear gloves in cold weather	Hand cream/lotion; hand exfoliator
Soft, weak nails that do not grow	Cut and file regularly to avoid splitting; avoid contact with harsh chemicals and detergents	Nail strengthener, emery board, nail food
Brittle nails that break easily	Keep nails short; take care to avoid further damage	Emery board; hand cream/lotion
Overgrown cuticles and/or hangnails	Do not pick; avoid contact with harsh detergents; have regular manicures	Cuticle massage cream; hand cream/lotion
Ingrowing toenails	Keep nails short and straight; can be corrected by a small 'v' cut into the nail	Emery board; orange wood stick
Athletes foot *(contra-indication)*	Dry thoroughly between the toes	Foot powder, anti-fungal preparations
Verrucae *(contra-indication)*	Do not pick; do not go barefoot, to avoid cross-infection	Specialist verruca preparations
Hard skin on feet	Remove daily and moisturise; regular pedicures to enhance circulation	Foot file, foot scrub, foot lotion

Contra-indications to manicure and pedicure:

Diseases and disorders of the nail	Diseases and disorders of the hands and feet
▸▸ Hangnail – dry, split cuticle	▸▸ Wart – viral infection
▸▸ Onycophagy – nail biting	▸▸ Verruca – painful ingrowing wart
▸▸ Onycholysis – separation of the nail from the nail bed	▸▸ Tinea – ringworm
▸▸ Abnormal discoloration of the nails	▸▸ Scabies – itch mite
▸▸ Beau's lines – deep horizontal depressions on all nails	▸▸ Eczema/dermatitis – dry, flaky, itchy skin
▸▸ Paronychia – bacterial infection of cuticle	▸▸ Melanoma – dark, irregular lesion
▸▸ Pterygium – overgrowth of cuticle	▸▸ Cuts, bruise and abrasions
▸▸ Onychomycosis – ringworm of the nail	▸▸ Recent scar tissue
▸▸ Onychogryphosis – thick, curved, ridged nails	▸▸ Undiagnosed lumps, bumps or swellings
▸▸ Onychocryptosis – ingrowing nail	▸▸ Broken or fractured bones

Assessment task 4.1

Describe the contra-indications to manicure and pedicure treatment. (M)

Basic product knowledge

There is a wealth of variety in the products available for the care of nails, hands and feet, which can be baffling for clients and trainee professionals. Many of the traditional skincare companies, such as Clarins and Clinique, and fashion labels, from French Connection to Chanel, have a nail care range alongside their established brands. Other cosmetic companies deal solely in nail care; Mavala and Jessica are two of the most popular, but the choice of nail products is almost as vast as the choice of skin care. As with skin care, most products have a basic formula which varies only slightly between manufacturers. As a beauty therapist, you should be aware of the main active ingredients in basic manicure and pedicure products, which are summarised overleaf.

Assessment task 4.2

Evaluate the main functions of products used for manicure and pedicure. Compare and contrast their function and effects of products with reference to active ingredients. (D)

Theory into practice

Research the costs of some basic nail care products from different product ranges, including coloured enamel, top/base coats, nail treatment preparations and hand cream. What factors do you think influence the retail prices?

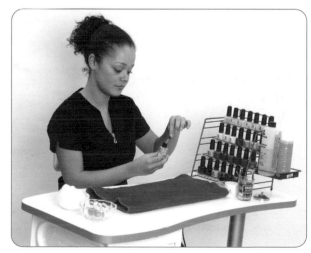

Manicure/pedicure products.

A summary of manicure and pedicure products:

Product	Main ingredients	Uses
Nail enamel remover	Acetone, perfume, colour	Removes nail enamel, dirt and oils
Cuticle massage cream	Emollient, e.g. lanolin; perfume, colour	Nourishes and softens cuticle
Cuticle remover cream	Strong alkali, e.g. potassium hydroxide; perfume, colour	Frees dry, dehydrated cuticle from the Nail plate
Nail bleach	Hydrogen peroxide or citric acid (natural bleach)	Whitens discoloured nails
Buffing paste	Abrasive particles, e.g. pumice, talc	Removes ridges, creates shine
Exfoliants	Detergent, abrasive particles	Removes dirt and hard skin
Hand cream/lotion	Emollient, e.g. lanolin; oil, e.g. almond oil; emulsifier, e.g. beeswax perfume; colour	Softens, nourishes and protects skin and cuticles; can be used as a massage medium
Nail strengthener	Formaldehyde	Hardens soft nails
Nail enamel	Formaldehyde, colour pigment, plasticisers, nitrocellulose; may contain pearlised particles	Enhances appearance, disguises discoloration
Foot spray	Antiseptic; perfume, and e.g. peppermint	Cleanses feet, gives feeling of freshness

Tools, materials and equipment

As well as gaining knowledge of the products used in manicure and pedicure, you must also be able to recognise, prepare and use correctly a range of specialist tools and equipment.

Manicure and pedicure tools:

Equipment	Method of use	Method of sterilisation
1 Emery board	Soft side for fingers, coarse side for toes; at 45° to nail filing from outside to centre	Disposable
2 Orange wood stick	Always cover tip with cotton wool; can be used to push back cuticle using small circular motions or to tidy nail enamel	Hot soapy water to sanitise; disposable
3 Hoof stick	Can be used to push back cuticle using small circular motions	Hot soapy water to sanitise

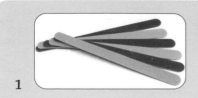
1

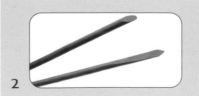
2

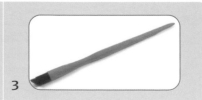
3

Equipment	Method of use	Method of sterilisation
4 Cuticle knife	Holding blade flat to the nail plate facing towards the centre of the nail; use to gently lift off adhered cuticle	Remove debris; autoclave
5 Cuticle nippers	Holding parallel to the nail, use to trim off hangnail and hard cuticle only	Remove debris; autoclave
6 Leather buffer	In conjunction with buffing paste, buff down the nail from cuticle to tip	Hot soapy water
7 3-way buffer	Starting with coarse side and progressing to finest grade, use in all directions across the nail plate	Hot soapy water; disposable
8 Nail scissors	Use curved edge to trim fingernails only	Remove debris; autoclave
9 Nail clippers	Hold in fist; can be used for fingers, toes and artificial nails	Remove debris; autoclave
10 Nail brush	To remove dirt and debris from fingernails and toenails	Hot soapy water; barbicide
11 Foot file	To remove hard skin and calluses	Nail brush to remove debris; hot soapy water to sanitise
12 Toe nail pliers	Use to trim toenails straight across only	Remove debris; autoclave

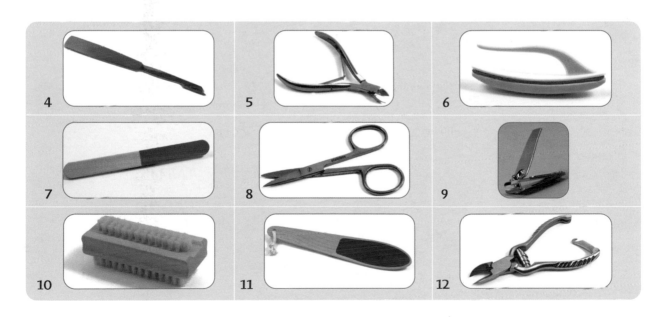

4

5

6

7

8

9

10

11

12

Techniques and procedure for manicure and pedicure
Step-by-step procedure for a manicure:

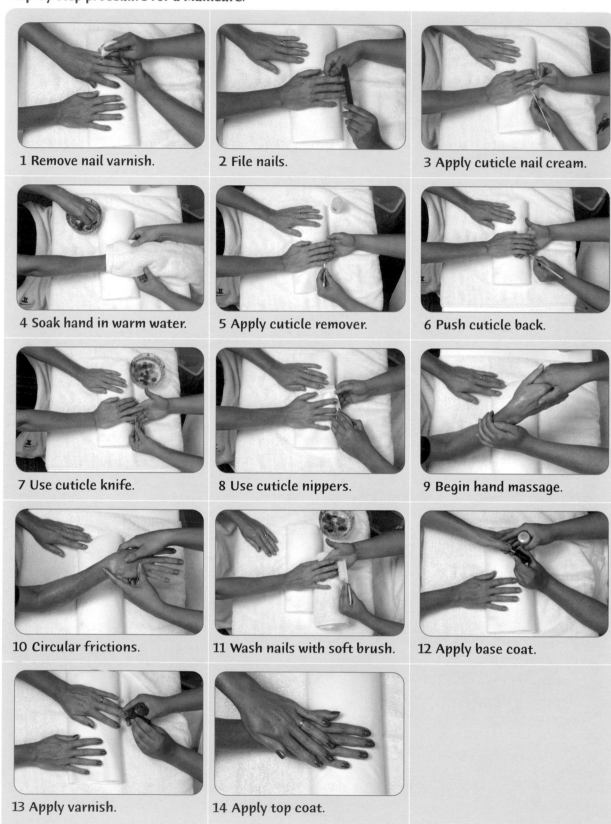

1 Remove nail varnish.

2 File nails.

3 Apply cuticle nail cream.

4 Soak hand in warm water.

5 Apply cuticle remover.

6 Push cuticle back.

7 Use cuticle knife.

8 Use cuticle nippers.

9 Begin hand massage.

10 Circular frictions.

11 Wash nails with soft brush.

12 Apply base coat.

13 Apply varnish.

14 Apply top coat.

More detailed instructions are given on pages 159–160.

Step-by-step procedure for a pedicure:

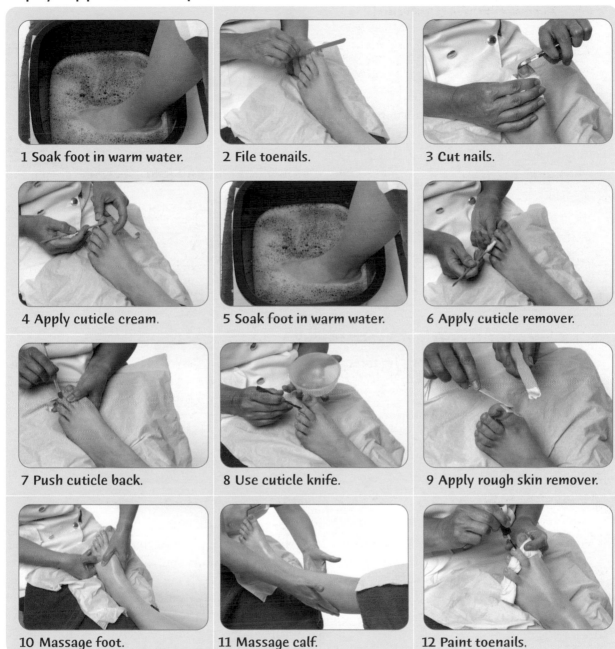

1 Soak foot in warm water.

2 File toenails.

3 Cut nails.

4 Apply cuticle cream.

5 Soak foot in warm water.

6 Apply cuticle remover.

7 Push cuticle back.

8 Use cuticle knife.

9 Apply rough skin remover.

10 Massage foot.

11 Massage calf.

12 Paint toenails.

Safe starting

Note: (M) = manicure; (P) = pedicure.

- Prepare work area and client.
- Complete record cards and check for contra-indications.
- Sanitise your hands using an anti-bacterial hand wash.
- Ask client to remove his or her jewellery and put it away (M).
- Sanitise the clients hands using an anti-bacterial hand wash (M).
- Spray the client's feet with anti-bacterial foot spray.
- **Practice point:** Always cut and file toenails straight across, to prevent onychocryptosis.

Safe working

1 Remove existing nail enamel.

2 Agree nail length and shape. Cut and file nails of left hand/foot, checking with the client throughout. Toenails should be cut straight across to avoid ingrowing nails.

3 Apply cuticle massage cream with an orange wood stick from the back of your hand.

4 Place tips of fingers in warm water and repeat to other hand (M).

5 Place feet in a bowl of warm soapy water and soak for 5 minutes (P).

▸ **Practice point:** As soon as you have finished with the water bowl, clear it away to prevent spillages.

6 Soften hard skin on the feet with a foot file and/or scrub (P).

7 Dry hands/feet thoroughly after soaking.

8 Apply a *small* amount of cuticle remover with an orange wood stick.

9 Use a tipped orange wood stick to *gently* push the cuticles back using small circular movements.

▸ **Practice point:** For hygiene reasons, always cover the end of the orange wood stick with cotton wool.

10 Use a *wet* cuticle knife to free any cuticle adhered to the nail plate. Always keep the blade flat to the nail and facing away from the nail groove.

11 Use cuticle nippers to remove hangnails *not* soft cuticle.

12 Remove debris with nail brush and repeat to the other hand/foot.

13 Buff the nails to remove ridges.

14 Perform a hand and arm/foot and leg massage.

15 Squeak nails with enamel remover before applying enamel. Always use a base coat followed by two coats of colour plus a top coat.

▸ **Practice point:** Massage procedures and benefits are explored in Unit 9: Body massage (pages 209–222).

Safe stopping

Give the client time and space to allow his or her nails to dry thoroughly.

▸ Help your client on with his or her coat and shoes.

▸ Check the client is satisfied with the treatment and with the end result.

▸ Offer home care advice and retail recommendations.

▸ Book your client's next manicure/pedicure appointment.

▸ **Practice point:** The treatment isn't complete until you have given your client home care and retail advice and booked his or her next appointment.

Assessment task 4.3

A client attends for manicure treatment. During the consultation you discover she has an allergy to lanolin. Her hands and nails are dry, with some splitting, and her cuticles are overgrown. Complete a record card for your client which contains accurate, precise and reliable information. (D)

Special hand and foot treatments

Warm oil manicure

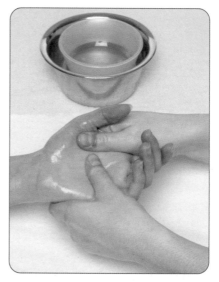

Application of warm oil to hands.

Oil can be warmed to aid its penetration into the skin. Ideal products to use for manicure are almond, olive, grapeseed or sunflower oils. Indications for warm oil treatments are overgrown or split cuticles, dehydrated and/or brittle nails, and dry or chemically dehydrated skin. This is an ideal treatment for softening the skin around the nail and is therefore performed prior to cuticle work. It is not advisable to carry out a warm oil treatment on the feet in the salon as the client could slip. However, warm oil could be used on dry feet at home as a massage medium. For additional benefit to the client, abrasive ingredients, such as bran or salt, could be added to the oil. When massaged over the skin this acts as an exfoliant, removing dry skin and staining, and allowing further penetration of the warm oil.

▸ **Practice point:** Warm oil and paraffin wax can be included as an intensive treatment for certain conditions or as a luxury treat for anyone!

Safe working

▸ Carefully place a small bowl of vegetable oil in a larger bowl of very hot water.

▸ Protect the work area and the client's clothing with towels and tissues.

▸ Test the temperature of the oil on yourself and your client.

▸ After cutting and filing the nails, immerse the fingertips in the warm oil to soak.

▸ Remove excess oil (or use it to massage) and carry out cuticle work.

▸ It is best not to paint the nails as squeaking would defeat the purpose of the treatment.

Paraffin wax

Paraffin wax is a traditional beauty therapy treatment still favoured by clients. In the salon it requires the use of specialist equipment which melts the wax and maintains it at a specific temperature of about 49°C. Paraffin wax causes a localised increase in heat which means it has far reaching benefits for a range of clients. Indications for use can broadly be divided into three categories: dry skin/nail conditions, relaxation, and sluggish physiological disorders; these are summarised below. Like warm oil, it is beneficial to use paraffin wax before cuticle work for dry skin conditions. As a relaxation or luxury treatment, paraffin wax can be used *after* the completion of cuticle work since it is usual in beauty therapy to perform the 'nice bit' at the end of the treatment. Once again, squeaking the nails in preparation for painting may be detrimental.

Safe starting

▸ Prepare all tools and materials.

▸ Prepare the work area with one small towel and one piece of couch roll for each hand/foot.

▸ Line a metal bowl with two or three layers of clingfilm.

▸ Complete the manicure up to/after completion of cuticle work.

▸ Apply a generous amount of hand/foot lotion to both hands/feet.

▸ Pour about three-quarters of a ladle of wax from the wax heater into the lined bowl.

▸ Test the wax on yourself (inner forearm) and your client (outer forearm) using a brush.

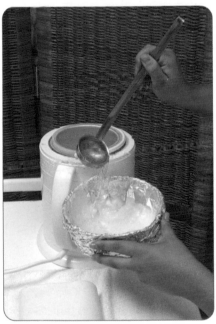

Ladling melted wax from the wax heater into a lined bowl.

Uses of paraffin wax treatment on hands or feet:

Indications	Benefits and effects
Cold hands/feet	Penetration of heat causes local increase in skin temperature
Sluggish circulation	Increases superficial blood circulation
Stiff, aching joints	Heat penetration provides relief from discomfort
Dry, cracked skin/cuticles	Aids penetration of nourishing products
Non-medical swelling	Increases lymphatic circulation and reduces congested fluid
Sluggish appearance to skin	Exfoliates dead skin cells and induces perspiration
Muscle tension	Heat penetration encourages muscle fibres to relax

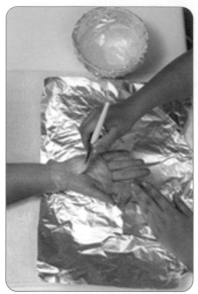

Apply paraffin wax to hand.

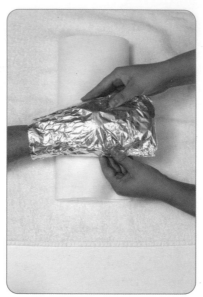

Wrap hand in tinfoil.

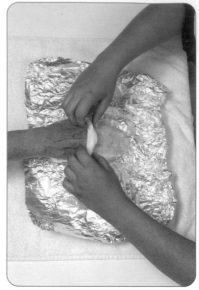

Removed cooled wax from hand.

Safe working

1 Using a brush, layer wax to the back of one hand/foot, from the tips of the fingers/toes to just above the wrist/ankle. Apply wax to the palm/sole.

2 Slip the hand/foot inside a plastic bag or wrap with clingfilm or tinfoil, then tissue and a towel.

3 Repeat to the other hand/foot.

4 Clean the bowl by removing the clingfilm and throwing away.

5 Clean the brush with a dry tissue.

6 Remove the wax like removing a glove after about 10 minutes or when it begins to cool.

7 Massage any residue lotion into the area and continue with the treatment.

Theory into practice

Design a treatment plan for a client who has split, dry cuticles, soft nails and dry skin, and who is getting married in six months' time. Think about basic/special techniques and appointment spacing as well as home care advice and retail recommendations.

Assessment task 4.4

Provide detailed and justified home care advice for the client in Assessment task 4.3 (on page 160) based on her consultation. Suggest three products suitable for retail with clear instructions for use. (D)

Temporary removal of body and facial hair

Most women in the UK choose to remove at least some body and facial hair using one of a variety of temporary methods. The reasons for doing this include social acceptance, enhanced appearance and personal comfort. Professional warm waxing can be described as the 'bread and butter' treatment for the beauty professional, so great is its popularity. It forms an integral part of any training programme, and competency in waxing can mean the difference between a successful and an unsuccessful trade test. Your future employment could, quite literally, depend on your ability to perform waxing treatments. Alternative hair removal methods are also available for salon or home use and you should be aware of these. The advantages/disadvantages of some of these methods are summarised in the table overleaf.

Methods of hair removal:

Method	Advantages	Disadvantages
Warm wax	Regrowth in 4–6 weeks; no stubble	Hair must be 1 cm prior to removal; slight discomfort felt by some; possibility of ingrowing hairs
Sugaring	Less skin irritation than for waxing	(As for waxing)
Hot wax	Heat opens hairs follicles so less discomfort in small areas	Can take up to twice as long as a warm wax
Shaving	Inexpensive; quick and easy to do at home	Stubble within hours, regrowth within days
Depilatory creams	Painless; can be done at home	Can be messy and hard to control; can cause skin irritation; regrowth within days
Tweezing	Inexpensive; ideal for small areas and stray hairs	Can cause hair breakage; not suitable for larger areas
Threading	No products and so no risk of skin irritation	An art form, with few practitioners
Electrolysis	Permanent removal; relatively established and proven	Slow to clear area; uncomfortable; relatively expensive
Laser	Long-term hair removal or permanent reduction	Only suitable for dark hair/pale skin; risk of scarring and/or burns; a relatively new treatment

---

Assessment task 4.5

Compare and contrast the various methods of temporary hair removal from the body and face. (D)

Pre-treatment preparation and procedure

Before the client arrives for treatment you should ensure that the work area is prepared with the appropriate products, tools and equipment, and with due regard to health, safety and hygiene (methods of sanitation and sterilisation are discussed in the Section 1, pages 12–13). As with all practical treatments, you should begin by carrying out a consultation to establish the client's history and requirements, which will enable you to develop a good professional relationship as well as provide suitable after care and retail recommendations. It is important to ask if the client has had waxing treatments done before and to establish the skin's reaction, the level of discomfort felt and the length of time for regrowth to appear. As always, all information should be recorded and kept confidential.

Indications

The main indication for warm waxing is the presence of unwanted hair. It is suitable for use on all areas of the body: legs, bikini line, abdomen, underarms and the face. Men may request warm waxing for the chest, shoulders and/or back. Waxing is preferable to other methods of temporary removal because it is longer lasting, usually about four to six weeks depending on the area and type of hair growth. Because the hairs are removed from the root, regrowth is softer as new tapered hairs grow through. The lack of stubble is one of the reasons why waxing is the preferred method of so many women. Waxing can feel uncomfortable at first but most clients get used to this sensation over time as the hairs become weaker. Most clients agree that the slight discomfort is a small price to pay for longer lasting hair-free skin without stubble.

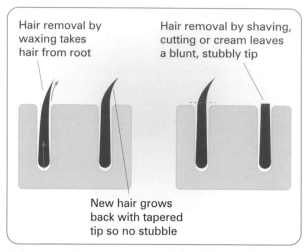

Hair removal by waxing takes hair from root

Hair removal by shaving, cutting or cream leaves a blunt, stubbly tip

New hair grows back with tapered tip so no stubble

Hair removed from the root and the skin's surface.

Contra-indications

You should be aware of and able to recognise common diseases and disorders of the skin, which are described in Unit 6: Dermatology and microbiology (pages 113–117). The contra-indications to waxing are any conditions that would be uncomfortable to the client or contagious. Small cuts, bruises or abrasions can be covered with petroleum jelly and worked around.

Contra-indications and cautions for waxing:

Contra-indications:	Cause for caution:
▸▸ Cuts, bruises, abrasions	▸▸ Eczema, dermatitis, psoriasis
▸▸ Raised moles	▸▸ Low skin sensitivity
▸▸ Skin infection	▸▸ Heightened skin sensitivity, e.g. vitiligo
▸▸ Varicose veins/ severe thread veins	▸▸ HIV
▸▸ Recent scar tissue	▸▸ Diabetes
▸▸ Contagious conditions, e.g. ringworm	

Assessment task 4.6

Explain the indications and contra-indications to warm waxing. (D)

Basic product knowledge

There is a great choice for the beauty professional when selecting wax products, but these can be roughly divided into three types: 'honey-style' wax, cream wax and organic wax. These are outlined overleaf, as well as hot wax and sugar, which may also be available in the salon. There is no 'best' type of wax and as a trainee beauty therapist you should try to work with and experience the different types and then choose the one that suits you best. The same is true of wax strips, where the choice is between paper and muslin cloth. Some therapists find the paper variety easier to work with because it is less floppy, but the exaggerated ripping sound it makes is often misconstrued as representing greater discomfort!

Other products required for waxing are pre-wax and after-wax lotions. As the name suggests, pre-wax lotion is used before waxing to ensure a clean, oil-free surface for the adhesion of wax. The active ingredients are ethanol – an alcohol used in cosmetic preparations for cleansing – as well as an anti-bacterial and anti-inflammatory ingredient such as camphor oil or tea tree oil. After-wax lotion is applied to soothe and cool the skin following wax depilation. It is an emulsion of oils and cooling agents, often fragranced with lavender, mint or tea tree to enhance its actions. After-wax oils are suitable for use on large areas of dry skin, such as the legs, while gel formulations are ideal for cooling facial and underarm areas. Tinted after-wax products are also available for use on facial areas.

Advice and recommendations

General advice:
If the area has an **erythema** it is more sensitive than normal. Avoid all perfumed or chemical products (soap, make-up, bath oils, lotions, chlorine), forms of heat (baths, showers, sunbeds, sauna, vigorous activity) and irritation (tight clothing, touching the area) until the redness subsides.

Assessment task 4.7

Provide detailed and justified home care advice for a client following her first half leg, bikini and underarm wax. Demonstrate an awareness of retail opportunities for the client. (D)

A summary of the basic product knowledge, treatment areas and equipment for waxing:

Type of wax	Characteristics
Traditional warm wax	Hard when cold and resembles honey when heated to temperatures of about 40°C. It consists of refined gum resin and chemicals called hydrocarbon tackifiers, which make it sticky.
Cream wax	More opaque than 'honey' wax and comes in a variety of colours. Contains moisturisers to soothe and azulene which is an anti-inflammatory. Has a slightly lower working temperature of about 35–40°C and so are more comfortable for some clients.
Organic waxes	Relatively new but gaining in popularity. Contain natural ingredients and do not set hard when cold. Many clients find organic waxes more comfortable and less irritating on the skin. This is often reflected in the higher price!
Hot wax	Solid pellets or blocks with a working temperature of 48–68°C depending on the manufacturer. Contains natural resins and microcrystalline wax. Less pliable and more brittle than warm wax.
Sugar paste	Resembles warm wax. Consists of sugar, lemon juice and water. Can be rolled over the skin as a ball of thick paste or performed using the strip method, like warm waxing.

Area treated	Home care advice	Retail recommendations
Legs	Exfoliate regularly and moisturise daily to prevent ingrowing hairs	Body scrub, body lotion, loofah
Bikini-line	Ingrowing hairs are likely; exfoliate regularly and do not pick	Gentle body scrub
Underarms	Do not wear deodorant or wash with soap for about 24 hours	Fragrance/chemical free deodorants
Facial area	Do not touch the area or wear make-up for up to 24 hours	Tinted after-wax lotion, cooling gel
Back	Exfoliate regularly and moisturise	Loofah, body lotion

Equipment	Method of use	Method of sanitation
Wax heater	Top up with wax and turn on to melt wax; maintain at correct working temperature prior to client's arrival	Clean outside of the heater with wax equipment cleaner and tissues
Spatula	A new wooden spatula should be used for each new area or new client	Disposable
Strips	Cut to size for different areas	Fold wax side in and dispose
Tweezers	To remove stray or short hairs after waxing	Autoclave
Scissors	To cut strips and trim long hairs to 1cm	Autoclave

Tools, materials and equipment

The treatment couch should be protected with a plastic sheet and/or couch roll as drips are inevitable when you begin to practise waxing techniques. You could also protect your uniform with a plastic wax apron or tabard. The client's clothing should be removed from the area being treated and stored out of the way. Underwear should be protected with tissues when waxing bikini line or underarm areas. Other equipment needed is summarised in the table at the bottom of page 165.

Techniques for hair removal:

Leg wax:

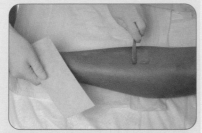

1 Apply in direction of hair growth.

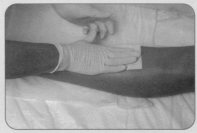

2 Press down firmly with wax strip.

▸▸ Practice point: Any oils, sweat, dirt or make-up on the skin will act as a barrier against the wax and could also lead to infected follicles.

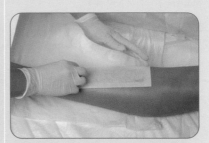

3 Peel back small edge to wax strip and stretch the skin.

▸▸ Practice point: Just because a client has been waxed before by someone else, it does not mean the procedure has been explained or performed well.

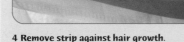

4 Remove strip against hair growth.

Bikini line wax:

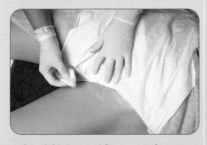

1 Clean bikini area with pre-wax cleanser.

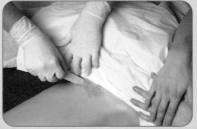

2 Apply wax to bikini area in direction of hair growth

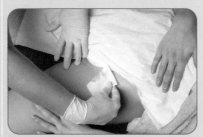

3 Remove against direction of hair growth.

Underarm wax:

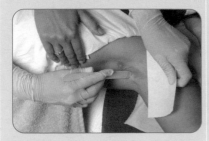

1 Apply wax to underarm area in direction of hair growth.

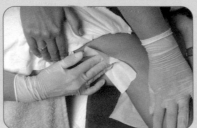

2 Stretch skin firmly.

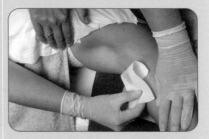

3 Remove against direction of hair growth.

Eybrow wax:

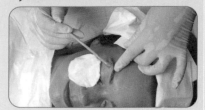

1 Apply wax to eyebrow area.

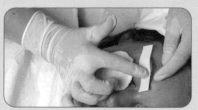

2 Apply small piece of wax strip.

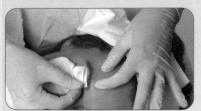

3 Remove against direction of hair growth.

Safe starting

- Prepare the couch with a plastic cover, towels and couch roll.
- Position clean wax heater with no trailing wires.
- Sterilise tweezers and scissors.
- Prepare tools, products and equipment.
- Position client on the couch and protect his or her clothing.
- Examine the area and check for contra-indications.
- Explain procedure and sensation to the client.
- Test the wax on yourself.

Safe working

- Prepare skin with pre-wax cleansing lotion.
- Test wax on the client.
- **Practice point:** The client can help to stretch the skin in fleshy areas like the thighs and bikini line. For the underarm she can help by pulling her bust away from the area being waxed.
- Apply wax *in the direction* of hair growth
- Stretch the skin.
- Remove strip *against* the direction of growth.

Safe stopping

- Make sure there is no wax left on the skin.
- Tweeze any stray hairs.
- Apply a soothing after-wax lotion, oil or gel.
- Explain the normal skin reaction and contra-actions.
- Provide home care and retail advice.
- Book the next waxing appointment for 4–6 weeks.
- **Practice point:** The area should be clean and dry, free from all hair, wax and stickiness, before the client dresses to leave.

Contra-actions

A contra-action is something that is not a normal or desirable reaction to treatment but is not uncommon. If any of the following occur during treatment stay calm and do not panic, it might not have been caused by poor technique. Do not worry the client, instead explain that this sometimes happens and deal with the situation in the appropriate manner. Contra-actions and how to deal with them are summarised below.

A summary of contra-actions to waxing:

Contra-action	Possible cause	Advice
Severe erythema	Ripping the hair from the follicle with hot wax	Avoid further irritation from heat, perfumed products or friction
Bruising	Pulling the strip upwards instead of backwards, or insufficient stretching	Can be covered with tinted lotion; avoid further pressure
Bleeding	More likely in bikini/underarm area where hair is more coarse	Apply pressure with dry cotton wool
Burns	Wax is too hot	Apply cold compress and soothing gel; avoid further heat
Ingrowing hairs	Hair breakage due to friction or bad waxing, dry skin or curly follicles; e.g. bikini line	Exfoliate regularly and apply moisturiser daily; do not wax too frequently

Assessment task 4.8

Design a record card suitable for waxing clients, including space for all relevant information. Complete the card, using yourself as client, with accurate and precise information. (D)

Eyebrow and eyelash treatments

Eyebrow shaping and eyebrow and lash tinting are popular salon treatments that require regular maintenance every 4–5 weeks. They are cost effective treatments for the salon, particularly if performed in conjunction with other treatments such as facials or waxing. A professional eyebrow or eyelash treatment can enhance the facial appearance in a subtle or dramatic way, and should be performed, to suit the client's needs.

Pre-treatment preparation and procedure

Before the client arrives for treatment you should ensure that the work area is prepared with the appropriate products, tools and equipment and with due regard to health, safety and hygiene. As with all practical treatments, you should begin by carrying out a consultation to establish the client's requirements; this will enable you to develop a good professional relationship and meet your client's needs. You should advise your client of the effects of tinting and help with the choice of colour.

For eyebrow shaping you should look together in a mirror to establish the required shape and thickness and agree the finished result. Make sure that your client has reasonable expectations about the treatment according to their existing eyebrow shape and hair colour. At least 48 hours before tinting the client should have a **patch test** to rule out the possibility of an allergic or adverse reaction to the chemical, even if he or she has had tinting at another salon in the past.

Patch test

» Should be carried out at least 48 hours before tinting.
» Cleanse the area either behind the ear or in the crook of the elbow.
» Mix a small amount of dark tint plus peroxide.
» Apply with an orange wood stick.
» Client should monitor the area for signs of irritation.

As with all treatments, details of the products used, reaction and finished result should be recorded for reference. There are a number of indications for eyebrow and eyelash treatments, which are listed below.

Indications for eyelash/eyebrow tinting:
» fair lashes and/or brows
» to enhance eye area
» allergy to make-up products
» no time to apply make up
» prior to holiday/special occasion.

Indications for eyebrow shaping:
» to frame the eyes
» to enhance facial features
» to correct distance between the eyes
» fashion shapes and trends.

Contra-indications to eyebrow and eyelash treatments

Skin diseases or disorders (see Unit 6: Dermatology and microbiology (pages 113–117) in or around the eye area could contra-indicate treatment. There are also several disorders of the eye area which should be avoided, including conjunctivitis, styes, eczema and bruising.

Contra-indications and cautions for eye treatments:

Contra-indications to eye treatments:	Caution required prior to eye treatments:
Positive reaction to patch test	Eczema, psoriasis
Conjunctivitis	Viral infections, e.g. cold or flu
Blepharitis (eyelid infection)	Hayfever – eyes may be watery
Recent operations or scar tissue	Sensitivity
Eyebrow tinting should be performed prior to and never after eyebrow shaping	

Assessment task 4.9

Describe the indications and contra-indications to eyelash and eyebrow treatments. (M)

Basic product knowledge

Tints are available in the form of creams, liquids and gels, depending on the manufacturer. They come in a variety of colours: (from lightest to darkest) brown, grey, black, blue and blue/black. Client colour choice is dependent on natural hair colour, colour and frequency of using make-up, and the desired result. Tints consist of a mixture of vegetable dyes and chemical dyes such as toluenediamine. Synthetic chemical dyes need to be oxidised in order to make them semi-permanent and are therefore mixed with hydrogen peroxide *just before* application. The molecules present in tints are small enough to enter the hair shaft and fill the spaces of the cuticle. When they are oxidised the molecules swell and become trapped in the cortex which makes the colour semi-permanent. Eyelash and eyebrow tint does not wash out, it gradually grows out or is lost as lashes are shed. The tint therefore *appears* to fade over time, lasting about four to five weeks. The client should be advised to cleanse the area gently to avoid losing excess lashes/brows.

Tools, materials and equipment

A wide range of tweezers is available for home and salon use, including manual, automatic and electrical tweezers. As always, it is best to try out as many types as you can and choose the type which suits you best.

Technique and procedure for eyebrow tinting

Safe starting

» Carry out a patch test 48 hours before tint.

» Wash your hands.

» Cleanse the area.

» Protect the skin around the eyebrow with petroleum jelly.

Safe working

1 Agree the colour with your client.

2 Mix and apply the tint.

3 Leave for 2 minutes only.

Safe stopping

» Remove tint with an orangewood stick.

» Use witch hazel to remove all traces of tint.

» Ensure client is satisfied.

» Provide home care and retail advice.

» Book next appointment for 4–5 weeks.

Technique and procedure for eyelash tinting

Safe starting

» Carry out a patch test 48 hours before tint.

» Wash your hands.

» Cleanse the area with eye make-up remover.

» Protect the skin around the eye with petroleum jelly and apply cotton pads.

Safe working

1 Agree the colour with your client.

2 Mix and apply the tint.

3 Cover the eyes with cotton pads.

4 Leave for 10–12 minutes only.

Safe stopping

» Remove tint with damp cotton wool.

» Ensure client is satisfied.

» Provide home care and retail advice.

» Book next appointment for 4–5 weeks.

Tools for eyebrow and eyelash treatments:

Equipment	Method of use	Method of sanitation
Tweezers	To remove individual hairs from the eyebrow	Autoclave or glass bead steriliser
Eyebrow brush	To brush hairs into shape	Hot soapy water
Orange wood stick	To align eyebrows prior to shaping	Hot soapy water
Orange wood stick or fine brush	To mix and apply tint	Disposable
Mirror	To check client's requirements	Cleaning spray
Glass dappen dish	To mix tint in	Hot soapy water
Damp cotton wool	To clean area and remove tint	Disposable

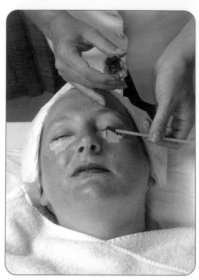

Mix and apply eyelash tint to upper and lower lashes.

Technique and procedure for eyebrow shaping

Guidelines for eyebrow shaping

1 Take an imaginary line from the corner of the nose to the inner corner of the eye and remove hairs from centre.

2 Take an imaginary line from the corner of the mouth to the outer corner of the eye and remove stray hairs.

3 Highest point of arch should be in line with the eye pupil.

Safe starting
▸▸ Prepare the work area and sterilise the tweezers.
▸▸ Wash your hands.
▸▸ Secure the client's hair in a head band or turban.
▸▸ Consult with the client using a mirror to agree the finished result.
▸▸ Cleanse the area.

Safe working
1 Grip hairs firmly and remove one at a time.
2 Remove in the direction of hair growth.
3 Work between left and right to maintain balance.

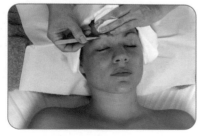

Shaping eyebrows using tweezers.

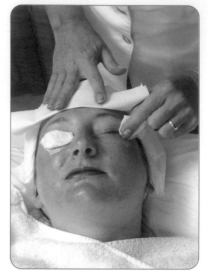

Remove eyelash tint with damp cotton wool pads.

4 Consult the client throughout.
5 Wipe the brow with witch hazel to remove hairs and cool the area.

Safe stopping
▸▸ Stand back and check the finished result.
▸▸ Ensure the client is satisfied.
▸▸ Place cooling pads on the brows to reduce erythema.
▸▸ Apply tinted bacterial lotion.
▸▸ Provide home care and retail advice.
▸▸ Book another appointment for 4–5 weeks.

Advice and recommendations

Whether eyebrows are shaped using warm wax or tweezers, post-treatment erythema will be present. For some clients this subsides within an hour or so while for others it might last longer, depending on skin sensitivity, hair type and the amount of hair removed. The advice is the same as for waxing: avoid all potential irritants such as heat, perfumed or chemical products and friction, and avoid touching the area while an erythema remains. The client might like to use an after-wax lotion or gel to mask redness and/or cool the area. You could also sell tweezers for removing stray hairs between salon visits as well as an eyebrow brush and/or pencil.

There is no specific advice when following lash or brow tinting other than to take care when cleansing the eye area to avoid the premature loss of hairs. The client might wish to use a clear mascara to enhance the appearance of the lashes, or tweezers to shape the brows. General make-up advice might be appropriate for some clients, to further enhance their appearance.

Assessment task 4.10

Describe the information that should be contained on a record card for a client who receives an eyelash tint and eyebrow shape. (M)

Assessment task 4.11

Evaluate treatments for the eyebrows and eyelashes. (D)

Basic make-up and simple camouflage techniques

A client may come to you for make-up for a number of reasons. She might be trying make-up for the first time or looking for ideas to update her usual look. She might need advice for corrective or camouflage techniques or require make-up for a special occasion. Bridal make-up is an enjoyable (and profitable) avenue for the beauty therapist to explore and often prompts further treatments in preparation for the big day, as well as obvious retail opportunities.

Theory into practice

Try preparing a bridal package which includes countdown treatments in the months leading up to the wedding day.

Some beauty therapists choose to specialise in make-up following their initial training and develop techniques suitable for film, theatre and television, special effects or fashion styling. In this section you will learn the practical skills and product knowledge necessary to create basic make-up, corrective and camouflage techniques.

Pre-treatment preparation and procedure

Before the client arrives you should prepare yourself and the working area for make-up. It is useful, both for you and the client, to have a selection of magazines, including bridal ones and those aimed at Asian, Indian or Caribbean women. Clients also like to see photographs of previous work and you could build a portfolio of different make-up looks you have created. If a client requests a special occasion make-up it is customary to carry out a trial run at the

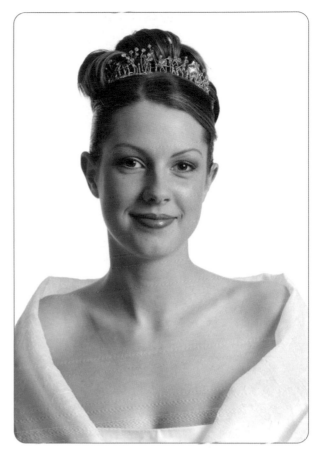

Bridal make-up and hair.

time of the consultation and this should be reflected in the price. Contra-indications to make-up are any skin or eye conditions which are contagious or cause discomfort to the client.

Ranges of products

The range of make-up products available is vast, including supermarket and chemist own brands, fashion labels, cosmetic and skin care companies and professional products. Most beauty therapists start with a small basic kit and add to it as they discover their own 'must haves'.

Theory into practice

Look through some magazines to familiarise yourself with the choice of make-up products and colours available.

Create a folder of different make-up looks using magazine images.

Some basic make-up products:

Make-up product	Uses	Application
Liquid foundation cream/ oil-based foundation	Lighter texture, good for combination and oily skins; heavier texture, good for dry, mature and dehydrated skins	With fingers or damp latex sponge, working outwards from centre of the face
Translucent powder	To set the foundation and reduce shine	Press onto skin with cotton wool, remove excess with large brush
Blusher – cream or powder	To add colour	With a brush to 'apple' of cheeks
Eyeshadow – cream, gel or powder	To add colour and enhance eyes	Disposable sponge applicator, brush or fingertips
Eyeliner pencil, pen or liquid	To define eye shape	From applicator to upper lid, from outer to inner corner
Mascara	To frame the eyes	Disposable applicator to take product from mascara wand
Lip liner pen/pencil	To enhance or correct lip shape	Just inside, just outside or on natural lip line
Lipstick	To add colour and enhance the lips	Take product onto spatula and apply with a brush, then blot and re-apply

Basic make-up

Basic make-up is suitable for day, evening or bridal wear, with slight variations to suit the occasion. Make-up should be applied in the same light in which the client will appear; thus, for day make-up natural light is best but for an evening look artificial UV light would be appropriate.

The foundation is the most important part of the make-up and should create a natural blank canvas rather than an artificial mask. Despite the amount of products available it is difficult to find a perfect match to each individual's skin colour straight from the shelves. Begin by deciding if the client's natural skin colour has a base which is brown, red or orange; this becomes easier with practice. Next, decide if the product you have selected is too dark or too light, and mix it with another product with the same base colour until you get a perfect match. Remember to mix enough product to cover the whole face and always test product on the jaw line line to avoid unsightly 'tide marks'.

As far as colour cosmetics go, the *tone* of colour and skill of application are more important than the actual colour. That said, clients requiring a natural looking make-up should choose colours from the warm spectrum that do not clash, e.g. brown, orange, amber and cream. Cool colours are more artificial and contrasting colours produce a more

Colour wheel.

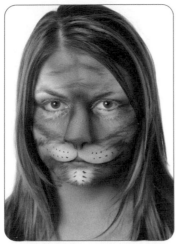

Lioness theatrical make-up.

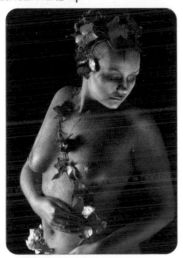

Statue theatrical make-up.

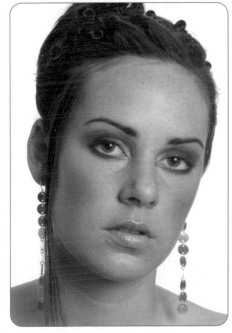

Evening make-up.

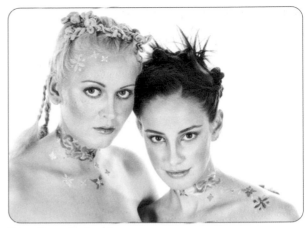

Fairy theatrical make-up.

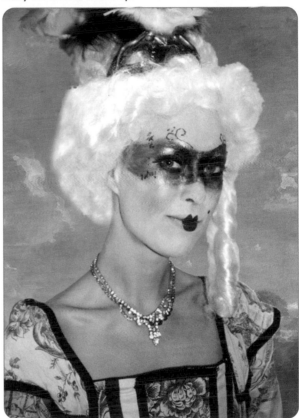

Victorian theatrical make-up.

striking effect, e.g. lavender and yellow or pink and orange. Colours used on cheeks, eyes, lips and nails should also be in harmony.

Make-up for a wedding day should enhance and define the natural features: the bride wants to look like herself, so find out how much make-up she usually wears. The make-up will need to be a *little* heavier than normal in order to show up in the photographs, and waterproof mascara (or an eyelash tint) is often requested as a few tears are almost inevitable on the day!

Make-up procedure

Safe starting

- Prepare self and work area with due regard to health and safety.
- Sanitise brushes and sponges.
- Carry out a client consultation.
- Secure hair with a head band or turban.
- Protect client's clothes with a cape or towel.

Safe working

1. Check for contra-indications and/or allergies.
2. Prepare the client's skin by cleansing, toning and moisturising.
3. Test the base colour on the jaw line in a good light.
4. Use disposable applicators where possible.
5. Never blow on brushes or the client.
6. Don't put brushes in pots.

Safe stopping

- Dispose of used tissues, cotton wool and disposable applicators.
- Make sure lids are tightly sealed. Sharpen pencils between clients to create a clean tip.
- Check client is satisfied.
- Summarise all advice given and retail products.
- Book follow up appointment.

Corrective make-up

There are a few simple rules to bear in mind when applying corrective make-up. Dark colours or matt finishes tend to make things appear smaller and detract attention away from them, whereas lighter colours or glossy finishes have the opposite effect – enlarging a feature and drawing attention to it. These rules don't just apply to make-up: the reason that black remains such a popular colour choice in women's clothing is its slimming effect; white has the opposite effect. Cleverly applied make-up following these basic rules can enhance the facial features.

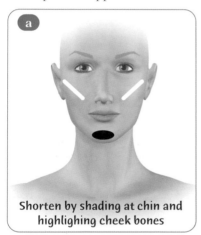

Shorten by shading at chin and highlighing cheek bones

Long

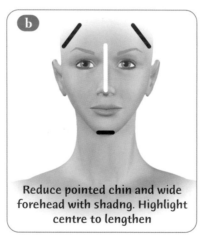

Reduce pointed chin and wide forehead with shadng. Highlight centre to lengthen

Heart shaped

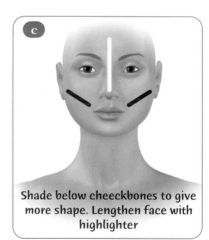

Shade below cheeckbones to give more shape. Lengthen face with highlighter

Round

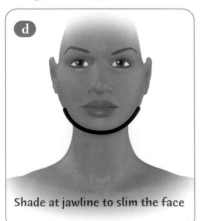

Shade at jawline to slim the face

Pear shaped

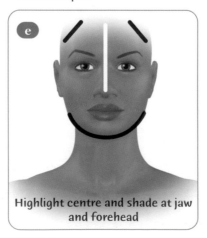

Highlight centre and shade at jaw and forehead

Square

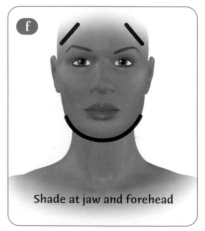

Shade at jaw and forehead

Rectangle

Face shapes.

Eye shapes

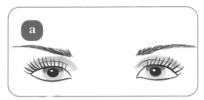

Deep-set eyes – use pale colours on eye socket. Mascara or artificial lashes will highlight further.

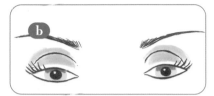

Heavy eyelids – use pale colours on eye socket. Artificial lashes at corners will help lift the eyes.

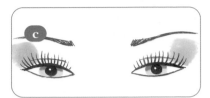

Narrow eyes – line upper lid only to avoid closing eyes further. Pale colours on outer part of lid give shape and definition; artificial lashes give fullness.

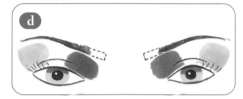

Wide-set eyes – darker colours on inner lid, pale colours on outer lid. Extend brows towards nose to narrow the gap between the eyes.

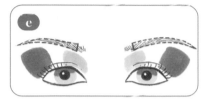

Close-set eyes – pale colours on inner lid, darker colours on outer lid. Shorten brows at nose to create wider gap between eyes.

Lip shapes

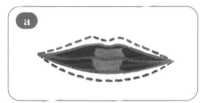

Thin lips – line lips just outside natural lip line. Apply lighter shade to centre.

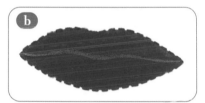

Full or thick lips – enhance with definition on the lip line.

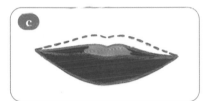

Thin or straight upper lip – re-define upper lip just outside natural lip line. Highlight centre of upper lip only.

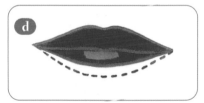

Thin lower lip – re-define lower lip just outside natural lip line. Highlight centre of lower lip only.

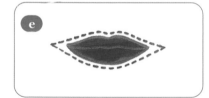

Asymmetric lips – create a lip line where required to achieve balance.

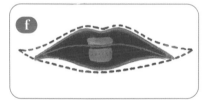

Droopy mouth – re-define at corners to give more upward lift. Highlight at centre.

Simple camouflage technique:

Problem	Technique
Dark circles under the eyes	Light application of skin coloured concealer under foundation
High cheek colour	Green tinted moisturiser under or powder over foundation
Isolated blemishes	Concealer one shade lighter than base under foundation
Sallow complexion	Violet-tinted powder over foundation

Simple camouflage techniques

Camouflage make-up can be used to disguise minor or major skin blemishes, ranging from dark circles under the eyes and high cheek colour to pigmentation disorders and birthmarks. There are specialist products available for camouflage make-up, which are used by specialists in this field, but regular cosmetics are suitable for the simple camouflage techniques applied by the beauty therapist. As the aim of camouflage make-up is to conceal, it is important to remember 'less is more' when applying products. Another tip is to refer to the colour wheel (on page 172) and remember the rule that opposite colours counteract each other, so green neutralises red and violet shades will neutralise a sallow (yellowy) skin tone.

Assessment task 4.12

Select six different tear sheets of make-up 'looks' from magazines. Analyse these images and describe the choice of products and the techniques used, explaining how they could be adapted for different skin colours or occasions. (D)

Cosmetic application of artificial lashes

There are two types of artificial eyelashes available, which should be selected according to client requirements. Strip lashes are temporary and can create a dramatic effect for a party or special occasion. They are available in natural and fantasy colours and some are decorated with jewels or diamantes. Individual lashes create a more subtle effect and are designed to blend in with the natural eyelashes to create a more defined appearance. They are available in brown or black and a variety of lengths, which should be selected to match the client's own eyelashes. A few individual lashes applied to the outer corners will help to 'open' the eyes while lashes applied across the whole upper lid will create a fuller effect. They are semi-permanent and fall out with the natural lashes.

Indications for use

- To add definition to the eyes and make the lashes appear longer and/or thicker.
- For clients whose natural eyelashes are sparse.
- As an alternative to mascara or eyelash tint in case of allergy.

- To correct the eye shape, making it appear wider and more open.
- To complete a fantasy or evening make-up.
- To enhance a natural or photographic make-up.

Safe procedure

- Patch test the eyelash adhesive 24 hours before application.
- **Practice point:** Check for diseases or disorders of the eye area which would contra-indicate application.

- *For individual lashes:*
  - cleanse the eye area with oil free cleanser
  - hold lashes with tweezers and dip bulb into adhesive
  - apply bulb as near as possible to the client's natural roots.
- **Practice point:** Check appearance frequently with client's eyes open to ensure you are achieving the desired result.

- *For strip lashes:*
  - apply adhesive to roots of strip lashes
  - place against the eyelid as close as possible to the client's lashes
  - press into place from inner to outer corner with an orange wood stick.

After care

- Apply eye make-up as normal.
- Do not use mascara as it will clog the lashes.
- Use oil-free make-up remover.
- Do not pick – have the lashes professionally removed.
- Avoid rubbing the eyes.
- Avoid saunas as the heat will melt the glue.

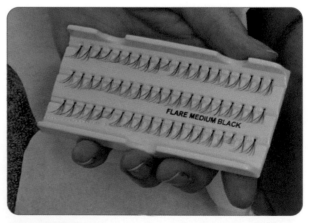

Individual lashes.

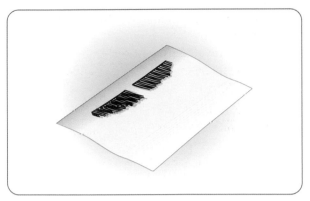

Strip lashes.

Knowledge check

1 Describe the treatment procedure for a pedicure.

2 Describe the pre-treatment preparations for a manicure.

3 What are the indications for a paraffin wax treatment?

4 Describe the main contra-indications to body waxing.

5 What are the safety procedures relating to warm wax treatment?

6 Compare and contrast warm wax with hot wax.

7 Explain the procedures for patch testing before tinting.

8 Describe the action of eyelash tint on the hair.

9 Explain the basic principles of corrective make-up.

10 What are the health and safety procedures relating to make-up application?

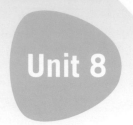

SECTION 4: PRACTICAL SKILLS IN BEAUTY THERAPY
Facial therapy

Unit 8

This unit introduces you to the knowledge and skills required to practise and apply beauty therapy treatments for the face. You will gain the theoretical knowledge associated with manual, mechanical and electrical facial therapy including revision of associated anatomy, physiology and scientific principles.

You will develop the practical skills required to apply treatment commercially, including procedures for manual cleanse and massage as well as the safe and effective use of mechanical equipment (vapour ozone, brush cleanse and vacuum suction) and electrical equipment (direct and indirect high frequency, galvanic disincrustation and iontophoresis, electrical muscle stimulation and microcurrent).

You will learn how to assess the needs of the client through accurate analysis and diagnosis of the skin and lifestyle through consultation, and will be able to offer justified home care advice and retail recommendations which are appropriate to the client and the treatment.

In order to achieve Unit 8 in Facial therapy you must complete the following learning outcomes:

LEARNING OUTCOMES

1 Describe and apply manual facial treatments.

2 Describe and apply manual facial massage.

3 Explore and apply mechanical facial treatments.

4 Investigate and apply electrical facial treatments.

Manual facial treatments

Pre-treatment preparation

Have a look at someone's face. It could be someone sitting close to you on the bus, a photograph of a friend or a picture in a magazine. It might be your own face in a mirror. What information does that face communicate to you about gender, age and ethnicity? Have another look. What other clues can you find about that person's health, lifestyle, even their job status? You could probably conjure up quite a lot of information about a person just by one fleeting glance at his or her face. Some people even believe that the face can be read, rather like the palm, and that it holds clues to a person's destiny.

What if you look even closer? What if you really analyse that face – what can it tell you about the person? As well as physical characteristics, the face can also act as a window onto the mental or psychological state of the individual. Does that face look relaxed, rushed, embarrassed, tired, stressed or elated?

The face is an incredible tool of communication between people. We can read volumes about a person's mood, state of mind and physical health from looking at his or her face, before ever starting a conversation. We can tell if the visitor at the door is a friend or a stranger, if he or she is comfortable and relaxed or shy and self-conscious. We can sense a sparkle in the eye, a flutter of the mouth or a blush, and from infancy we can learn to judge a person's emotions simply by the look on his or her face. Although our faces are roughly the same shape and size and contain similar features, every face looks different and tells a different story.

The beauty professional interested in facial therapy must learn the skills of facial analysis and diagnosis. This does not involve making superficial judgements or predictions for the future but informed decisions based on experience and detailed knowledge. In order to offer the best possible service to our clients, beauty professionals should take an holistic approach to therapy which considers the **physical** – what can be seen and touched, the **physiological** – what is happening inside the body, and the **psychological** – the mental well-being and feeling state. This begins with the consultation.

Consultation for facial therapy

A consultation is a sharing of information between the professional and the client which enables treatment to be carried out safely and effectively.

There are many environmental and lifestyle factors which affect the skin that may not be visually apparent to the professional. Exposure to environmental factors such as pollution, ultraviolet light, air conditioning and central heating should be considered as well as the client's levels of stress, smoking, alcohol and sleep. These may vary from month to month, week to week, or even from day to day, and so it is important to carry out a consultation and analysis of the client's skin prior to each and every facial treatment. In this way, the professional can monitor progress and assess any changes while making informed decisions about their causes. Consequently, the client can be best advised of the most suitable course of action on each salon visit.

Theory into practice

Some suggestions are made overleaf for areas of discussion with the client under the headings of Client Concerns, Skincare and Lifestyle. Practise preliminary facial consultations with a friend or colleague and think of what advice you would offer him or her. Can you think of any other areas for discussion?

FACIAL TREATMENT CARD

Name: Jane Mellor	D.O.B.: 26.2.1970
Address: 72 Carlton Road, Hatfield	Occupation: Teacher
Postcode: 0ZF XEJ	Doctor: Dr. Calahan
Tel. Day: 07851 623571 Evening:	Medication (The Pill, Steroids, etc.): Pill

MEDICAL HISTORY Pregnancy-birth february 2004, currently breastfeeding

Other comments:

SKIN DIAGNOSIS			Notes:
Mature ○	Dehydrated ☑	Dry ○	Previously oily skin, very dehydrated
Sensitive ○	Oily ○	Dry Patches ☑	
Normal ○	Milia ○	Dilated Capillaries ○	
Comedones ○	Moles ○	Open Pores ☑	

NECK AREA:

EYE AREA: Fine lines, milia below left eye

TREATMENT: Hydrating facial

Facial record card.

Date	Treatment(s)	Products Used	Results	Advised for Home Use	Purchased
30/5/04	Hydrating facial	Gentle exfoliator, massage oil, nourishing day cream	Clearer, more even texture	Products for skin type, 2l water daily	Serum, eye cream

Facial record card (reverse).

Possible areas of discussion prior to facial therapy:

Client concerns	Skincare	Lifestyle
Can these be addressed by looking at the client's current lifestyle?	Is this the best skincare routine for the client?	Is the client exposed to indoor pollution?
Is the client concerned about the signs of ageing?	Does the client cleanse in the evening to prevent blocked pores and/or comedones?	Air-conditioned or centrally-heated environments cause dehydration, resulting in a sallow, sluggish appearance.
Are the visible signs due to premature ageing?	Does the client cleanse in the morning to remove dust and perspiration?	Is the client exposed to outdoor pollution?
Is the client's lifestyle of sunbathing/alcohol/smoking/stress/lack of sleep a factor?	Is soap and water disturbing the pH and drying the skin?	Conditions such as wind or sunlight are damaging to the skin without adequate protection. Is the client under stress?
		Skin reacts to stress in a number of ways. Heightened sensitivity can result in skin imperfections such as eczema, rashes, allergies, acne, etc.

Skin analysis and diagnosis for facial treatment

Close examination of the skin under a magnifying lamp can tell us much about the skin's condition: the water and sebum content, the condition of superficial capillaries, the condition of the pores and the presence of furrows, lesions or superfluous hair growth. If you look at a photo of skin under ultraviolet light, any disorders are more visible. It is possible to see areas of pigmentation and blemishes, as well as oily patches and dry patches. In order to conduct an analysis and subsequent diagnosis of skin, the beauty professional requires a detailed knowledge of its structure and function. This knowledge will enable the therapist to accurately diagnose skin type and to select and prescribe the most suitable products and treatments for the client at that particular time.

When something is described as 'normal' it is often implied that it is typical, common or average. The normal facial features which the majority of humans possess are two eyes, two ears, a nose and a mouth. What about a 'normal' skin type? Is normal skin typical or average? Unfortunately, the answer is 'no'. The beauty professional who refers to a normal skin type is describing an ideal – a skin without imperfections that is healthy, glowing fresh and vibrant. In other words, a normal skin type is one that we hope to achieve through proper skin care rather than one which we automatically acquire.

Normal skin type:

Appearance	Possible causal factors	Advice
Smooth and soft to the touch	Good general health	Client should be advised how best to maintain his/her skin with regard to:
Even-textured with no areas of flaking skin or rough patches	Good **metabolism**	▸▸ lifestyle factors ▸▸ product selection and use ▸▸ type/frequency of facial therapy.
Has a healthy glow	Balanced diet which contains all the essential nutrients	
Has an even colour with no visible broken **capillaries** or **erythema**	Limited consumption of alcohol and fatty or spicy foods	
Does not appear shiny or dull and is neither too oily nor too dry	Low/managed stress levels	
Looks and feels firm, suggesting good elasticity	Correct skincare routine	
No lines or furrows	Good product choice including UV protection	
No areas of sagging or crêpey skin	Limited exposure to ultra-violet light and extremes of temperature	
Unblemished	Not smoking	
Rarely develops spots	Adequate sleep	
No visible lesions or abnormalities	Possible hereditary influences	
	Good fortune!	

Most individuals will have some idea of their own skin type and this will influence the type of cosmetic products and treatments that they buy. However, the non-professional may be ill-informed and his or her self-diagnosis is likely to be inaccurate, so the job of the beauty professional is to perform a detailed, clinical analysis and diagnosis based on a number of factors, including skin colour, texture, elasticity and general health.

An analysis is made by close examination of the skin under a magnifying lamp, by touch and by considered questioning during the consultation. Only after a thorough analysis is the professional able to make an accurate diagnosis of skin type and client needs and thus provide detailed and justified product and treatment recommendations. Information gained during pre-treatment consultation and analysis is said to inform the therapist of the **indications** for treatment.

For the purpose of beauty therapy, professionals identify four basic skin types which are determined primarily by the water and sebum content. These are:

» normal
» oily
» dry
» sensitive.

The comprehensive checklists for each skin type (on pages 181–183) include the main characteristics of each skin type to assist in the process of analysis. Combination skin is discussed on page 184. Also included are a list of possible causes for each skin type as well as basic skincare advice which should be offered to the client during facial therapy.

Sensitive skin type
Sensitive skin could be more accurately described as 'sensitised' skin because it has usually been made sensitive by other factors. These fall into three broad categories; outdoor pollution, indoor pollution and lifestyle.

Oily skin type:

Appearance	Possible causal factors	Advice
Shiny appearance	Over-production of **sebum**	Client should be given skin care advice with regard to: » likely cause of his/her skin condition » lifestyle factors » year-round UV protection » basic skincare routine should be explained, and including cleanse, tone and moisturise » specialist product choice, including exfoliation, rebalancing masks and deep cleansing » type/frequency of facial therapy
Oily to the touch	Over-secretion by the **sebaceous** glands	
Open/blocked pores	Diet may be high in fatty or 'junk' foods	
Comedones	Diet may be high in carbohydrates which are converted by the body into fat	
Tendency towards blemishes, **papules** and/or **pustules**	Incorrect skincare	
Sallow or dull appearance	Poor skin hygiene	
Tendency towards coarser texture	Medical condition/medication	
Possible **acne vulgaris** or scarring	Age-related conditions which lead to increased glandular activity, such as puberty	

Dry skin type:

Appearance	Possible causal factors	Advice
Feels taut, especially after cleansing	Under-production of sebum	Client should be given skin care advice with regard to:
Possible tendency towards sensitivity	Incorrect skincare	▸ likely cause of his/her skin condition
May appear dull and/or sallow and lack a healthy glow	Over-use of alkaline substances and astringents – such as soap or facial scrubs	▸ lifestyle factors ▸ year-round UV protection ▸ basic skincare routine should be explained, including cleanser, tone and moisturise
Uneven colour/possible erythema	Insufficient nourishment from under-use or wrong choice of moisturiser	▸ specialist product choice, including exfoliation, rebalancing masks and deep cleansing
Uneven texture with rough or flaky patches	Over-exposure to sunlight	▸ type/frequency of facial therapy
Possible dandruff in the eyebrows	Over-exposure to central heating or air conditioning	
Possible **milia**	Poor diet	
Appearance of premature lines and wrinkles	Low water intake	
	Illness/medication	
	Stress	
	Smoking	

Sensitive skin:

Appearance	Possible causal factors	Advice
Often dry/flaking	Outdoor pollution	Client should be given skin care advice with regard to:
Uneven texture	UV/sun damage	▸ likely cause of his/her skin condition
Erythema	Traffic fumes, smoke	▸ lifestyle factors including year-round UV protection
Reactive to temperature, products and/or touch	Indoor pollution: central heating, air conditioning	▸ specialist product choice, including minimal exfoliation, and soothing masks
May be allergic to products	Lifestyle: smoking, stress alcohol, drugs, illness	

Combination skin type

A combination skin type will display a combination of characteristics in different areas. It is not an 'in-between' skin type, for example, normal *to* oily, but rather a combination of skin types, for example, normal *and* oily. The most typical example of a combination skin type will display an oily 'T-zone', i.e. oily forehead, nose and chin with dry cheeks.

Possible causal factors will be as for the individual skin types.

As far as possible, different areas of skin should be treated according to their skin type. Always choose products which will not exasperate either condition.

Contra-indications to facial therapy

In addition to the generic considerations, there are a number of non-treatable conditions which are specific to manual facial therapy. Some are localised disorders which should be avoided even though the treatment may proceed.

Technical Procedure

Preparation

Prepare yourself and your work area before your client arrives. All tools and equipment should be sterilised or sanitised according to professional guidelines. You should obtain the client's record card from your file or have a new one ready to fill in.

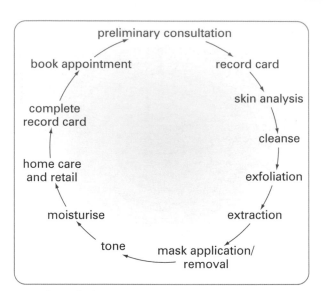

Procedure clock.

Your couch should be made up with towels and/or blankets and your trolley should be neatly presented with the consumable and semi-consumable stock you need for manual facial treatment.

Stock for manual facial treatment:

Consumables	Semi/non-consumables
Facial products for all skin types	Large towels/blanket
Mask ingredients	Small hand towel
Tissues	Headband/turban
Damp and dry cotton wool	Spatula
Couch roll	Mask brush
Sponges/wash cloths	Equipment

Cleansing

A step-by-step cleansing routine is shown overleaf.

Extraction

Extraction is the term used to describe a professional technique for the removal of comedones. The skin should be prepared for extraction by cleansing and/or by mechanical techniques. The safest way to extract comedones is to use a metal extractor which will have been correctly sterilised prior to use.

A step-by-step cleansing routine:

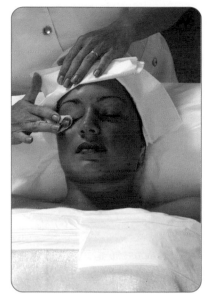

1 Apply eye make-up remover.

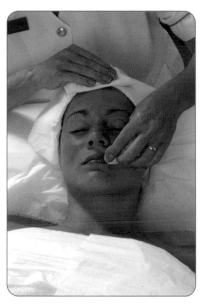

2 Using cotton wool, remove lipstick.

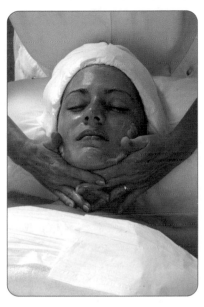

3 Using upward movements from the jaw, cleanse the face.

If this is not available, you can use tissues to cover the fingertips and apply gentle pressure around the comedone until it wriggles free. Whichever method is used, you should avoid squeezing or applying too mush pressure as this can cause bleeding and/or facial scarring. Because you will come into contact with body fluids, sebum and/or blood, you should wear disposable gloves to protect yourself and your client from cross-infection.

Post-treatment
After the treatment it is important to record the effects of any products or equipment you have used, how the skin has reacted and the reaction of the client. Also make a note of the home care advice and retail recommendations you have offered. Try not to be too ambitious here; if you offer the client a couple of retail items he or she is more likely to purchase them than if you recommend an entire range. You can always give samples of the other products but never use samples in place of retailing: the idea is to try *before* you buy – not instead of. Also discuss with your client the benefits of having regular facial treatments and aim to book follow-up appointments for every client before he or she leaves the salon. Most skins will benefit from a facial once a month but over-stimulation or under-stimulation brought about by the incorrect frequency of facial therapy can be counter-productive.

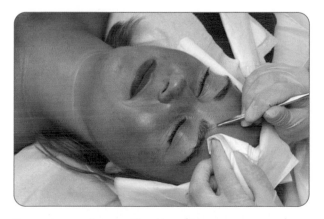

Extraction – using sterilised metal extractor.

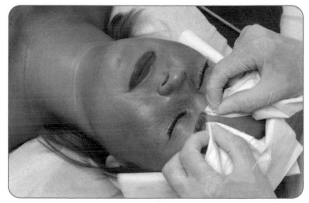

Applying gentle pressure to ease out comedone.

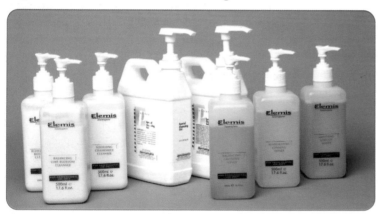

Theory into practice

Try role-playing the end of a treatment. How easy is it to sell a range of products to a client? Practise some retailing techniques to improve your confidence.

Product knowledge

Cleansers

Cleansing products contain ingredients that form an emulsion with oily substances and so dissolve make-up and sebum on the surface of skin, which can then be removed with tissues or cotton wool. Cleansers are alkaline substances so the use of harsh cleansers, such as soap and water, or the use of an incorrect cleanser for the skin type, can disturb the acid mantle and leave skin prone to blemishes and bacterial infection. All cleansing products contain **active ingredients** dissolved in water which enables the product to spread on the skin. Most products also contain preservatives which extend the shelf life, as well as colours and fragrances. Cream cleansers have a higher oil/water content and are therefore suitable for dry or mature skins, while cleansing lotions and wash-off cleansers have a higher water/oil content and are better for more oily skins. It is important to select the correct product for skin type to be used in the facial treatment as well as for home care.

Toners

Toners are used to remove any traces of dirt, sebum or make-up left behind after cleansing and also to rebalance the pH of skin. Toners have astringent properties which help to shrink pore size and some may contain alcohol which makes their effect more astringent. They also contain **humectants**, which attract moisture to the skin and prevent loss of water through evaporation. Toners designed for use on dry or sensitive skins also contain ingredients which help to cool and soothe.

Exfoliants

Exfoliants are abrasive cleansing products which are used to aid **desquamation** and improve the skin's texture. They are stimulating to the circulation and so encourage cell renewal. While mild erythema is

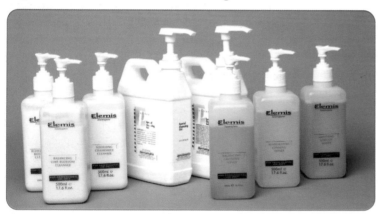

Different cleansing products.

Facial cleansing products:

Cleansers	Active ingredients	Method of use	Skin type
Cleansing cream	Mineral oil, e.g. paraffin wax	Apply with fingers, remove with damp cotton wool	Dry, mature
Cleansing lotion	Mineral oil, e.g. beeswax detergent	Damp cotton wool	Normal, oily, combination
Face wash/gel	Detergents, foaming agents	Apply with fingers, rinse with water	Oily, combination, young
Facial wipes	Detergent	Wipe over skin	Removal of superficial make-up only

Toning products:

Toners	Active ingredients	Method of use	Skin type
Low alcohol toner	Chamomile, azulene	Damp cotton wool	Sensitive
Mid-alcohol toner	Rose water, orange blossom	Damp cotton wool	Dry, normal
High alcohol toner	Witch hazel, allum	Dry cotton wool	Oily

Exfoliating products:

Exfoliant	Active ingredients	Method of use
Face scrub	Detergent, pumice, ground fruit stones, oatmeal	Massage over damp skin, remove with water
Mechanical peel	Clay-based cleansing agents	Apply thin layer, leave to dry, friction off with dry hands
Fruit acid peel	Alpha hydroxy acid (AHA)	As lotion or mask

likely on dry or sensitive skins, over-use can cause dehydration and **hyperaemia**. While most skins will benefit from the weekly use of an exfoliating product, the type and frequency of use should be adapted according to skin type, with sensitive skins requiring less frequent application than oily skins. The quality of ingredients used in facial scrubs can be dramatically altered by the cost of the product, with cheaper brands using crushed fruit stones or pumice which can be too harsh for use on more sensitive skins. Other manufacturers use detergent chips, pearlised particles or oil encapsulated in synthetic beads, which dissolve on the skin. There are also a number of mechanical and chemical peels available for salon and home use.

Moisturisers

Moisturisers are oil and water emulsions which attract water to the skin and prevent moisture loss by evaporation. They also act as a protective barrier against pollution and many contain UV sunscreens. Moisturisers described as 'day creams' are a lighter formulation than those designed to be used as 'night creams'. Moisturisers should be used by all skin types (even oily) to protect, nourish and even out texture and/or to provide a base for make-up. They should be applied with clean hands to a cleansed face and neck, avoiding the delicate eye area. Specialist eye creams or balms should be used to add moisture and protect the eye area, and some clients also prefer to use a separate neck cream which may contain richer products. Tinted formulation can be used in place of a foundation, to cover minor blemishes.

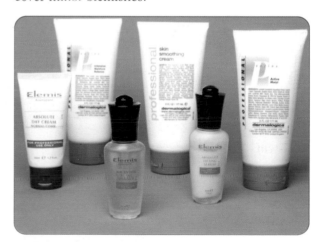

Different moisturising products.

Details of different types of moisturising products are given in the table overleaf.

Moisturising products:

Moisturiser	Active ingredient	Skin type
Cream: 40% oil, 60% water	Oil, e.g. paraffin or jojoba; humectant, e.g. glycerine, collagen/elastin, anti-oxidant vitamins A,C,E	Dry, mature, skin requiring protection
Lotion: 15% oil, 85% water	Oils, humectant, vitamins	Dry, base for make-up
Neck cream	Vitamin E, collagen, elastin	All skins
Eye cream	Oils, collagen, vitamins; chamomile to soothe	Cream – dry, mature; balm – oily, normal

Face masks

Face masks have different functions depending on their formulation and can therefore be used to treat a range of skin types and conditions. They can be applied with a brush or fingers to clean skin at the end of a facial treatment or as maintenance between salon visits. You should use and retail the most appropriate mask for your client and be able to explain its actions, main active ingredients and methods of application and removal. Mask therapy can be divided into three categories: setting, non-setting and specialised.

Setting masks

Setting masks are clay based. They have a deep cleansing action which absorbs excess sebum and sweat and aids desquamation. Setting masks are prepared in the salon by combining active powders in equal parts with active liquid ingredients to form a soft paste. They are applied with a brush to the face and neck, avoiding the delicate eye area, and should be removed with a warm compress after 10 minutes, making sure that no powdery traces of product are left on the skin.

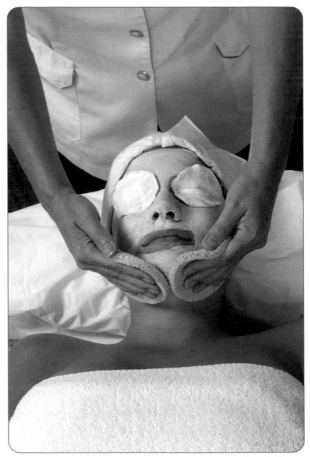

Removing a face mask.

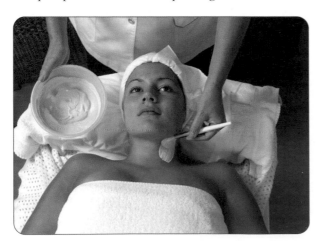

Face mask application.

Masks and skin types:

Skin type	Active ingredients
Normal	Kaolin & fullers earth + witch hazel
Dry	Kaolin & magnesium carbonate + rose water/orange flower water or almond oil
Oily	Fullers earth + witch hazel
Sensitive	Calamine & magnesium carbonate + rose water
Mature, dehydrated	Calamine & magnesium carbonate + almond oil
Acne, excess oiliness, seborrhea	Sulphur, oatmeal & magnesium carbonate + warm water

Mask ingredients – powder:

Powder ingredient	Characteristics	Effects
Calamine	Fine pink powder	Calming, soothing, reduces erythema
Magnesium carbonate	White powder	Mild astringent, used as a bulking agent
Kaolin	Dirty white powder	Deep cleansing
Fullers earth	Greenish powder	Stimulates circulation, deep cleansing, can cause erythema
Sulphur	Yellow powder	Reduces sebaceous activity, dissolves surface sebum

Non-setting masks

Non-setting masks form a thin film over the skin which remains flexible when dry. Unlike setting masks, they do not alter the moisture content of the skin. Professional non-setting masks contain natural ingredients used to treat a variety of skin conditions. Non-setting masks can also be made at home using fresh kitchen ingredients. They are applied using fingers or a brush and left for 10–15 minutes. Masks are then peeled or rinsed off with warm water.

Mask ingredients – liquid:

Liquid ingredient	Action
Distilled water	None
Rose water	Very gentle toning
Orange flower water	Mild astringent
Almond oil	Nourishing, humectant
Witch hazel	Stimulating astringent, drying action

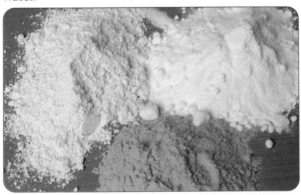

Face mask ingredients – powder.

Non-setting masks:

Type of mask	Active ingredients	Action
Biological	Honey, egg white, egg yolk, natural yogurt	Refining, nourishing
Fruit extract	Crushed avocado,	Re-balancing
Vegetable	Cucumber, oatmeal	Astringent

Specialised masks

Specialist masks commonly used in beauty therapy, which use heat to enhance their actions, are paraffin wax masks and warm oil masks. Some product ranges also include self-heating thermal masks which should be used according to manufacturer's instructions. Specialised masks can be used to treat a variety of skin types. Extra precautions should be taken to check for any contra-indications to specialist mask therapy before use.

Paraffin wax mask

Paraffin wax can be used to treat all areas of the body but is most commonly applied to face, hands and feet. At room temperature, paraffin wax is a solid form of petroleum jelly which is heated to a working temperature of 49°C in a special heater. It is applied to the face over gauze and left to work for 10–15 minutes, until it starts to cool.

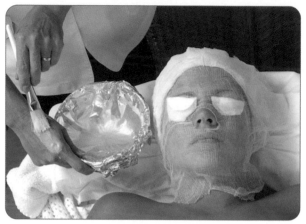

Checking the temperature of paraffin wax prior to its application over gauze.

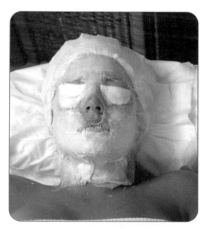

Paraffin wax face mask in place.

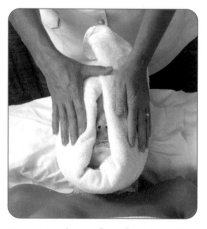

Warm towel over face for up to 15 minutes.

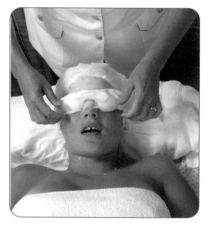

Removing the face mask.

Indications, actions and contra-indications of paraffin wax masks:

Indications	Actions	Contra-indications
▶ dry, dehydrated skin	▶ stimulating, rebalancing	▶ claustrophobia
▶ mature skin	▶ regenerating, cell renewal	▶ vascular conditions
▶ uneven skin texture	▶ desquamating, deep cleansing	▶ infection, irritation
▶ seborrhoea	▶ desquamating, deep cleansing, remove surface adhesions, remove skin blockages	▶ nervous, tense client

Warm oil mask

Warm oil masks are suitable for dry, dehydrated and mature skins. They combine the nourishing effects of the product with the penetrative effects of radiant heat. Gauze is soaked in warm vegetable oil such as almond or grapeseed and then placed over the face, making sure that the eyes are protected and breathe holes are not obstructed. An infrared lamp is positioned for 10–15 minutes to aid absorption of the oil, after which time the remainder of the oil, can be massaged into the skin.

> **Assessment** task 8.2
>
> Design a prescription card which includes suitable skincare products for dry, normal, oily and sensitive skin types. For each type you should include day and night care products, treatment masks and suitable massage mediums. (M)

Manual facial massage

Facial massage techniques

Facial massage is the most enjoyable part of facial therapy for most clients. When performed correctly, it is extremely relaxing and can benefit the client in a number of ways. There are four classical massage movements which are adapted to suit the face. These are **effleurage**, **petrissage**, **tapotement** and **vibrations**. Different movements have different effects which can be either relaxing or stimulating. Effleurage movements are used to start and finish a routine and for linking. They can be either deep or superficial. Petrissage movements are more stimulating. They are rhythmic movements used over relaxed areas of muscle bulk to reduce tension. Tapotement movements are light, brisk and

stimulating and are used on fleshy areas, never over bone. Vibrations provide gentle stimulation for more sensitive skins. Facial massage should take about 15–20 minutes of the one hour treatment time.

Effects of facial massage

These effects can include the following:

- client relaxation
- stimulates blood circulation
- transport of oxygen and nutrients to skin and removal of carbon dioxide and waste
- localised heat in tissues aids the absorption of products
- stimulates desquamation
- retention of moisture in collagen and elastin fibres improves elasticity
- improved muscle tone
- improved lymphatic drainage reduces local puffiness.

Step-by-step facial massage procedure

Repeat each movement three times; images of some of the techniques are shown overleaf.

1 Prayer movement effleurage up the neck and around the jaw line to finish at the base of the ear.

2 Supporting left side of the neck, effleurage neck from left to right, then repeat to the other side.

3 Knuckling up the sides of the neck and across the jaw using both hands.

4 Supporting left side of neck, palmar vibrations across the neck from left to right, then repeat to the other side.

5 Supporting head, effleurage across the jaw line from left to right, then repeat to the other side.

6 Tapotement under the chin and across the jaw line.

Facial massage movements:

Effleurage	Petrissage	Tapotement	Vibration
finger stroking	knuckling	percussion	shaking.
palmar stroking	compression	tapping	
prayer movement.	finger kneading	light pinching.	
	deep pinching		
	scissoring		
	wringing.		

Facial massage movements (cont.):

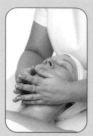
1 Prayer movement effleurage.

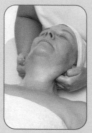
3 Knuckling to the sides of the neck.

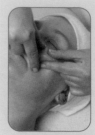
8 Finger kneading to the cheeks.

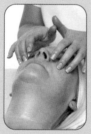
12 Ring finger kneading around the nose.

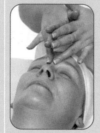
14 Supporting the left side of the head, small finger circles at the temple and stroking under the eye.

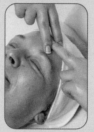
16 Ironing movement across the forehead.

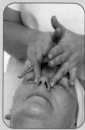
18 Tapotement to the face.

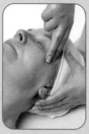
20 Ring finger stroking up centre of the face.

7 Finger kneading across the chin and jaw line.

8 Finger kneading to cheek muscle.

9 Prayer effleurage across jaw line.

10 Prayer effleurage across cheeks.

11 Ring finger kneading around the mouth.

12 Ring finger kneading around the nose.

13 Ring finger kneading around the eyes.

14 Supporting left side of the head, three small finger circles at the left temple and stroking under the eye; repeat to the other side.

15 Finger kneading across the forehead.

16 Ironing movement across the forehead.

17 Effleurage across forehead with and without vibrations.

18 Light tapotement to the whole face.

19 Prayer effleurage across neck, face and forehead.

20 Ring finger stroking up centre of the face to finish.

Product knowledge

Massage medium is chosen according to skin type. Most clients (and therapists) prefer to use a massage cream as it provides a good level of slip. You should not be concerned about using creams on normal and combination skins as they will only absorb the required amount of moisture. However, very oily skins and some male clients might prefer the use of an ampoule which has a lighter texture. Extremely dry and/or mature skin might benefit from massage with oil, possibly in conjunction with a warm oil mask treatment.

Manual massage is often the most enjoyable part of the facial treatment. Describe the additional benefits of facial massage in a way that clients would understand. (M)

Mechanical facial treatment

Manual facial treatments are relaxing both for the client and for the practitioner and can produce significant skin enhancing results if performed regularly. Mechanical facial equipment can be used to further enhance the effects of manual techniques. In this section you will learn the skills necessary to administer vapour, mechanical exfoliation and mechanical lymph drainage. Because mechanical treatments are used as well as not instead of manual facial treatments, pre-treatment preparation should be carried out as before. There are some additional contra-indications to be considered for mechanical work and, because of the particular benefits of each piece of equipment, you also need to familiarise yourself with the specific indications for use.

Vapour

The steamer remains one of the most popular pieces of mechanical equipment to be used by beauty therapists as it can benefit all, except very sensitive skin types. It works by heating distilled water in a large 'kettle' to produce water vapour which is applied directly to the skin. Some steamers also produce **vapour ozone** by passing oxygen from the steam over an ultraviolet bulb, which has an anti-bacterial effect. Guidelines provided by local government departments and examining bodies means that the use of ozone has become tightly regulated and in some areas is prohibited due to the minor risk of respiratory problems. Your tutor will be able to advise you on local legislation for the safe use of vapour ozone.

Vapour treatments:

Indications for use	Recommended timing	Benefits and effects
Tight, blocked pores	15 minutes	Heat causes pores to relax and encourages sweating to deep cleanse
Comedones	15 minutes	Become softer and easier to extract after steaming
Dry, flaky skin	10 minutes	Increased circulation aids desquamation
Dry, dehydrated skin	10 minutes	Sebaceous glands are stimulated
Dull, sallow skin	10 minutes	Desquamation, increased circulation, erythema
Dry, mature	5 minutes	Increased circulation stimulates cell renewal
All clients		Warmth aids relaxation as well as the absorption of products that are later applied

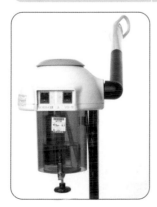

Steamer.

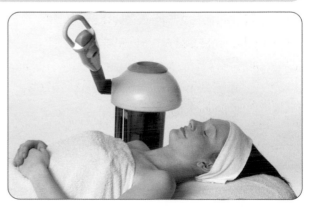

Steamer in use.

Any infectious skin conditions will flourish in moist conditions and so contra-indicate treatment with vapour. What other conditions do you think should be avoided?

Safe starting

» Prepare the work area and client. Check for contra-indications to vapour.
» Make sure the machine is stable with no trailing wires.
» Check the water level and top up with distilled water only.
» Ensure the nozzle is pointing away from client and turn on to heat the water.
» Check that the machine is working.
» Practice point: Do not use tap water in steamers as this will cause them to spit.

Safe working

» Explain the treatment effects and sensation to the client.
» Cover the client's eyes with damp cotton pads and protect his or her hair with a towel.
» Position the machine 30–40 cm away and direct the nozzle onto the client's face.
» Stay with your client throughout to monitor his or her comfort.
» Do not exceed the treatment time (see table on page 193).
» Practice point: Stay close to the client in case he or she feels claustrophobic. Remove the steamer at once if it becomes uncomfortable for him or her.

Safe stopping

» Move vapour nozzle away from client before switching off, to avoid spitting.
» Switch off at mains socket and return machine to storage area with leads neatly wrapped.

» Blot skin dry with tissue and continue with facial procedure.

Mechanical exfoliation

Exfoliation can be performed in a number of ways. Brush cleansing can be incorporated into a facial treatment as a mechanical method of exfoliation to increase the circulation and assist the natural process of desquamation.

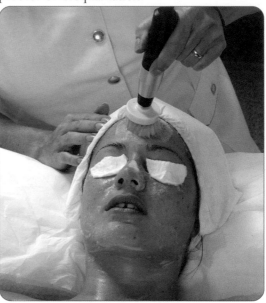

Brush cleanser in use.

Contra-indications to mechanical exfoliation:

» sensitive skin
» skin infections
» pustular acne
» eczema/psoriasis/dermatitis
» vascular conditions.

Safe starting

» Make sure all brushes are sanitised prior to use.
» Prepare the work area and client. Check for contra-indications to brush cleansing.
» Test machine by holding away from the client and turning on.

Brush cleansing:

Indications for use	Recommended timing	Benefits and effects
Tight, blocked pores	8–10 minutes	Deep cleansing
Comedones	8–10 minutes	Softens and loosens to aid extraction
Dry, flaky skin	5–10 minutes	Aids desquamation
Dull, sluggish skin	5–10 minutes	Increases circulation, produces erythema

Safe working

▸ Explain the treatment effects and sensation to the client.

▸ Apply appropriate product, e.g. foaming cleanser or facial scrub, to create slip.

▸ Keep the brush parallel to the skin and cover the area in small circular motions.

▸ Use an appropriate brush size for the area.

Do not overstimulate the skin (see treatment timings on page 194).

▸ **Practice point:** Avoid delicate eye area and hairline to prevent discomfort to the client.

Safe stopping

▸ Remove brush from skin and switch off.

▸ Wash and sanitise brushes and leave to dry.

▸ Wipe down machine and store neatly.

▸ Remove all the product from your client's skin with damp sponges and continue with facial procedure.

▸ **Practice point:** Brushes should be washed with hot soapy water and can be sanitised in a solution, such as Milton, between use.

Assessment task 8.4

Evaluate the use of brush cleanse and vapour treatments with reference to health and safety procedures, contra-indications and indications to use. (D)

Mechanical lymphatic drainage

The lymphatic system carries waste products to drainage points which enables them to be secreted. A sluggish lymphatic system can lead to the build up of toxins, swelling and medical oedema. Vacuum suction is a mechanical method of increasing the flow of lymph towards the drainage points, which enhances manual massage and mirrors natural lymph flow.

Contra-indications to vacuum suction:

▸ loose, crêpy skin

▸ hypersensitivity

▸ undiagnosed swellings

▸ high/low blood pressure

▸ skin infections

▸ pustular acne

▸ recent scar tissue

▸ dilated capillaries

▸ bruises.

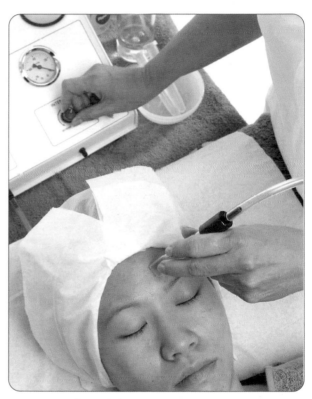

Vacuum suction unit in use.

Vacuum suction:

Indications for use	Effects and benefits
General cleansing for normal, dry, oily and combination skins	Speeds up removal of waste and circulation of essential nutrients
Deep cleansing for seborrhoeic skin	Loosens comedones for extraction
Improvement of dry, dehydrated skin	Aids desquamation, increases circulation of blood and nutrients to skin, stimulates sweat and sebaceous activity
Improvement of mature skin	Stimulates cell metabolism, temporarily puffs out fine lines and wrinkles

Safe starting

» Make sure that the venteuses are clean and dry before use.

» Prepare the work area and client. Check for contra-indications to vacuum suction.

» Make sure the machine is stable with no trailing wires.

» Turn all dials to zero before switching on.

» Test machine on yourself to make sure it is working.

» **Practice point:** Make sure the venteuses are not cracked or damaged as this will break the vacuum and may scratch the client.

Safe working

1 Explain the treatment effects and sensation to the client.

2 Use sufficient product to prevent dragging.

3 Use the correct size venteuse for the area.

4 Check the intensity at the forehead and adjust as necessary.

5 Use gentle gliding movements in direction of the lymph to the nearest lymph nodes.

6 Use 6 to 8 strokes depending on the skin's reaction, then move on half the width of the venteuse.

7 Full face should take 10 minutes. Do not over-stimulate.

» **Practice point:** Never allow the venteuse to become more than one-third full.

  - Always break the vacuum before removing venteuse from the skin to avoid bruising.

  - Glass attachments can be sterilised in Barbicide or Milton solution.

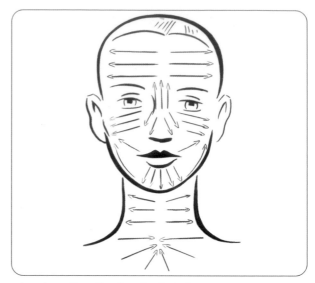

Direction of application for facial vacuum suction.

Safe stopping

» Turn all dials to zero.

» Wash venteuses with hot soapy water.

» Wipe down machine and return to storage.

» Remove product from face and continue with facial treatment.

Theory into practice

Using the information on indications for and effects of mechanical treatments, prepare a facial treatment plan for each of the following skin types, to include manual cleanse, at least two mechanical treatments, massage, mask and moisturise:

(a) dry/dehydrated
(b) oily with comedones
(c) sensitive
(d) mature

What home care advice and retail recommendations would you offer each client?

Assessment task 8.5

Explain how you would combine the benefits of manual and mechanical facial treatments. Design a suitable treatment for Emma (Assessment task 8.1 on page 184) with reference to skin type, timing and frequency. (D)

Assessment task 8.6

Provide detailed and justified home care advice and retail recommendations for Emma. (D)

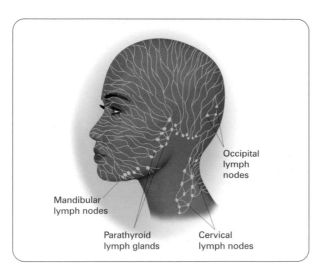

Occipital lymph nodes

Mandibular lymph nodes

Parathyroid lymph glands

Cervical lymph nodes

Lymph nodes of head and neck.

Electrical facial treatments

Mechanical facial treatments tend to mimic natural physiological processes and/or manual techniques, for example, mechanical exfoliation to aid desquamation, mechanical lymph drainage to aid lymph flow, and vapour to stimulate circulation. However, the electrical equipment used in facial therapy, or **electrotherapy**, tends to be more specialised and involves highly specialist scientific principles. In this section you will learn the underpinning theory and skills necessary to administer high frequency treatments, galvanic treatments, electrical muscle stimulation and microcurrent. In order to understand fully how the equipment works and how to use it safely, you should revisit the section on electricity in Unit 1, pages 24–6.

Contra-indications to direct and indirect high frequency:

- skin infections
- epilepsy
- sunburn/windburn
- pregnancy (indirect high frequency)
- pustular acne
- nervousness
- asthma
- excessive number of fillings.

High frequency treatment

The high frequency machine uses an alternating (ac) electrical current at a high frequency of 200,000–250,000 hertz. A small flow of current passes from the equipment via a wire to an insulated handle which holds a glass **electrode**. The effects of the current are local to the point of contact of the electrode to the skin and so are relatively superficial compared to other pieces of electrical equipment. There are a number of different electrodes available for use in electrotherapy, to be used for different areas of the face, head and body.

There are two methods of applying high frequency to the client: direct and indirect. Both have the effect of increasing circulation, bringing essential nutrients to the skin and aiding the removal of waste products. The skin feels warm, assisting the absorption of products, and an erythema will be visible. As well as these general effects, a soothing or stimulating effect can be achieved depending on the method used.

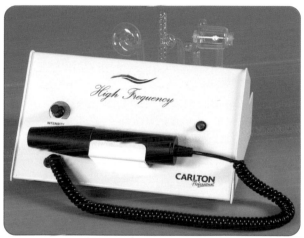

High frequency machine.

High frequency treatments:

Indication for use	Application	Timing	Physiological effects
Oily, acne skin	Direct HF using mushroom electrode over talc or gauze	5–15 minutes depending on skin condition and reaction to treatment	Aids desquamation, has a drying effect, is mildly germicidal
Papules, pustules	Sparking with mushroom electrode	3–5 minutes	Increased local effects, germicidal, aids healing
Dry/mature skin	Indirect HF applied via manual massage	5–15 minutes depending on reaction to treatment	Stimulation of sweat and sebaceous glands
Fine lines	Sparking using manual tapotement	3–5 minutes	Immediate temporary removal of fine lines
Scar tissue	Indirect method	Within treatment	Aids healing

Technique for indirect high frequency

Safe starting

- ▸ Prepare work area and client and remove client's jewellery.
- ▸ Check for contra-indications.
- ▸ Make sure machine is stable with no trailing wires.

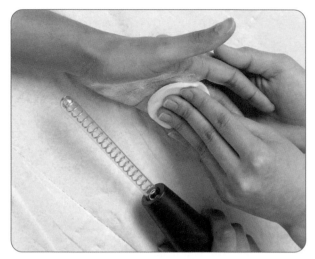

Attach saturator electrode to insulated holder and give to client to hold.

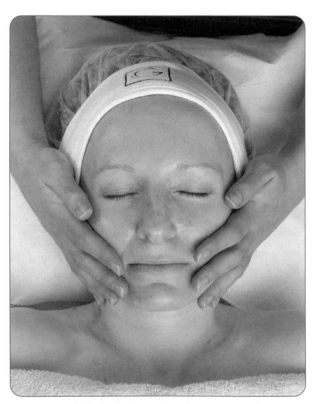

Treatment with indirect high frequency.

- ▸ Test the machine on yourself.
- ▸ Check intensity dials are at zero.
- ▸ Cleanse skin thoroughly but do not tone.
- ▸ Attach saturator electrode to insulated holder and give to client to hold.
- ▸ Apply sufficient massage cream to face and neck.
- ▸ **Practice point:**
  - Make sure that the saturator electrode is not in contact with any body piercings or metal fasteners.
  - Maintain a comfortable position with feet firmly on the floor – not on metal frames of stool or couch, which would divert the current.

Safe working

- ▸ **Practice point:** Superficial movements are more stimulating than deep movements.

1. Explain sensation and effects of indirect high frequency to your client.
2. With one hand make contact with the client's forehead.
3. With the other hand gradually increase current intensity until you can both feel a slight tingling sensation.
4. Apply facial massage routine for recommended time according to skin type.
5. Maintain contact at all times and reduce current over bony areas.
6. To treat fine lines, use horizontal tapotement movements.
7. Monitor skin's reaction and cease treatment if it becomes uncomfortable or sensitised.

Safe stopping

- ▸ Bring hands back to forehead to finish.
- ▸ With one hand in contact, gradually turn down intensity to zero and switch off machine.
- ▸ Remove electrode from holder, sanitise and put away.
- ▸ Continue with the facial treatment.

Theory into practice

Why do you think that pregnancy is a contra-indication to the indirect method of application but not the direct method?

Technique for direct high frequency

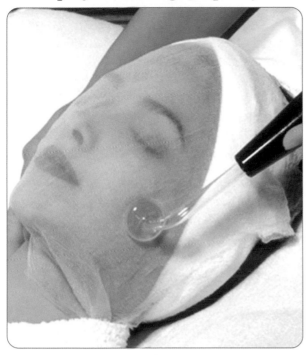

Treatment with direct high frequency.

Safe starting
- Prepare work area and client and remove client's jewellery.
- Check for contra-indications.
- Make sure machine is stable with no trailing wires.
- Test the machine on yourself.
- Check intensity dials are at zero.
- Cleanse skin thoroughly but do not tone.
- Apply gauze or talc to the face (your tutor will advise you about this).
- Attach the mushroom electrode to the insulated holder.
- **Practice point:** One hand holds the electrode; place the other hand flat on the couch or use it to hold the cable away from the client.

Safe working
1. Explain the sensation and effects of direct high frequency to your client.
2. Place the electrode on the client's forehead and increase the intensity slowly until he or she feels a comfortable tingling sensation.
3. Using small circular movements, cover the face, neck and decolletage area according to the recommended treatment times for skin type.
4. To treat papules and pustules, use 'sparking' technique.
5. Monitor the skin's reaction and cease treatment if it becomes uncomfortable or sensitised.

- **Practice point:**
  - Avoid 'sparking' around the delicate eye and lip areas.
  - Keep the electrode in even contact with the skin to prevent unwanted 'sparking'.

Safe stopping
- Finish with electrode on forehead.
- Gradually turn down intensity to zero and switch off machine.
- Remove electrode from holder, sanitise and put away.
- Continue with the facial treatment

Assessment task 8.7

Describe in detail the use of direct and indirect high frequency with reference to benefits, techniques and health and safety. (M)

Galvanic treatment

Before you start this section, I would like to acknowledge the fact that most students (and some lecturers!) struggle at first with the underpinning science of galvanic treatment. My advice is to take it slowly, refer to the appropriate sections in the Scientific Principles section (Unit 1) and use the summary tables and glossary to help you. It will all make sense – eventually!

The galvanic unit uses direct current (dc) which produces a chemical change in the tissues by reacting with sodium chloride (salt). Galvanic treatment requires two electrodes in order to make a complete circuit. The inactive electrode is held by the client while the active electrode is applied to the skin by the therapist. Polarity of the electrodes is determined by a switch on the galvanic unit which can be positioned at positive (+) or negative (−). The positively charged electrode is called the **anode** and the negatively charged electrode is called the **cathode**. Note that the active electrode can be

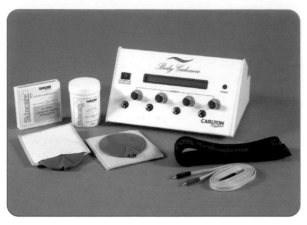

Galvanic unit.

positive or negative, i.e. the anode or the cathode. Many students mistakenly think of positive/negative as synonymous with active/inactive, until they fully comprehend the scientific principle of galvanism.

You should refer to the manufacturer's instructions and the polarity of product for directions on polarity of active electrodes.

There are two methods of galvanic application to the face. **Disincrustation** is a deep cleansing treatment and **iontophoresis** is used for the application of specialist treatment products.

Contra-indications to disincrustation and iontophoresis:

- lack of skin sensitivity
- metal pins, plates or excess fillings
- highly nervous client
- pustular acne
- cuts or abrasions
- hypersensitive skin, acne rosacea
- low blood pressure
- first three months of pregnancy.

Galvanic treatment:

Indications for use	Method	Effects	Timing
Oily skin	Disincrustation (-)ive	Deep cleansing	5–10 mins
Congested, sluggish skin	Disincrustation	Stimulating, cleansing, softening of comedones	5–10 mins (-)ive, then 2–5 mins (+)ive after extraction
Combination skin	Disincrustation (-)ive	General cleansing	5–10 mins
Dry, dehydrated skin	Iontophoresis	According to product	10–15 mins
Sensitive skin	Iontophoresis	According to product	8–10 mins depending on skin reaction
Mature skin	Iontophoresis	According to product	10–15 mins

Safety precautions for galvanic treatment:

Pre-treatment precautions	Post-treatment precautions
▸ Make sure unit is stable with no trailing wires	▸ Avoid massage on treated areas
▸ Remove all jewellery	▸ Avoid drying or stimulating face masks
▸ Test the machine on yourself first	▸ Use non-setting cream masks to soothe
▸ Make sure all dials are set at zero	
▸ Check polarity of machine	

Disincrustation

Disincrustation, which is sometimes referred to as **electrophoresis**, is used as a deep cleansing treatment for oily, congested or combination skin types. It works by passing a direct current through an **electrolyte**, such as saline solution, on and within skin tissue. Electrolytes are electrically charged atoms which contain (+)ive and (-)ive **ions** that move around freely in the solution. Positively charged ions are called **cations** and negatively charged ions are called **anions**. When direct current is applied via the anode and cathode, the ions will move away from one electrode and towards the other. This is because similar charges repel each other (like two magnets) and opposite charges attract. In disincrustation treatment, the negative cathode (-) is the active electrode and the positive anode (+) is the inactive electrode.

▸▸ **Practice point:** (+)ive cations move towards the (-)ive cathode; (-)ive anions move towards the (+)ive anode.

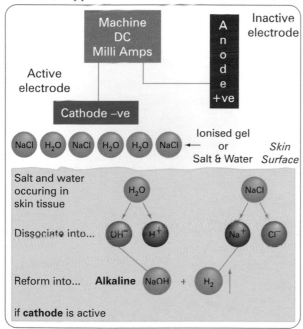

The action of galvanic current on saline solution.

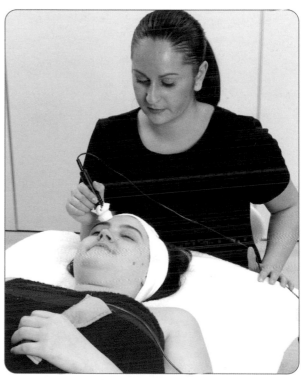

Treatment with galvanic disincrustation.

Disincrustation – polar effects:

Polar effects at the (-) cathode:	Polar effects at the (+) anode when polarity is reversed:
▸▸ alkali NaOH is formed which saponifies sebum, softens skin and breaks down keratin	▸▸ formation of HCl acid
▸▸ vasodilation and erythema improves appearance of sluggish skin	▸▸ slight vasodilation and erythema
▸▸ increased circulation brings nutrients to surface and aids removal of waste	▸▸ HCl has a firming effect and refines pores after cleansing and extraction
▸▸ increased metabolism stimulates cell renewal	▸▸ release of O_2 has a revitalising and nourishing effect
▸▸ fluid drawn towards (-) cathode has temporary hydrating effect	▸▸ fluid moves away from the anode (+)
▸▸ NaOH alters skin's pH and destroys acid mantle.	▸▸ HCl restores the acid mantle and increases the skin's resistance to infection.

Technique for disincrustation

↦ **Practice point:** cathode is active electrode.

Safe starting

↦ Check for contra-indications.

↦ Explain sensation and effects of disincrustation to your client (-)ive cathode is active.

↦ Prepare disc-shaped electrode by securely wrapping it with several layers of damp lint.

↦ Prepare the inactive electrode by securely wrapping it with moist lint/cotton wool.

Safe working

1 Cleanse the client's skin and moisten with saline solution or disincrustation gel.

2 Place cathode on the client's forehead and gradually turn up the intensity to suit his/her level of tolerance (usually between 0.5 and 2.0 milli amps).

↦ **Practice point:** Concentrate on areas of congestion but avoid pustules because the current will feel more intense.

3 Using small circular movements, cover the face and neck.

4 Treatment time is 5 to 10 minutes depending on skin type and tolerance.

5 Gradually reduce intensity and turn off.

6 Wipe over face with damp cotton wool and proceed with extraction of comedones.

7 Reverse polarity by switching machine to (+)ive.

8 Apply for 2–5 minutes depending on skin's reaction.

↦ **Practice point:** Polarity is reversed in order to restore acid mantle.

Safe stopping

↦ Finish with electrode on forehead, gradually reduce intensity and switch off machine.

↦ Dispose of lint/cotton wool and put away electrodes and machine neatly.

↦ Wipe over skin with damp cotton wool to remove product.

↦ Follow with a light massage concentrating on neck and shoulders.

Iontophoresis

Iontophoresis literally means 'the movement of ions'. It is used to introduce beneficial products into the skin. It is recommended for dry, dehydrated, mature and sensitive skins, but can be used on all skin types depending on the active ingredients of the products used. Like disincrustation, it works according to the scientific principle that similar charges repel and opposite charges attract. Specialist products for use with iontophoresis come in the form of gels, ampoules or serums. The products carry a (+)ive or (-)ive charge which informs us of the correct polarity setting for the treatment. If the product has a (-)ive charge then the active electrode is (-)ive, so that the product is 'pushed' and 'pulled' into the skin.

↦ **Practice point:**
  – (-) ive charged product: active electrode is (-) cathode / inactive electrode is (+) anode
  – (+) ive charged product: active electrode is (+) anode / inactive electrode is (-) cathode

Effects of iontophoresis:

Polar effects:	**Interpolar effects:**
↦ depends on product used, therefore correct skin analysis is imperative to ensure correct product choice.	↦ increased blood and lymph circulation ↦ increased metabolism ↦ lowering of blood pressure.

Theory into practice

Discuss the difference between a polar and an interpolar effect. What are the treatment implications of these differences?

Technique for iontophoresis

↦ **Practice point:** Skin type influences product choice, which dictates polarity. (-) product = (-) active electrode.

Safe starting

↦ Check for contra-indications.

↦ Skin analysis and product selection.

↦ Select correct cathode or anode as active electrode, according to product selection.

↦ Explain the sensation and effects of iontophoresis to your client.

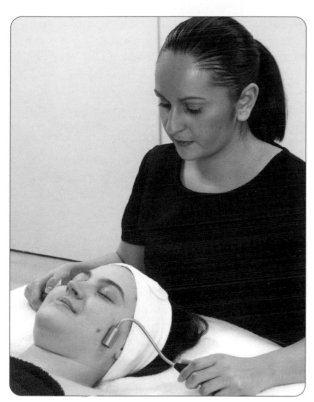

Treatment with galvanic iontophoresis.

Safe working

1 Cleanse client's skin and apply product.

2 Begin rolling one electrode on the chest area and gradually turn up intensity until comfortable. Apply second roller.

▸▸ **Practice point:** Re-apply product during treatment if rollers start to drag.

3 Using the pair of roller electrodes, follow the sequence below for 10 to 15 minutes.

4 Keep both rollers in contact with the skin.

5 Make sure that the rollers do not come into contact with each other.

▸▸ **Practice point:** Do not reverse polarity for iontophoresis.

Safe stopping

▸▸ Finish with both electrodes on the chest.

▸▸ Put down one electrode. Gradually turn down intensity to zero and switch off.

▸▸ Remove second electrode and wipe over skin to remove any remaining product.

▸▸ Sanitise electrodes and put equipment away neatly.

▸▸ Continue with the facial treatment.

▸▸ Give correct aftercare advice to the client.

Aftercare advice following disincrustation and iontophoresis

Galvanic treatment is highly stimulating and the skin will continue to excrete waste products post-treatment. As a consequence of the deep cleansing effect, the skin may look blotchy and some papules may appear. You must advise your client of these contra-actions prior to galvanic treatment.

Roller electrode sequence for iontophoresis:

	Movements are slow and rhythmic. Repeat each movement three times in sequence.
1	Starting on the neck, slide up sterno-cleido-mastoid from clavicle to ear. Slide down and repeat.
2	Work horizontally across platysma, one roller following the other.
3	Dive rollers at chin, glide along jawline to ear. Slide down and repeat.
4	Circle mentalis, one roller following the other around the chin.
5	Slide from corners of mouth to temples, working over lower cheek area. Slide down and repeat.
6	Glide up to zygomaticus and repeat as above. Do not go too close to the eyes.
7	Circle temporalis at corner of eye.
8	Work horizontally across frontalis, one roller following the other.
9	Between the eyebrows, work in small figure of eight movements.
10	Repeat movements in reverse order to finish on the neck.

Clients should also be advised not to have galvanic treatment immediately prior to a special occasion. It is best to leave at least a week between treatment and a special event.

Home care

- Make-up should not be applied for the rest of the day.
- Lightly cleanse in the evening but avoid stimulating products.

- Avoid heat treatments such as sunbeds, sauna or epilation for 24 hours.
- Do not use self-tan products for at least 24 hours.

Theory into practice

Imagine that a client has returned to the salon post-galvanic treatment for advice after suffering a reaction to the sun. What would be the implications for you as her therapist if you had not advised her correctly? What advice would you offer her now? Discuss the importance of giving after-care advice and the implications if you don't.

Assessment task 8.8

For each of the following three clients (see table overleaf), plan a course of four facial treatments to include manual mechanical and electrical techniques. (D)

Assessment task 8.9

Provide detailed and justified home care and retail recommendations for each of the three clients described on page 205. (D)

A summary of terms used in galvanic treatment:

Galvanic current	Direct current (dc) in one direction between two poles
Active electrode	In direct contact with the skin
Inactive electrode	Held by the client
Cathode	(-)ively-charged electrode
Anode	(+)ively-charged electrode
Electrolyte	Chemical compound that carries an electrical current
Ion	Electrically-charged atom
Cation	(+)ively charged ion
Anion	(-)ively charged ion
Saline solution	An electrolyte containing sodium chloride (NaOH) and water (H_2O)
Effects at cathode	Na reacts with OH to produce NaOH alkali and H gas
Scientific principle	Similar charges repel, opposite charges attract
Effects of alkali	Dries skin, saponifies sebum, loosens comedones, desquamating, destroys acid mantle
Effects at anode (reversed polarity)	Cl reacts with H to produce HCl acid and O_2 gas
Effects of acid	Tightens pores, nourishes skin, restores acid mantle
Saponification	Production of soap-like substance in pores when sebum and ingredients in galvanic gel mix together
Interpolar effects	Increased blood/lymph circulation, increased cell metabolism, reduced blood pressure

Three clients for Assessment task 8.8:

Client name:	Camilla Rushby	Esmin Shah	Andrew Crisp
Lifestyle considerations:	Busy office worker and mother of two. Aged 45. Occasional smoker. Drinks 2–3 glasses of wine each evening.	Degree student aged 18. Lots of studying, lots of late nights. Does not drink or smoke.	Landscape gardener aged 30. Smokes 20 cigarettes a day, drinks most evenings.
Current skincare:	Cleanse, tone and moisturise twice daily. Facials every 3 weeks.	Facial wipes to cleanse. Astringent toner. Never had a facial.	Washes in evening with soap and water.
Skin analysis:	Dry, dehydrated skin, acne rosacea. Fine lines around eyes and mouth.	Oily skin, some papules and acne scarring.	Dull, sallow and congested. Comedones and ingrowing hairs.
Medical/other considerations:	Irregular periods, occasional hot flushes.	Nervous client, self-conscious. Superfluous facial hair.	None.

Electrical Muscle Stimulation

Electrical muscle stimulation or EMS is a treatment which stimulates superficial facial muscles. It is used as a preventative measure to delay the visible signs of ageing or premature ageing. EMS uses a low frequency, interrupted direct current (dc) between 10–120 Hz, which is applied to the motor point of the muscle to cause a contraction. Current is applied to the facial muscles via either a metal mushroom electrode or a plastic facial electrode. The mushroom electrode consists of a metal disc on a handle which can be placed on the motor point of individual small muscles. An **indifferent** (inactive) electrode is required to complete the circuit, which can be placed behind the client's shoulder. The (newer) facial electrode consists of a plastic block which contains both the active and inactive electrodes and no indifferent electrode is required. It is used to stimulate groups rather than individual muscles, which some clients find less intense and therefore more comfortable. Clients should be advised that while there may be some immediate skin improvement and improvement in the appearance of facial contours, these effects may be temporary and a course of treatment is necessary to achieve a more sustainable result.

▸▸ Practice point: **Effects of electrical muscle stimulation include**:
  - increased circulation improves condition of epidermis and underlying muscle tissue
  - improved muscle tone
  - vasodilation and erythema
  - stimulates sensory nerve endings
  - temporary reduction of puffiness.

Contra-indications to microcurrent:

▸▸ hypersensitive skin

▸▸ nervousness

▸▸ high blood pressure

▸▸ epilepsy

▸▸ migraine or headache

▸▸ bony areas

▸▸ vascular conditions/ rosacea

▸▸ sinus congestion

▸▸ metal plates/pins/ excess fillings

▸▸ diabetes.

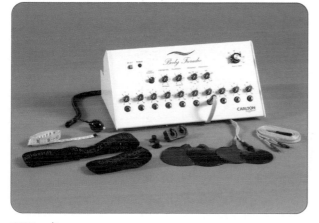

EMS unit.

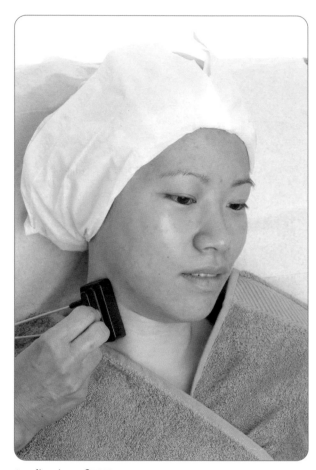

Application of EMS.

Technique for electrical muscle stimulation

Safe starting

▸ Prepare work area and client and remove client's jewellery.
▸ Check for contra-indications to EMS.
▸ Make sure machine is stable with no trailing wires. Test machine on yourself.
▸ Check intensity dials are at zero.
▸ If mushroom electrode is used, cover with lint soaked in saline solution and position indifferent electrode behind client's shoulder.

Safe working

1 Cleanse skin to remove all traces of oil and product.
2 Explain the sensation and effects of EMS to your client.
3 Place the electrode in position and increase the intensity slowly until a tingling sensation is felt.
4 Continue to increase intensity slowly during 'surge' period until a contraction is obtained.

5 After 6–8 contractions, gradually reduce intensity to zero during 'rest' period.
▸ **Practice point:** Turn up during surge period and turn down during rest period to maintain client comfort.

6 Repeat on other areas. Repeat to entire face, up to three times.
▸ **Practice point:** Do not exceed treatment time as this will cause muscle fatigue. Treatment time should be no more than 10–15 minutes.

Safe stopping

▸ Gradually turn intensity down to zero and switch off.
▸ Sanitise electrodes and put equipment away neatly.
▸ Tone the face and continue with facial treatment.

Theory into practice

Sometimes contractions are poor. Try to establish some of the reasons for this.

Microcurrent

Microcurrent is a relatively new treatment compared to other forms of electrotherapy. The equipment uses a pulsed direct current (dc) at a very low intensity as an anti-ageing treatment. The intensity is measured in microamps, the smallest unit of electricity used in electrotherapy, which are much smaller than milliamps and are barely perceptible to the client. (One microamp is equal to a thousandth of a milliamp.) Microcurrent is modified by waveforms which are interrupted by varying pulses. Pulses have a duration (or width)

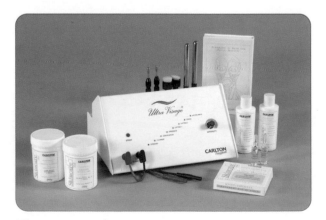

Microcurrent unit.

Waveforms:

Waveform	Effects
Sine	Most gentle effect, similar to body's electrical wave form. Improves circulation and colour, has toning effect on skin.
Ramp	Rises sharply and gradually decreases after peak. Mimics a rolling wave to stimulate and move lymph fluid. Aids muscle relaxation.
Rectangle	Has a rapid rise, a long duration and a sharp decline. Has an intensive lifting effect.
Square	Similar to rectangle but the rise and intensity duration are equal. Has a lifting effect.

varying from one millionth of a second (1 mu) to 2 seconds. Microcurrent signals vary in pulses per second and pulse widths to achieve different results. Waveforms may be sine, ramp, square or rectangle (see table above).

Effects of microcurrent

There is some controversy about the effects of microcurrent treatment with debate between manufacturers and scientists. As beauty therapists we are stuck somewhere in the middle! Some companies claim that microcurrent stimulates muscle tissue but scientists disagree. The effects listed below are scientifically recognised and the client should be advised that any effects are temporary and that only regular courses of treatment will achieve sustainable results.

Technique for microcurrent

Microcurrent units have set programmes which achieve different results, so you should consult the manufacturer's instructions and your tutor's advice. Remember to follow the standard safety procedures for electrotherapy.

The effects of microcurrent treatment:

Physiological effect	Benefit to client
Stimulates fibroblasts in the connective tissue which encourages renewal of collagen and elastin fibres.	Temporary removal of fine lines and improved elasticity.
Stimulates tissue repair and regeneration.	Aids the healing process, refines pores and reduces visible scar tissue.
Increased blood and lymph circulation.	Immediate freshness and 'glow' and removal of puffiness.
Oxygenation.	Improves texture and appearance of epidermis.

Contra-indications to microcurrent:

- heart conditions/pacemaker
- recent facial surgery/scarring
- eye or skin infections
- diabetes
- migraine
- pregnancy

- circulatory disorders
- recent heat treatment
- epilepsy
- metal plates/pins or excess fillings
- recent laser or chemical dermabrasion
- cancer/treatment for cancer.

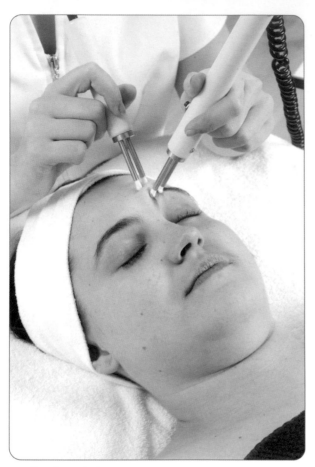

Application of microcurrent.

Theory into practice

Collect information from magazines, trade journals and manufacturers on microcurrent treatment. Are you convinced by their claims? How would you explain these claims, scientifically or otherwise? How do you think microcurrent compares to EMS?

Assessment task 8.10

Evaluate the use of facial EMS with due regard to timing, frequency, health and safety. (D)

Knowledge check

1 List the consumable and non-consumable stock required for a manual facial and describe the procedures for sanitation.

2 List the lifestyle factors that can affect the condition of skin.

3 Describe four basic skin types and the possible causal factors for each.

4 Compare and contrast three types of cleanser, toner and moisturiser.

5 List, with specific examples, the four classical massage movements.

6 Evaluate the benefits of manual facial massage.

7 Compare and contrast manual and mechanical exfoliation procedures.

8 Describe the procedures for safe working with vacuum suction.

9 Name and locate the main lymph nodes of the head and neck.

10 Compare and contrast the indications for direct and indirect high frequency treatment.

11 Evaluate the use of 'sparking' in high frequency treatment.

12 Explain the main scientific principle underlying galvanic facial treatment.

13 Describe pre- and post-treatment health and safety precautions for galvanic treatment.

14 Describe the polar effects at the cathode during disincrustation treatment.

15 Describe the polar effects at the anode during disincrustation when polarity is reversed.

16 Evaluate the polar and interpolar effects of iontophoresis.

17 Explain the use of active and indifferent electrodes in a facial EMS treatment.

18 Explain why microcurrent treatment is thus called.

19 Evaluate the scientific effects of microcurrent.

20 Provide retail recommendations to a client following 'anti-ageing' electrotherapy treatment.

Body massage

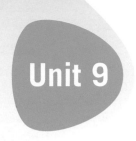

Unit 9

The purpose of this unit is to introduce the knowledge and skills required to practise and apply manual body massage. You will discover the history of body massage and explore the physical, physiological and psychological effects as well as the indications and contra-indications to treatment. You will learn the benefits and effects of classical massage techniques and through practical work will develop an awareness of the human body which will consolidate your theoretical knowledge of anatomy (Unit 5) and human physiology (Unit 2).

There is an emphasis on good practice especially in relation to health, safety and hygiene. You will learn to assess client's needs through analysis and diagnosis and lifestyle consultation in order to develop suitable treatment programmes for manual body massage. You will learn how to provide homecare advice and make appropriate retail recommendations.

The knowledge and skills required to perform advanced body treatments are developed from the theory and practice of body massage. It is necessary, therefore, to complete this unit successfully before attempting Unit 10: Body therapy.

In order to achieve Unit 9 in Body massage you must complete the following learning outcomes:

LEARNING OUTCOMES

1 Demonstrate effective body massage treatment.

2 Explore the effects of body massage manipulations and indications of their use.

3 Investigate underlying anatomical structures in relation to safe and effective massage treatment.

4 Explore alternative forms of manual massage treatments.

Body massage treatment

The history of body massage

Body massage is one of the oldest forms of medical treatment; it has been practised throughout history by all cultures and in all countries as a preventative and remedial treatment for injury and disease. Ancient Greek and Roman literature refers to massage as a treatment for asthma, digestive disorders and even sterility, but the oldest recorded reference to massage was found in a Chinese book dated around 2700BC. Body massage, as we know it, grew in popularity due to the influence of a Swedish man, Per Henrik Ling (1776–1839). His system of 'Swedish massage' spread throughout Europe and remains in our classification system to the present day. During World War I, massage was used extensively for the treatment of nerve injury and shell shock but its popularity waned with the development of modern medicine and technology. The perception of massage changed and it became associated with self-indulgence, pampered luxury and even sleaze.

> **Ancient Chinese writing**:
> 'Early morning stroking with the palm of the hand, after the night's sleep, when the blood is rested and the tempers relaxed, protects against colds, keeps the organs supple and prevents minor ailments.'

In more recent years the image of massage (and its practitioners) has changed again. Experience has shown that conventional medicine treats the symptoms of illness rather than the cause and that prescription drugs can be accompanied by side effects almost as unpleasant as the symptoms themselves. Thus, once again, the therapeutic properties of body massage are being recognised and valued, along with a host of other 'complementary therapies', because of the physical, physiological and psychological benefits they can offer. Also, of course, body massage can be enjoyed by men, women and children of all ages for the simple purpose of pure indulgence!

▶▶ **Practice point:** As always, it is important to remember that the job of the massage therapist is not to diagnose illness or to offer, or interfere with, medical advice. It is worth thinking of body massage as a therapy which is *complementary to* rather than an *alternative to* conventional medicine.

Pre-treatment preparation

Before the client arrives for a body massage treatment you should ensure that the work area is prepared with the appropriate products and equipment and with due regard to health, hygiene and safety. All towels should be clean and dry, massage oil should be in a bottle with a lid, and there should be a place for clients to leave their clothes (but not their jewellery, which should be their own responsibility). You should remove your own jewellery and sanitise your hands. If possible, the lighting may be dimmed. The room must be kept warm since the client's body temperature will drop during treatment; feeling cold can spoil a good massage. Soothing music can also help to create a pleasant ambience for body massage, although you should remember that musical preferences vary and what one client enjoys another may find annoying.

Check before you begin that the music choice and volume, as well as the lighting and temperature, are suitable for your client. Check throughout the treatment that he or she still feels warm enough.

▶▶ **Practice point:** The client will cool down as he or she relaxes while you will feel warm because of the physical effort you put into the massage. Supply a duvet or electric blanket so that the client is warm enough without the room temperature being too high for you to work comfortably.

Consultation

It is necessary to carry out a thorough consultation before body massage treatment because, as you have seen from the brief introduction, massage has an effect on the physical, physiological and psychological well-being of the client. You should refer to the discussion of consultation procedures and generic contra-indications in Section 1: Professional basics (pages 7–9) as well as considering the indications and contra-indications outlined below. There are countless reasons why clients choose body massage and the reason for each visit, as well as the client's expectations, should be ascertained during the consultation.

Indications for body massage:

▶▶ emotional stress
▶▶ physical stress
▶▶ general fatigue
▶▶ general aches and pains
▶▶ persistent headaches
▶▶ later stages of pregnancy
▶▶ to feel nurtured
▶▶ insomnia/other sleep problems
▶▶ poor circulation
▶▶ stiffness in joints
▶▶ muscle tension
▶▶ feeling of lethargy
▶▶ general relaxation
▶▶ as a treat.

Once you have identified the indications for body massage, you will be able to devise a suitable treatment plan. Massages are usually booked by time: half hour, one hour, one and a half hours, even two hour treatments, so you will need to agree with your client how you are going to divide up the time to meet his or her specific needs.

BEAUTY RECORD CARD

Name: Patrick Brooker Age: 43 Tel. No.: 07842 398490

Address: 27, Church Lane

PERSONAL DOCTOR	DETAILS OF PRESCRIBED DRUGS
Name: Dr. Sehra	None
Address: Medical Centre, Bridge Rd	
Tel. No.:	

MEDICAL HISTORY

Height: 6'1"   Weight: 14st   Chest: Waist: Hips:

Heart Disease: Yes ☐ No ☑   Varicose Veins: Yes ☐ No ☑

Details of Operations: _____

_____   Other Comments: Plays football

_____   2-3 times per week

_____   Active lifestyle,

_____   balanced diet.

BEAUTY RECORD CARD

Date	Treatment	Remarks
21/3/04	1 hour body massage	Tension backs of legs and lumbar region of back.
27/5/04	1 hour body massage	As before

Body massage record card.

Contra-indications

You should refer to the generic contra-indications listed in Section 1: Professional basics (page 9) and record a detailed medical history which considers previous as well as current conditions. As with all treatments, some conditions will only contra-indicate massage in a localised area, whereas others mean that massage should be avoided completely. There are other conditions which do not contra-indicate body massage but should be treated with caution and/or require a doctor's note. Contra-indications for body massage fall roughly into two categories: things you cannot see or physiological conditions, and things you can see or contagious conditions.

Contra-indications:
- recent or major operations
- early stages of pregnancy
- circulatory disorders
- nervous disorders
- broken/fractured bones
- lymphatic disorders
- cancer
- contagious skin conditions
- undiagnosed swelling
- high temperature/feeling unwell.

Considerations:
- epilepsy
- diabetes
- later stages of pregnancy
- migraine
- previous injury
- thread veins
- painful areas
- menstruation
- diarrhoea.

Consumables

Body massage requires very little preparation with regard to tools, materials and equipment. An important consideration for the massage therapist is that the couch is at the correct height to maintain good posture. Leaning over a couch that is too low, or having to stretch over one that is too high, will cause back pain and over time may lead to irreversible damage. The couch should be prepared with enough clean, dry towels to cover the client fully as well as to keep him or her warm. You might want to use cushions or bolsters for support at the ankles or shoulders when working on those areas of the body. The trolley should be prepared with massage mediums, cotton wool and cologne.

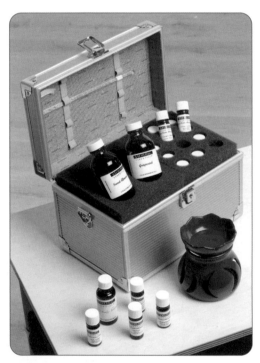

Body massage oils.

Massage materials:

Product	Application	Uses
Eau de cologne	With cotton wool	To wipe over areas, e.g. feet prior to massage; to remove oil after massage if client desires
Massage oil	With hands, warm first	Creates slip and is suitable for all except very oily skin types or excessively hairy areas
Talc	With cotton wool	Preferred by some men or for very oily skins or excessively hairy areas

Procedure

The procedures used in body massage are based on those introduced by Per Henrik Ling and known as Swedish massage. The movements and procedures are the same for each area of the body and are adapted to suit, so that a fleshy area such as the back of the thighs will demand deeper kneading and wringing movements while a flat area such as the back will require more gliding or stroking movements. Bony areas are never worked over but should be worked around with small finger kneading movements to relieve tension. Some massage therapists like to finish with a back massage because it is the most relaxing, while others start with the back since it often holds the most tension and therefore requires the most work. Some clients may have a particular area they want you to avoid, perhaps the abdomen, or another area they particularly enjoy being massaged, such as the hands or feet. It is important to establish the client's requirements as well as his or her likes and dislikes so that you can plan your treatment time accordingly. Massage can be performed as often as the client wishes. Some clients have regular massages while others see it as an occasional treat. If your client has a specific indication, such as muscular shoulder tension, you might advise him or her to have regular treatments.

As with all treatments, body massage is not complete until you have given home care advice and retail recommendations to your client. The list opposite includes general advice and retail recommendations suitable for most clients, as well as specific advice for some more common individual needs.

Home care advice
▸ Step down from the couch carefully, you might feel a little dizzy.
▸ Take it easy after a treatment, if possible just go home and relax.
▸ You might need to go to the toilet immediately after body massage.
▸ Try not to eat a heavy meal immediately after (or before) a massage.
▸ Drink plenty of fluid, preferably water.

Specific advice
▸ Swollen ankles – sit with your feet raised whenever possible in the evening.
▸ Varicose veins – avoid hot baths, do not cross your legs, practise ankle/knee rotations.
▸ Cold hands/feet – keep moving, try not to stand or sit in one position for too long.
▸ Back/neck tension – practise good posture always, carry weights equally, do not hold the phone between chin and shoulder.
▸ Pins and needles – common symptom of poor circulation, keep moving, dry body brushing.
▸ Hollow back – abdominal exercises.
▸ Cellulite – regular massage at home and salon, drink plenty of water, dry body brushing.
▸ Overweight – body massage cannot help with weight loss.

Retail recommendations
▸ Body lotion – for all clients to nourish skin and stimulate circulation.
▸ Bath oil – for very dry skin and/or relaxation.
▸ Body brush – to stimulate circulation and aid desquamation.
▸ Body exfoliator – to aid desquamation.
▸ Cellulite creams – to facilitate absorption of cellulite.

Theory into practice

What other indications would prompt you to suggest regular body massage treatments for your client?

Design a suitable body massage treatment for each of the following four clients, including home care advice and retail recommendations with regard to timing, frequency and client's needs. (D)
(a) Mother of two infants, has lower back strain, often tired, no time for herself.
(b) Middle-aged businesswoman, works at a computer all day, neck strain and headaches.
(c) Older gentleman, swollen joints, often feels cold.
(d) Young client, cellulite on backs of thighs, cold feet, slightly overweight.

Procedure

For a general one-hour body massage the timing may be as follows, but remember that each massage should be adapted to suit the client's needs and requirements:

- consultation
- client prepares   2 minutes
- back massage   20 minutes
- back of legs   5 minutes each
- front of legs   5 minutes each
- abdomen   5 minutes
- arms   3 minutes each
- neck and chest   5 minutes
- client dresses   2 minutes
- home care and retail advice.

Safe starting
- Prepare work area with regards to health, safety and hygiene.
- Prepare client in correct position.
- Complete consultation and record card.
- Sanitise your hands with anti-bacterial hand wash.
- Ask client to remove all jewellery and put it away.
- **Practice point:** Make sure that both you and the client are as comfortable as possible.

Safe working
1 Perform the massage according to the agreed treatment plan.
2 Apply a suitable massage medium.
- **Practice point:** Only expose the area being treated, to maintain client dignity.

3 Ensure that you maintain good posture throughout.
4 Keep the client warm and encourage him or her to relax.
5 Be aware of underlying anatomical structures.
6 Adapt manipulations according to your client's needs.
- **Practice point:** Check that the depth of pressure is comfortable on each new area.

Safe stopping
- Tell the client you have finished.
- Allow the client a few minutes to adapt and get dressed.
- Offer home care advice and retail recommendations.

Body massage techniques

Classical massage movements are classified into four categories: effleurage, petrissage, friction and tapotement. These movements can be adapted into techniques to suit different areas of the body, different body shapes and individual client requirements.

Back and shoulders procedure

Apply massage medium with superficial stroking. Repeat each movement three times. Photos of certain techniques are shown on page 215.

1 'T' effleurage from sacrum to occipital groove, from sacrum to 12th thoracic vertebra (bra strap level) and from sacrum around the waist (photo 1).
2 Palmar kneading to cover the back and shoulder area.
3 Reinforced palmar kneading in figure 8 around scapulae (photo 2).
4 'T' effleurage as for step 1.
5 Wringing across shoulders to trapezius and sides of back to latisimus dorsi (photo 3).
6 Skin rolling to sides of back (photo 4).
7 'T' effleurage as for step 1.
8 Single-handed wringing to back of neck.
9 From head downwards, reverse effleurage with hands either side of the spine.
10 Finger frictions around each scapula.
11 Finger/thumb frictions around sacro-iliac joint (photo 5).

Back and shoulders procedure

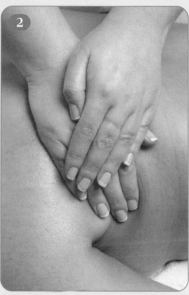

'T' effleurage from sacrum around the waist.

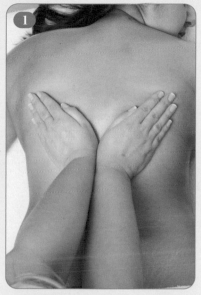

Reinforced palmar kneading around the scapula in a figure 8 movement.

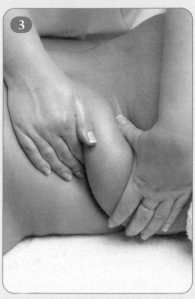

Wringing along sides of the back to the latisimuss dorsi muscle.

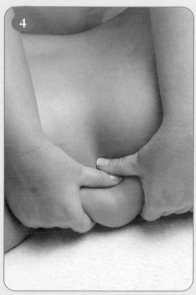

Skin rolling to the latisimuss dorsi muscle.

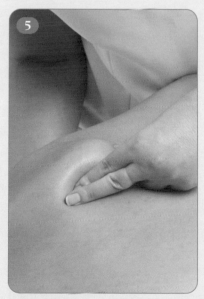

Finger frictions around the sacro-iliac joint.

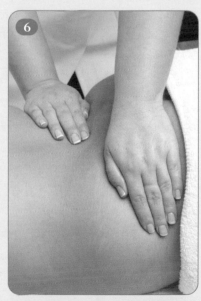

Transverse stroking to the lumbar region.

12 Reverse effleurage.

13 'T' effleurage as for step 1.

14 Finger frictions around gluteals.

15 Finger kneading up erector spinae.

16 Transverse stroking in lumbar region (photo 6).

17 Hacking and/or cupping to back.

18 Pounding to buttocks only.

19 'T' effleurage.

20 Light downwards stroking to finish.

Back of legs procedure

Photos for this procedure are shown on page 217.

1 Efleurage to cover inner, outer and upper aspects of whole leg.

2 Effleurage to thigh and buttocks only.

3 Reinforced 'V' kneading to hamstrings muscles (photo 7).

4 Kneading and wringing to outer thigh and buttocks.

5 Effleurage thigh and buttocks.

6 Knuckling to back of knee.

7 Picking up to calf muscle (gastrocnemeus).

8 Light hacking to lower leg.

9 Hacking and cupping to thigh and buttocks (photos 8 and 9).

10 Pounding to buttocks only (photo 10).

11 Effleurage as for step 1.

12 Light downwards stroking and hold the ankle to finish.

Front of legs procedure

1 Effleurage to cover sides and front of whole leg.

2 Effleurage to the thigh.

▶ Practice point: The inner thigh is more sensitive than the outer thigh; adapt the depth of pressure accordingly.

3 Reinforced 'v' kneading to front of thigh.

4 Kneading and wringing to outer and inner thigh.

5 Hacking to thigh muscles.

6 Finger kneading around the patella.

7 Thumb kneading between tibia and fibula.

8 Finger kneading around tarsals and metatarsals.

9 Deep thumb kneading to sole of foot (photo 11).

10 Effleurage to foot.

11 Effleurage to whole leg.

12 Light downwards stroking and hold foot to finish.

Abdomen procedure

Photos for this procedure are shown on page 218.

1 Effleurage around ribs to umbilicus and around waist to top of pubis bone (photo 12).

2 Gentle transverse stroking, first one way and then the other.

3 Wringing to waist.

▶ Practice point:
 – Avoid working over the abdomen of a client of the opposite sex if you or the client feels uncomfortable with this.
 – Always work anti-clockwise over the abdomen, following the direction of the digestive tract.

4 'Caterpillar' kneading over the colon (photo 13).

5 Circular finger kneading over the colon (photo 14).

6 Effleurage as for step 1.

7 Rest hands in region of solar plexus to finish.

Arms procedure

Photos for this procedure are shown on page 218.

1 Effleurage to cover posterior and anterior aspects of whole arm.

▶ Practice point: The inner arm is usually more sensitive than the outer arm; adapt depth of pressure accordingly.

2 Single-handed picking up to biceps.

3 Single-handed picking up to triceps and deltoid (photo 15).

4 Knuckling to crook of elbow.

5 Thumb kneading to posterior aspect between radius and ulnar.

6 Thumb kneading between carpals and metacarpals.

7 Turn hand over – deep thumb kneading to palmar surface (photo 16).

8 Thumb kneading to anterior aspect between radius and ulna.

9 Effleurage as for step 1.

10 Light downwards stroking and hold hand to finish.

Back of legs procedure

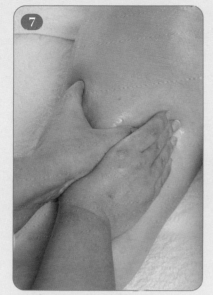

Reinforced 'V' kneading to the hamstrings.

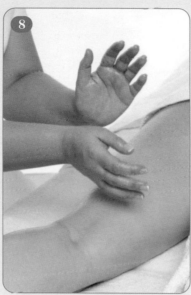

Hacking to the thigh.

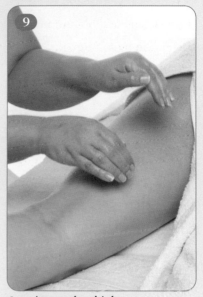

Cupping to the thigh.

Front of legs procedure

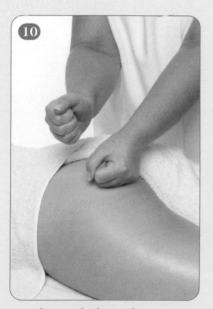

Pounding to the buttocks.

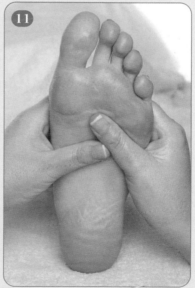

Deep thumb kneading to the sole of the foot.

Abdomen procedure

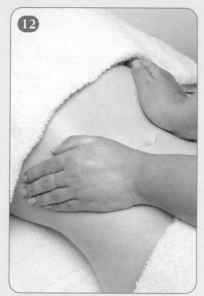

Effleurage around the ribs to the umbilicus.

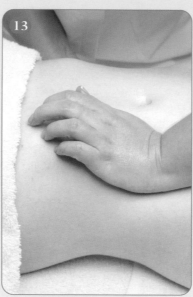

'Caterpillar' kneading over the colon.

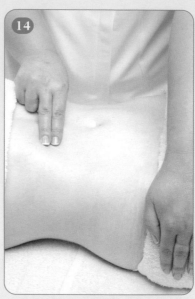

Circular finger kneading over the colon.

Arms procedure

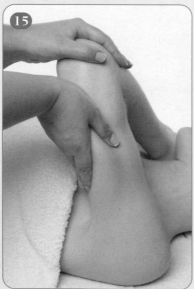

Single-handed picking up, to triceps.

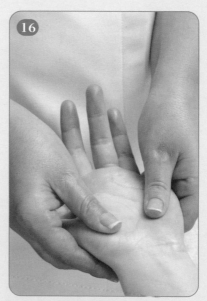

Deep thumb kneading to the palmar surface.

Neck and chest procedure

1 Effleurage out from centre of chest around back of neck and up to occipital process.
2 Knuckling out from centre of chest around back of neck and up to occipital process.
3 Deep thumb kneading along trapezius from shoulders to occipal process.
4 Effleurage.
5 Stroking to one side of neck with alternate hands, then to the other side of neck.
6 Gentle effleurage and hold shoulders to finish.

Basic knowledge in relation to techniques

Think about what you can physically do with your hands. You can rub, you can press, you can knead and you can stroke. We rub things better when they hurt, or stroke the arm of a friend in distress. These very basic instinctual reactions illustrate some of the healing powers of touch. Massage manipulations are based around just a few 'instinctual' techniques which are adapted according to the underlying anatomical structures. There are a few fundamental ground rules to ensure safe practice but other than that you should try to develop and trust your instinct – learn to 'see' with your hands what lies beneath the skin.

Ground rules for massage:

▸▸ use stroking movements to start, link and complete an area
▸▸ warm the tissues with gentle movements before using stimulating techniques
▸▸ calm the tissues with gentle techniques after stimulation
▸▸ work in the direction of blood and lymph flow
▸▸ never apply pressure over bones
▸▸ when kneading, make sure you are working on the underlying muscle not just the skin
▸▸ don't try to work miracles in one session, be realistic about what you can achieve and re-book your client for a follow up treatment if necessary
▸▸ if in doubt – don't do it!

Theory into practice

The best way to learn about good (and not so good) massage techniques is to experience them for yourself. In training, aim to work with as many other people as possible and ask for and offer constructive feedback.

Effects of body massage

The effects of body massage can be categorised according to physical, physiological and psychological benefits. Physical effects are those sensations that the client feels, such as relaxation. Physiological effects are those changes which take place internally in the body's systems, such as an increase in circulation. Psychological effects are those which alter the client's mood or emotional state, such as relief from stress. These effects are summarised below.

Physical effects of body massage:

▸▸ temporary pain relief
▸▸ stress relief
▸▸ tension release
▸▸ relaxation
▸▸ erythema
▸▸ lower body temperature.

Physiological effects of body massage:

▸▸ lowers blood pressure
▸▸ lowers heart rate
▸▸ release of lactic acid
▸▸ increased blood flow to tissues
▸▸ increased lymph flow
▸▸ desquamation
▸▸ stimulates digestive system
▸▸ stimulates urinary system
▸▸ stimulates small muscle fibres.

Psychological effects of body massage:

▸▸ pampering
▸▸ feeling of being nurtured
▸▸ mental relaxation
▸▸ client feels better and therefore looks better
▸▸ relief from day-to-day pressure
▸▸ healing power of touch.

In addition to these general effects, body massage manipulations are categorised into four basic techniques which may be relaxing or stimulating according to the pressure used. These are: effleurage, petrissage, friction and tapotement.

Theory into practice

Some massage movements, particularly petrissage and tapotement, are best practised on a cushion until you get the hang of them!

A summary of massage techniques:

Manipulation	Technique	Effects
Effleurage	A slow rhythmic, stroking movement using the palmar surface. Pressure may be deep or superficial as required.	Client relaxes and becomes accustomed to your hands; used to start, link and end the massage.
Petrissage, e.g. kneading, wringing, rolling	Tissues are grasped and released rhythmically following muscle shapes.	Contracted muscles relax, tone of small muscles is improved; increased circulation and heat to the area.
Friction	Deep movement with fingers or thumbs to muscle or around bone.	Releases muscle knots, eases stiff joints, releases fluid, creates localised heat.
Tapotement, e.g. hacking, cupping, pounding	Co-ordinated and rhythmic technique using loose wrists to 'strike' an area with sufficient muscular or fatty tissue. Also known as percussion.	Localised heat, erythema, invigorating, tones small muscles, increased circulation.

Underlying anatomical structures

Anatomical systems

In order to perform a safe body massage treatment it is vital that you have a good understanding of human anatomy and physiology. Massage techniques can have deep and general effects which you must be aware of and you should consider the underlying structures for each area of massage, as summarised below. Refer also to Unit 2: Human physiology and Unit 5: Anatomy.

Back

Concentrate on these areas:
- trapezius
- erector spinae
- around the scapula
- around the sacrum and coccyx
- gluteal muscles.

Be cautious in these areas:
- region of the kidneys
- avoid working over the scapula
- avoid working over the vertebral column
- take care on the neck
- avoid heavy tapotement in the lumbar region.

Back and front of leg

Concentrate on these areas:
- thighs which tend to be fleshy and muscular
- gastrocnemeus

- around ankle joint
- around knee joint
- don't forget the feet.

Be cautious in these areas:
- avoid upper thigh and groin on opposite sex clients
- less pressure over thread veins
- avoid varicose veins
- cellulite can be painful
- avoid working over the patella
- medical oedema/arthritis.

Abdomen

Concentrate on these areas:
- work clockwise (when facing client) in the direction of the digestive system.

Be cautious:
- during pregnancy
- prior to or during menstruation
- when suffering from diarrhoea or constipation.

Arms

Concentrate on these areas:
- apply more pressure on triceps
- between radius and ulna
- don't forget the hands.

Be cautious in these areas:
- apply less pressure on the biceps
- avoid swollen joints (medical oedema)
- avoid areas of arthritis
- avoid pressure over bony areas.

Neck and chest

Concentrate on these areas:
- apply pressure according to client's needs.

Be cautious:
- prior to or during menstruation
- when feeling tired or unwell
- over areas of local swelling.

Theory into practice

Using your knowledge of anatomy and physiology, explain why the cautions listed above and on page 220 are necessary during massage. Can you think of any other precautions related to the underlying structures of the human body?

Assessment task 9.4

Define the anatomical systems and underlying structures of the body, describing how massage techniques are adapted to the needs of the underlying structures. (M)

Alternative forms of manual massage treatments

These can include Aromatherapy, Baby Massage, Bowen Technique, Chiropractice, Deep Tissue, Hawaiian, Holistic, Indian Head Massage, Manual Lymph Drainage, Osteopathy, Physiotherapy, Pressure Point Massage, Reflexology, Remedial, Shiatsu, Sports Massage, Swedish Massage, Thai Massage, Therapeutic Massage, Tui Na.

Special knowledge

There are countless forms of manual massage, mostly originating from Eastern techniques, which are gaining popularity in the Western world. Aromatherapy is one of the best known alternatives and is explored in Unit 13. Indian head massage is a method available in many hair, health and beauty salons and is explored in Unit 19. Other popular treatments include lymphatic drainage and shiatsu.

Lymphatic drainage

The lymphatic system is explored in Unit 2: Human Physiology (pages 56–7). Its main functions are to remove waste from the tissues, help fight infection and maintain fluid homeostasis. Lymph fluid is transported through the vessels to the lymph nodes which are present at sites where infection might occur. The lymphatic vessels lie superficially in the human body so they are stimulated by even the gentlest manipulation. Manual lymphatic drainage (**MLD**) therefore consists of light stroking towards the lymph nodes and gentle friction or pressure in the area of the nodes. The lymphatic system is stimulated indirectly in all forms of massage but specific drainage techniques can also be used on facial and body areas.

Indications for use:
- diagnosed swelling
- tenderness around joints
- sinusitis
- tonsillitis
- bronchial conditions.

Contra-indications:
- undiagnosed swelling
- arthritic conditions
- cancer of the lymphatic system
- mastitis
- pregnancy.

Theory into practice

Find out about alternative forms of massage you are not familiar with.

The role of manual massage in the beauty therapy industry

Manual massage has a key role in the beauty therapy programme. As you have discovered, the indications for use are vast, ranging from the complementary treatment of illness or injury to general relaxation and pampering. Some beauty therapists choose to specialise in massage techniques because of an interest in health or fitness – or they might see it as hard work and just a necessary part of their job! However *you* feel about performing body massage, your client will pick up on those feelings. Try to be as relaxed and focused as possible in order to deliver the best results. Some therapists develop their interest in massage further still and train as sports therapists in order to help sportsmen and women prepare for events and recover afterwards. Others might have an interest in aromatherapy for the treatment of physical and emotional ailments in conjunction with gentle massage techniques.

Clients can be introduced to massage after receiving other treatments. Most clients agree that the massage is the most enjoyable part of a manicure, pedicure or facial treatment, so this can be used as a selling point for a longer body massage treatment. In addition, any details about physical or emotional stress gained during consultation for a treatment can be used to recommend massage.

Assessment task 9.5

Select three alternative forms of manual massage and evaluate their role within the beauty therapy industry. (D)

Knowledge check

1 Why might a client decide to have a manual body massage?

2 Describe the pre-treatment health and safety procedures.

3 Name the classical body massage movements, with examples of each.

4 How would you choose a suitable massage medium?

5 Describe the physical effects of manual body massage.

6 Describe the physiological effects of manual body massage.

7 Describe the psychological effects of manual body massage.

8 Explain the effects of massage on the circulatory system.

9 What is manual lymph drainage?

10 What general advice would you offer to a client following a body massage?

Body therapy

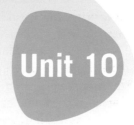
Unit 10

The purpose of this unit is to introduce the knowledge and skills required to practise and apply a range of mechanical and electrical body treatments. It builds on the knowledge and skills gained from studying manual body massage and it is therefore necessary that you complete Unit 9: Body Massage before starting this unit.

The unit will guide you through analysis and diagnosis for body therapy, including figure and posture analysis, and will build on the theoretical knowledge of human physiology and anatomy gained from studying Units 2 and 5.

This unit will help you to explore mechanical body treatments (gyratory vibration, vacuum suction and audio sonic); and electrical body treatments (electrical muscle stimulation (EMS)), and galvanism. You will be made aware of the indications, contra-indications and contra-actions to body therapy as well as the procedures, product knowledge, home care and retail advice appropriate to each treatment.

In order to achieve Unit 10 in Body therapy you must complete the following learning outcomes:

Learning Outcomes

1 Investigate figure and posture analysis in relation to mechanical and electrical body therapies.

2 Describe and apply mechanical body treatments.

3 Describe and apply electrical body treatments.

4 Examine light irradiation and describe and apply sun tanning and self-tanning treatments.

Figure and posture analysis

Procedures

Consultation

Before starting a body therapy programme it is essential to conduct a thorough visual assessment of the client followed by a verbal and manual analysis. Through consultation with the client, the body therapist is able to devise the most suitable treatment plan based on health and lifestyle, existing figure and posture, and desired results. The client who attends for body therapy is likely to have concerns about his or her shape and/or size, which fall into one of three categories: overweight, underweight or out of proportion. The client might be nervous, apprehensive or embarrassed and may feel intimidated by a therapist whom he or she perceives as younger, slimmer or more attractive. It is imperative that you conduct the consultation with sensitivity and in a non-judgemental way and do all that you can to put the client at ease. Take your time to listen and show empathy in your responses.

Bear in mind that the majority of the UK population are overweight and most of us have at least one area of our body that we are unhappy about. Remember also that an individual looking in the mirror can often see things that those who observe him or her cannot. Assure the client that there is nothing abnormal or unusual about his or her concerns. As you gain experience in body therapy, you will meet and treat clients of all shapes and sizes and learn to approach each one with professionalism and discretion.

Observation

Notice the overall height, shape and size of the client – is he or she in proportion? Be aware of posture as the client walks, stands and sits. Observe any attempts to disguise figure faults through style of dress, clever positioning or tensing muscles to flatter the body shape. Do perceived figure faults actually exist or is poor posture to blame? Does the client look well groomed or slovenly?

Questioning

You've heard the phrase, 'it's not *what* you say but *how* you say it that matters'. In fact both are important when listening to the client's responses to verbal questioning. Notice the client's body language and mannerisms. Does he or she appear fidgety, tense or embarrassed? Does he or she maintain eye contact or look away nervously? Is it difficult to gain the information you seek or does the client chatter incessantly, and if so what about? These observations are indicative as to the client's frame of mind and will help you to build a mental picture of his or her personality. You will need to question the client about medical history and lifestyle, as for all treatments (see Section 1: Professional basics, pages 7–10) and also to take into consideration specific factors, which are described overleaf.

Client questionnaire:

Objective	Yes/No	Details
Achieve inch loss		(Where, how much?)
Achieve weight loss		(How much, what timescale?)
Improve health and vitality		(How will this make you feel?)
Improve muscle tone		(Which area?)
Improve postural defects		(Specify)
Promote relaxation		(Stress, lifestyle factors)
Reduce cellulite		(Where, what type?)
Develop self-confidence		(In what context?)
Improve circulation		(General/specific)
Alter poor eating habits		(Usual dietary concerns)
Reduce smoking		(How much?)
Reduce drinking		(How much?)
Encourage exercise		(How often, what type?)
Treatment recommendations		(Electrical, mechanical, manual)
Diet recommendations		(Portion size, cooking methods)
Exercise recommendations		(Type, frequency)

Specific factors for consideration:

- **lifestyle:** occupation, interests, personality
- **general concerns:** body condition, health, vitality, weight gain/loss
- **fat:** cellulite/soft fat distribution
- **identify causal factors:** posture, lifestyle, diet
- **diet:** balanced, regular meals, over-/under-eating, eating disorders
- **exercise:** what, how often, fitness level
- **medical:** medical history, medication, contra-indications
- **pregnancy:** now or previous, dates
- **health:** smoking, alcohol, sleep patterns.

It might be helpful to use a simple questionnaire to establish your client's short- and long-term goals. As you gain more experience, you will develop your own style of questioning which will be more informal and less rigid. The format on page 224 would provide you with suitable prompts. Don't just hand the questions to the client – read them out and discuss the client's objectives before making recommendations for treatment, diet and/or exercise.

Touch

Tactile touch can be used to assess types of fatty (adipose) tissue, which are described on page 228, or to assess the tone, shape and condition of muscles. When observing the client's figure and posture it is less disconcerting if you place your hands firmly on each area in turn, e.g. shoulders and hips to assess their level, rather than just observe from a distance. Make sure your hands are warm before you do so!

Figure analysis

It is necessary to analyse the client's figure before body therapy in order to prescribe the appropriate treatment plan and achieve the most positive results. Ideally, any observations should be made when the client is naked as even underwear can give a false impression of body shape. However, very few clients, particularly on their first visit, will feel comfortable undressing completely. It is worth asking them, therefore, not to wear enhanced or supportive underwear, e.g. 'tummy tamers', when they attend the salon for body therapy, so that you can make accurate observations and measurements without the client undressing fully.

Body types

Different body types can be categorised as endomorph, ectomorph or mesomorph.

The endomorph
Physical traits:

- short and plump
- padded contours
- fatty deposits on shoulders, hips, abdomen
- prone to weight accumulation
- small hands and feet
- wide hips.

Common personality traits:

- placid
- easy-going
- often shy
- slow, deliberate movements
- poor eating habits.

The ectomorph
Physical traits:

- slim
- long slender bones
- little muscular bulk
- lack of curves
- may be underweight.

Common personality traits:

- easily flustered
- unusual eating habits
- highly strung/neurotic
- lacks strength and stamina
- lacks vitality.

The mesomorph
Physical traits:

- athletic build
- well-developed shoulders
- boyish hips
- well-developed musculature
- inverted triangular shape.

Common personality traits:

- competitive
- courageous
- sporty but likes to win
- domineering
- can be aggressive.

Height and weight

The height of the client should be measured (without shoes) so that the height and weight ratio can be ascertained. This will enable the therapist to decide if the client is carrying excess or insufficient weight and will influence the course of body treatments to follow. The client should be weighed wearing the minimum amount of clothing, just

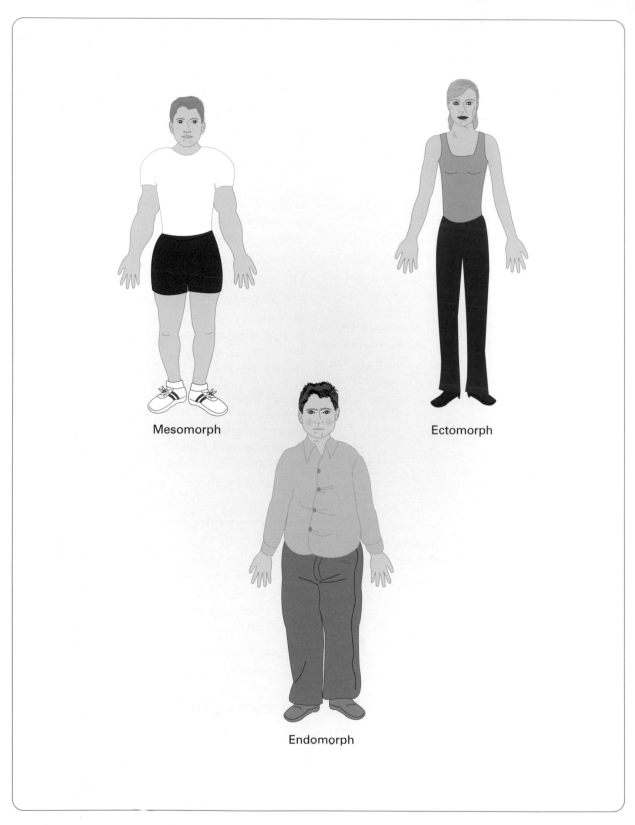

Mesomorph

Ectomorph

Endomorph

Body shapes: Mesomorph, ectomorph and endomorph.

underwear is ideal, as clothes can add an average of 3–5 lbs. The client who needs to monitor his or her weight, as part of a weight loss programme, should be weighed at regular intervals, not too close together and always at the same time of day.

▶▶ **Practice point:** *We weigh more towards the evening than in the early morning. Women can weigh up to 10 lb (4.5 kg) more when they are pre-menstrual, due to water retention.*

Theory into practice

Explain why the client should be weighed only once a week and at approximately the same time of day on each occasion.

Ideal height to weight ratios are included in the table below. These should be used as a rough guide only and it is not necessary to adhere to them rigidly to achieve a healthy and attractive figure. Ideal weight is an individual matter and therefore a reasonable weight can fall within 6 kg (1 stone) of that indicated on the table. Frame size is determined by measuring the circumference of the wrist (see below).

▶▶ **Practice point:**
Frame size:
small frame: 4½ – 5½"
medium frame: 5½ – 6¼"
large frame: 6¼ – 6¾"

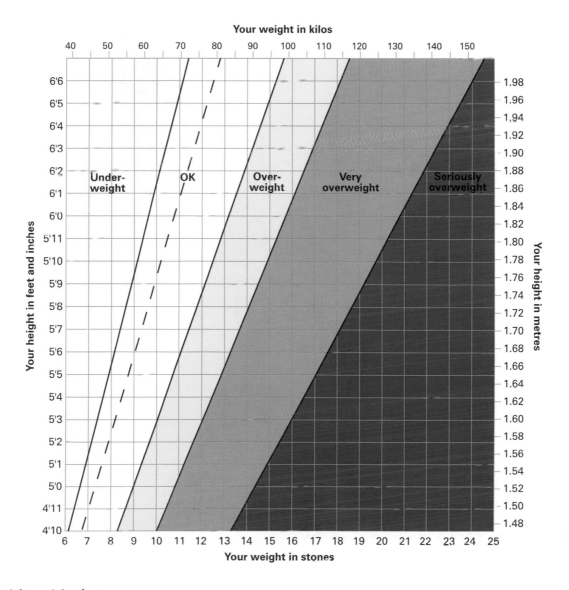

Ideal height: weight chart.

Body measurements

Some clients will be uninterested in individual body measurements while others may want to monitor them as a guide to how the treatment programme is progressing. It is important that measurements are read accurately; ideally they will be taken by the same body therapist each time with the client wearing just his or her underwear, which should be neither restricting nor uplifting. The tape measure should fit snugly over the area; not so tight that it creates an indentation and not too loose that it hangs down. All measurements must be taken from a fixed point, that is a bone such as the knee or hip, so that true readings are observed. Also, remember to measure both left and right limbs and observe any fluctuations.

▸ **Practice point:**
   Ideal proportions:
   waist: 8–10″ smaller than bust
   abdomen: 1–2″ smaller than bust
   hips: 1–3″ larger than bust
   calf: 4–5″ larger than ankle
   thigh: 10–12″ larger than ankle

Measurements:

1 Bust – at fullest part of the bust.

2 Middle – at xiphoid process of the sternum.

3 Waist – at narrowest point.

4 Hips – at pubis symphysis.

5 Top thigh – at widest point (L&R).

6 Mid-thigh – 6″ up from patella (L&R).

7 Lower thigh – 3″ up from patella (L&R).

8 Calf – at widest point (L&R).

9 Ankle – above ankle bone (L&R).

10 Leg – from anterior iliac spine to ankle bone (L&R).

11 Top arm – level with top of axilla and insertion of deltoid (L&R).

12 Wrist – below styloid process (L&R).

13 Neck – at widest point.

14 Suprasternal notch to right nipple.

15 Suprasternal notch to left nipple.

16 Right nipple to umbilicus.

17 Left nipple to umbilicus.

18 Umbilicus to symphis pubis.

Adipose tissue

Body fat, or **adipose** tissue, may be of different types: hard adipose, soft adipose, trapped adipose and cellulite. The type and location on the body should be noted.

Hard adipose tissue

This is solid, well-established fatty tissue. It cannot be picked up easily and is therefore difficult to distinguish from muscle. Care should be taken to correctly identify hard adipose tissue which may lie directly over well-toned muscle. Hard fat is more difficult to shift than soft fat.

Soft adipose tissue

This can be picked up easily and separated from the muscle layer beneath. A suitable programme of diet and exercise will shed soft fat fairly easily.

Trapped adipose tissue

This describes deposits of fat found between bundles of muscle fibres and is common in people who used to train regularly but no longer do so, such as ex-dancers or ex-athletes. Trapped fat is slow to respond to diet or exercise.

▸ **Practice point:** Muscle cannot turn into fat and fat cannot turn into muscle but adipose tissue can become deposited between slack muscle fibres.

Cellulite

Cellulite consists of fatty tissue and waste products. Because adipose cells have a poor blood circulation, toxins within them stagnate and cause water retention which causes the typically 'orange peel' appearance. The skin appears lumpy and dimpled, typically around the thighs, buttocks and backs of the upper arm. Cellulite is much more common in women than men and can be observed on even the slimmest of figures.

Causes of cellulite:

▸ poor metabolism
▸ an uneven distribution of fat
▸ fluid retention
▸ long-term medication
▸ sedentary lifestyle
▸ sleep deprivation
▸ long-term stress
▸ hormonal fluctuations
▸ poor diet
▸ lack of exercise
▸ dehydration
▸ smoking/alcohol.

Hard cellulite

The skin's surface may be smooth but has hard, lumpy pockets of fat. It may be painful to touch and prone to bruising. Hard cellulite is most common in mature women since it is built up over time. It is also seen in dancers and athletes. Long-term treatment is required to de-congest the tissues, break down fatty deposits and re-establish the healthy circulation of blood and lymph.

Soft cellulite

The skin appears dimpled and is spongy to the touch. Soft cellulite is most common in younger women and can be more prominent pre-menstrually or at times of increased stress. It is less difficult to treat than hard cellulite because it is not so developed and therefore less solid.

▸ Practice point:

Cellulite treatment
Cellulite should be treated with a combination of diet, exercise and body therapy. The aim of treatment is to improve the circulation and metabolism in the affected areas so that toxins and waste products can be drained away. Body massage and therapies can help to soften cellulite while a balanced diet and suitable exercise programme will prevent further fat from forming, as well as helping to invigorate the body's systems. There are no miracle cures!

Theory into practice

Find out about some of the products and treatments available for the reduction of cellulite. How do they work and are you convinced by the manufacturer's claims?

Posture analysis

You should refer to Unit 5: Anatomy (see pages 92–5) for a discussion of the anatomical features of posture as well as the chief anti-gravity and postural muscles. In order to make accurate postural observations for the purpose of body therapy, the client should be clothed in underwear. Use a plumb line to create an imaginary line down the centre of the body and note any inbalances.

▸ Practice point: You can make your own plumb line by tying a weight to a long piece of string.

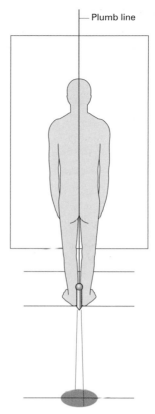

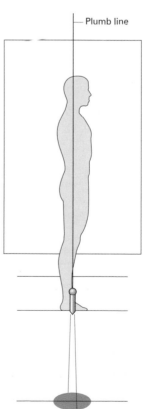

Postural analysis using a plumb line; posterior and lateral views.

Posture analysis – imbalances:

Postural imbalances	Position	Conditions to note
Head and neck	Lateral view	Forward tilt due to rounded shoulders
	Posterior view	Flexion to one side due to tension
Shoulders	Lateral view	Rounded shoulders may be due to a heavy bust, self-consciousness, habitual or work-related poor posture
	Posterior view	Uneven due to carrying heavy weights
Pelvis	Lateral view	Anterior tilt (common during pregnancy) or posterior tilt
	Posterior view	Uneven with uneven distribution of adipose, poor posture or spinal deformity such as scoliosis*
Abdomen	Lateral view	Protrusion may be due to muscle weakness (can it be sucked in?)
Spine	Lateral view	Exaggerated thoracic curve (kyphosis*) exaggerated lumbar curve (lordosis*)
	Posterior view	Winged scapula, lateral curvature (scoliosis*)
Legs	Lateral view	Forward or backward tilt
	Posterior view	Less than 3 gaps may be due to bow legs, knock knees, or excess adipose

Abnormal spinal curvatures

Scoliosis is a spinal deformity which causes a lateral curvature of the spine. It might take the form of a single 'C' shaped curve or have a primary curve in one direction with a compensatory curve in the opposite direction forming an 'S' shape. Scoliosis can develop in people whose legs are of unequal length, after significant trauma or following a stroke.

Lordosis is a spinal deformity characterised by an exaggerated curvature in the lumbar region. This causes the abdomen and buttocks to protrude and the back to appear hollow. Lordosis can be caused by obesity and hip deformities, and is common during pregnancy.

Kyphosis is a spinal deformity characterised by an exaggerated curvature in the thoracic region. This causes a hunch back or **dowager's hump**. Kyphosis

can have a congenital cause but is more often the result of poor posture and weak back muscles.

▸▸ Practice point:
SC – oliosis = 'S' shaped or 'C' shaped curvature of the spine.
L – ordosis = L – umbar curve is exaggerated, hollow back.
kyp- H – osis = Hump backed, exaggerated thoracic curve.

Procedures

Record card completion

The record card for body therapy should include the client's personal details as well as details of the figure and posture analysis and any measurements you have taken. It might also be useful to have a body treatment log book and/or a summary sheet which includes treatment aims and short-/long-term goals. The first consultation will provide a great deal of information while measurements made on consecutive visits should also be recorded to monitor progress. Some suggestions for recording are included overleaf.

Assessment task 10.1

Working with a partner, identify and describe in detail the main figure and posture problems and suggest possible causal factors based on a lifestyle questionnaire. (M)

Body therapy summary sheet:

Observations		Date:	Date:	Date:	Date:
Figure analysis	Height				
	Weight				
Posture analysis	Lateral view				
	Posterior view				
Adipose tissue	Type				
	Distribution				
Condition of muscle	Tone				
	Distribution				
Treatment recommendations					
Diet recommendations					
Exercise recommendations					

Assessment task 10.2

Design a body therapy record card and then complete it with clear and coherent information based on your findings in Assessment task 10.1 on page 230. (M)

Mechanical body treatments

Mechanical body treatments performed by the beauty therapist include gyratory massage, audio sonic and vacuum suction. The principles of these treatments are the same as for facial therapy, which was explored in Unit 8. Mechanical body treatments are administered in conjunction with manual massage and therefore the pre-treatment preparations are the same as for body massage discussed in Unit 9. The generic contra-indications for body massage should be considered as well as the specific considerations listed for each mechanical treatment.

Gyratory Massage

Mechanical massage describes the manipulation of body tissues using a machine, such as the gyratory massager. This is a heavy, vibrating machine which is used to provide a deep, powerful massage. The effects are similar to manual massage but the sensation is less personal and much heavier. The equipment uses an electric motor to control the head, which the therapist holds.

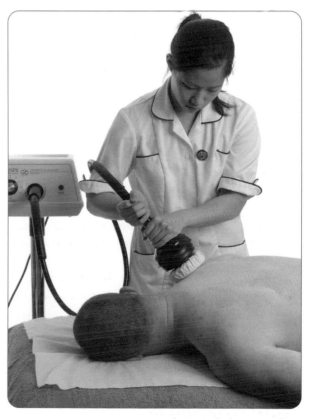

Gyratory massager in use.

Heads of a gyratory massage unit (G5):

Head	Uses	Effects	Caution
Sponge head	To start and finish an area	Same as effleurage but much deeper	Can cause an itching sensation
Horse shoe	To start and finish treatment on the thigh	Same as effleurage but much deeper	Only use if the applicator fits the area
Prickle head	Good for hips and gluteals	Same as deep petrissage	Only use on fleshy areas
Egg box	Can be applied to the back by straddling each side of the spinal column	Same as deep petrissage, may be more comfortable than prickle head applicator	Do not use on bony areas
Concave discs	Commonly used over cellulite	Same as deep petrissage	Do not use over bony areas
Pin cushion	Can be used on all areas	Same as tapotement, causes erythema	Avoid hairy areas or sensitive skin
Lighthouse	Can be used down sides of spine or around scapula to relieve tension	Depending on the pressure used, can mimic effleurage or petrissage	Always work around bones, never over them

When the machine is in operation, the head turns, or gyrates, round and round to provide a deep massage. A series of different applicators are attached to the head to provide specific effects and sensations in different areas of the body.

Contra-indications to gyratory massage:
- bruises
- dilated capillaries
- varicose veins
- recent scar tissue
- recent operations
- abdomen during menstruation
- abdomen during pregnancy
- back if spinal conditions
- sensitive skin prone to bruising
- skin diseases and disorders.

Gyratory massage:

Indications for use	Benefits and effects
To reduce fatty deposits	Hard adipose tissue is softened and dispersed
To reduce cellulite	Cellulite is softened and dispersed
To relieve general aches and pains	Increased blood supply will warm tissues and promote relaxation of the muscles and nerves
To relieve muscular tension	Deep pressure will remove lactic acid from muscles and relieve tension nodules
To improve a sluggish circulation	Stimulation of blood and lymphatic circulation
For male clients	A heavier and less personal treatment than manual massage
To improve the appearance of the skin	Creates erythema and stimulates cell metabolism

Technique
Safe starting
- **Practice point:** cover applicator heads with plastic food bags to maintain good hygiene.
- Prepare and sanitise equipment and work area.
- Prepare client and check for contra-indications to treatment.
- Ensure equipment is stable with no trailing wires.
- Select suitable applicator head for the area and wipe over with surgical spirit or cover.
- Attach head and switch on away from the client, to make sure it is secure.

Safe working
- **Practice point:** keep applicator heads parallel to the area.
- Explain the treatment effects and sensation to the client.
- Apply talc to the area; oil will damage sponge heads.
- Use sponge heads to warm the area, then start the routine.
- **Practice point:** monitor skin erythema throughout treatment.
- Apply long effleurage strokes using your other hand to lead.
- Use petrissage heads in a kneading motion using your other hand to feed the tissues towards the applicator.
- **Practice point:**
  - Treatment of a specific area should not normally exceed 30 minutes but this may be reduced depending on skin/client reaction.
  - For spot reduction it should be incorporated into a treatment programme of twice weekly for 4–6 weeks.
  - For relaxation, gyratory massage can be used as required.

Safe stopping
- Switch off machine.
- Wash applicators with hot soapy water (not sponge heads).
- Wipe down machine and return to storage.
- Apply manual effleurage to complete the treatment and continue with body therapy.

Assessment task 10.3

Describe the contra-indications and indications to gyratory massage. (M)

Assessment task 10.4

Describe pre-treatment preparation procedures related to gyratory massage with due regard to health and safety. (M)

Describe the benefits and uses of gyratory massage with due regard to timing, frequency, health, safety and client's needs. (M)

Audio sonic vibrator

The audio sonic vibrator is a small, hand-held appliance which creates gentle stimulation through sound waves. Sound waves are transmitted by all media – solid, liquid and gaseous – with varying degrees of efficiency. The molecules in human tissues will resonate when struck by sound waves: they absorb the sound waves which travel through the tissue until the energy is absorbed and then it stops. It is believed that lymph fluid, cartilage, muscle and bone can conduct audio sonic pulses.

The audio sonic vibrator contains a coil which is controlled by an electro-magnet. When electrical current moves one way, the coil moves forwards. When it moves the other way, the coil moves backwards. This forward-backward movement is transmitted to the head of the appliance but, unlike percussion massagers, the head remains static so the treatment is less stimulating on the surface and more relaxing for the client. When applied to the body, the vibration of the coil compresses and decompresses the tissues. Sound waves penetrate deep into the tissues at a cellular level and are therefore beneficial in relaxing tension nodules.

Contra-indications to audio sonic treatment:
- metal or plastic pins or plates
- intrauterine devices, e.g. coil
- undiagnosed pain
- thrombosis
- back or abdomen during pregnancy
- headache or migraine
- highly vascular or inflammatory conditions
- skin diseases and disorders.

Describe the contra-indications/indications to audio sonic treatment. (M)

Technique

Safe starting
- Prepare and sanitise equipment and work area.
- **Practice point:** some appliances are dual purpose, make sure it is set for audio sonic.
- Prepare client and check for contra-indications to treatment.
- Select flat or ball applicator.

Safe working
1. Explain the treatment effects and sensation to the client.
2. Apply talc or oil according to skin type, or use over clothes.
3. Use stroking or circular movements, to suit the area.
- **Practice point:** treatment time is 5 to 15 minutes depending on degree of erythema.

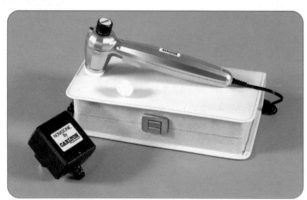

Audio sonic vibrator.

Audio sonic treatment:

Indications for use	Benefits and effects
To relieve tension nodules, muscle spasm and overworked muscles	Compresses and dilates deep in tissues at a cellular level
To promote relaxation	Produces local warmth, erythema and relaxation of tissue fibres
To improve the appearance of dry, dehydrated or sensitive skin	Increases cell metabolism and circulation; aids desquamation; stimulates sebaceous activity

Safe stopping

» Switch off machine.
» Wipe applicator heads with surgical spirit and return to storage.
» Remove oil if desired and continue with body therapy.

Assessment task 10.7

Describe pre-treatment preparation procedures related to audio sonic treatment, with due regard to health and safety. (M)

Assessment task 10.8

Describe the benefits and uses of audio sonic treatment with due regard to timing, frequency, health, safety and client's needs. (M)

Medical applications

Audio sonic vibrators are used to successfully treat certain conditions which contra-indicate treatment by the beauty therapist. These include: rheumatic and arthritic conditions, swellings, sprains, migraine, neuralgia and painful sinus conditions. While this might be frustrating, it is important that you recognise your own professional limitations and refer the client to a medical specialist where appropriate.

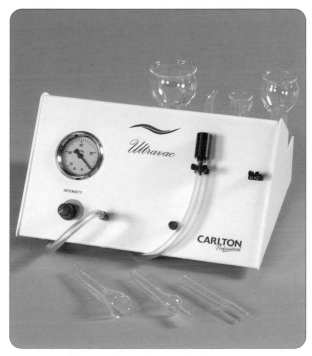

Vacuum suction.

Vacuum suction

Vacuum suction equipment creates a negative pressure which stimulates the lymphatic system. A motor sucks skin and subcutaneous tissue into a cup (venteuse) which is manually stroked across an area towards the nearest lymph node. A sluggish lymphatic circulation can result in a build up of toxic waste, swelling, discomfort and medical oedema. Vacuum suction is a method of increasing the flow of lymphatic fluid which mimics natural lymph flow. It is used in conjunction with manual massage or other mechanical treatments, such as gyratory massage.

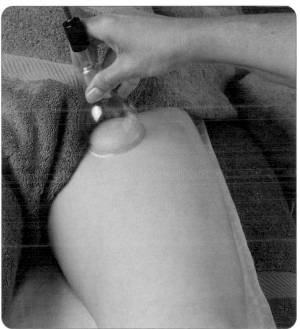

Vacuum suction in use.

Contra-indications to vacuum suction:
» disorders of the lymphatic system
» undiagnosed swelling
» broken capillaries
» varicose veins
» recent scar tissue
» bruises
» breast tissue
» sunburn
» bony or excessively hairy areas
» thrombosis
» loose, thin skin.

Assessment task 10.9

Describe the contra-indications/indications to vacuum suction. (M)

Vacuum suction:

Indications for use	Benefits and effects
To reduce areas of fluid retention such as gravitational oedema	Lymph flow is stimulated which reduces stagnation and increases drainage
To reduce fatty deposits	Areas of soft adipose tissue are carried in the lymph towards the lymph nodes
To reduce areas of cellulite	Waste products carried in the lymph are drained away as circulation is stimulated, and the overall appearance of the skin is improved
To reduce the appearance of dowager's hump	Fatty deposits below the neck can be drained in the lymphatic system
To help prevent varicose veins	Venous circulation is stimulated to prevent stagnation
To improve the appearance of the skin	Aids desquamation, creates erythema, stimulates cell metabolism

Vacuum suction technique

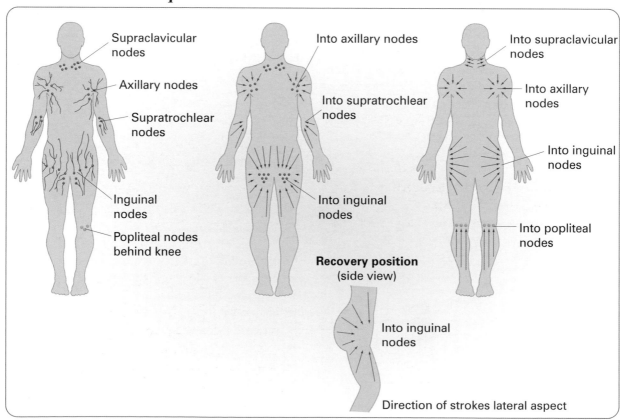

Direction of application for vacuum suction.

Safe starting

▸ Prepare and sanitise the equipment and work area.

▸ Prepare client and check for contra-indications.

▸ Place machine on a stable base with no trailing wires.

▸ Turn all dials to zero before switching on.

▸ Test machine on your forearm.

▸ Select suitable size venteuse for the area and wipe over with surgical spirit.

> ↠ **Practice point:** always pre-heat the area with gyratory or manual massage.

Safe working

- ↠ Explain the treatment effects and sensation to the client.
- ↠ Apply a sufficient quantity of oil to the area.
- ↠ Place the venteuse on the area and turn up the intensity.
- ↠ Slide venteuse in direction of lymph flow to nearest lymph node.
- ↠ Break the vacuum by removing your finger from the hole or depressing the client's flesh.
- ↠ Overlap the previous stroke by half and repeat until the area has been covered.
- ↠ Repeat to the entire area 5 to 8 times.
- ↠ **Practice point:** never allow volume of flesh in venteuse to exceed 20%.
  - Treatment of a specific area should not normally exceed 30 minutes but this may be reduced depending on skin/client reaction.
  - For relaxation, gyratory massage can be used as required. For spot reduction it should be incorporated into a treatment programme of twice weekly for 4–6 weeks.

Safe stopping

- ↠ **Practice point:** always take care when breaking contact with the client.
- ↠ Turn all dials to zero and switch off.
- ↠ Wash venteuses and tubes with hot soapy water.
- ↠ Wipe down machine and return to storage.
- ↠ Apply manual effleurage to complete the area.
- ↠ Remove oil if desired and continue with body therapy.

Assessment task 10.10

Describe pre-treatment preparation procedures related to vacuum suction with due regard to health and safety. (M)

Assessment task 10.11

Describe the benefits and uses of vacuum suction with due regard to timing, frequency, health, safety and client's needs. (M)

Generic mechanical procedures

As with all treatments, it is necessary to record the details of body therapy applications. Make a note of the intensity, duration and frequency of any equipment used, as well as observations on skin reaction and client sensation. This will help you to plan consecutive treatments as part of a body therapy programme. It is also important to provide home care advice to the client to support the effects of the treatment, and you should be fully aware of retail opportunities. Refer to Section 1: Professional Basics and Unit 9: Body Massage for further guidance.

Specific home care advice:

- ↠ Weight loss – diet and exercise recommendations to support body therapy.
- ↠ Cellulite – drink plenty of water to flush the body of waste; practise dry body brushing to stimulate circulation.
- ↠ Postural defects – try to ascertain the cause and advise accordingly about the importance of good posture and postural exercises.
- ↠ Swollen ankles – sit with feet raised whenever possible in the evening.
- ↠ Varicose veins – avoid hot baths, do not cross legs, practise ankle/knee rotations.

Retail recommendations:

- ↠ Body brush – to stimulate circulation and aid desquamation.
- ↠ Body exfoliator – to aid desquamation.
- ↠ Cellulite creams – to stimulate the metabolism and improve skin condition.
- ↠ Body lotion – for all clients, to nourish skin and stimulate circulation.
- ↠ Bath oil – for very dry skin and/or relaxation.

Assessment task 10.12

Provide detailed home care advice and retail recommendations for the client in Assessment task 10.1 (on page 230) based on your suggested treatment plan. (M)

Electrical body treatments

Electrical body treatments performed by the beauty therapist are **faradism** or electrical muscle stimulation (**EMS**) and **galvanism** (**cellulite polarity**). The principles of these treatments are

Electrical body treatments – product knowledge:

Product	Benefits and effects	Use
Saline solution	A salt and water solution used in electrotherapy to conduct electrical current into the tissues	EMS, cellulite polarity
Galvanic gels	Electrically-charged preparations used to enhance the effects of treatment	Body galvanism
Body exfoliants	Granular preparation used to aid desquamation and increase circulation	Home use between salon visits
Body lotions	to hydrate and nourish the skin and improve appearance	Home use between salon visits
Body brush	Use dry on a daily basis to improve circulation	Home use to support anti-cellulite and slimming treatments

the same as for facial therapy, which was explored in Unit 8. Electrical body treatments are administered in conjunction with manual massage and therefore the pre-treatment preparations are the same as for body massage (discussed in Unit 9). The generic contra-indications for body massage should be considered as well as the specific considerations listed for each electrical treatment.

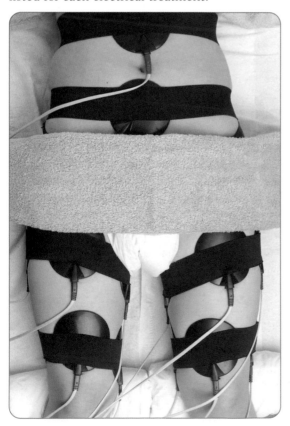

EMS in practice.

Faradism

Electrical muscle stimulation (EMS) is also known as faradism because the original equipment used a faradic current. Modern equipment uses a surged or interrupted direct current but EMS is still known by the alternative name of faradism. An electrical current is used to stimulate muscle fibres in electrical muscle (EMS) treatments. Muscles contract in response to stimuli transmitted by the brain. In EMS, an electrical pulse is generated by the equipment which initiates muscular contraction. The best contractions are produced when electrical pulses are applied at the point where a motor nerve enters the belly of the muscle, which is called the **motor point**.

Electrical impulses and stimuli

A constant flow of current will not produce a contraction since the muscle adapts to the current. Direct current must therefore be used which produces electrical impulses that rise and fall at regular intervals. It must be applied at a high enough intensity (I) and for a long enough duration (D) to produce a contraction. The electrical impulses are grouped together with rest periods in between so that when the current flows the muscle contracts (C) and when it stops the muscle relaxes (R). Machine settings can be altered to create different programmes which either rise gradually and stop or rise gradually and fall gradually. These patterns may be familiar to those of you who use gym equipment such as treadmills or ski machines.

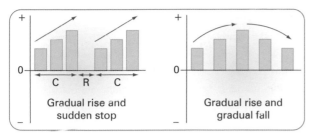

Gradual rise and sudden stop

Gradual rise and gradual fall

Illustration of surged intensity.

Placement of electrodes

The most common form of body electrode are round, rubber pads. Accurate placement of electrodes, or 'padding up' as it is known, is essential if EMS is to be effective. Muscle fibres will respond to stimulus no matter where the pads are placed but the sensation is likely to be uncomfortable and less effective than if it is stimulated at the motor point. Motor point padding is therefore the most precise

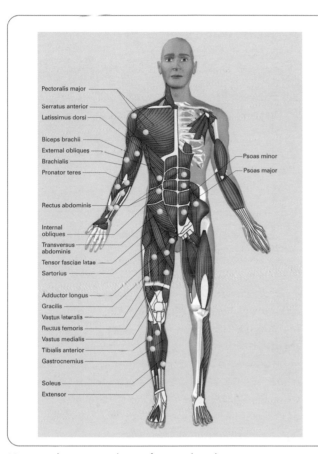

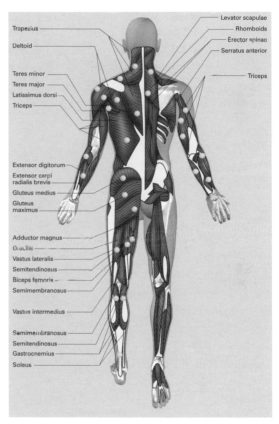

Motor points – anterior and posterior view.

Faradism – alternative method of application:

Type of padding	Method	Suitable muscles
Longitudinal padding	Padding on the upper and lower motor points of long muscles, to gain maximum contraction with minimum intensity	Rectus abdominus, rectus femoris, gracilis, trapezius, triceps
Duplicate padding	A pair of pads is placed on the motor points of adjacent muscles with similar actions	Gluteus medius with tensor fascia lata; adductor longus with gracilis; external oblique with rectus abdominus
Split padding	One pair of pads is split between the motor points of the same muscle on opposite sides of the body	Right and left pectorals; right and left triceps; right and left gluteus maximus

and effective method of treatment. Alternative methods of application include longitudinal padding, duplicate padding and split padding (see table on page 239).

> ▸▸ **Practice point**: the main disadvantage of duplicate and split padding is that adjacent muscles or muscles on opposite sides of the body cannot be individually controlled.

Reasons for poor contractions

Visible contractions might not be possible, especially on the first visit, if the client has poor muscle tone or excess fatty deposits. Clear contractions give the best results, but client comfort is of the utmost importance. Use the checklist below to ensure the best possible contractions and also be guided by your client.

Poor contractions can be caused by:
▸▸ incorrect positioning of pads
▸▸ current intensity is too low
▸▸ straps are not tight enough to maintain contact between pads and the skin
▸▸ pads are too dry
▸▸ too much fatty tissue in the area.

Contra-indications to EMS:
▸▸ muscle injury or spasm
▸▸ heart conditions; pacemaker
▸▸ metal pins or plates
▸▸ recent scar tissue
▸▸ varicose veins
▸▸ high or low blood pressure
▸▸ epilepsy
▸▸ thrombosis
▸▸ thin, frail frame
▸▸ nervous conditions
▸▸ abdomen during menstruation
▸▸ recent pregnancy or lactation.

Indications for use:
▸▸ figure reshaping and/or inch loss
▸▸ tones out-of-proportion thighs and buttocks
▸▸ to restore waistline after pregnancy
▸▸ to firm pectorals after pregnancy
▸▸ to tone muscles after prolonged disuse
▸▸ to tone abdominals and improve posture
▸▸ to maintain a firm figure.

Benefits and effects:
▸▸ causes muscle fibres to contract and so improves the tone of specific muscles or muscle groups
▸▸ circulation and metabolism are stimulated to improve the condition of muscle fibres.

Technique

Safe starting

▸▸ Prepare and sanitise the equipment and work area.
▸▸ Place machine on a stable base with no trailing wires.
▸▸ Turn all dials to zero before switching on.
▸▸ Test the machine on yourself.
▸▸ Prepare the client and check for contra-indications.
▸▸ **Practice point**: pre-heat the body to improve muscle action.
  - cover small abrasions with petroleum jelly.

Safe working

1 Explain the treatment effects and sensation to the client.
2 Select a suitable padding layout and secure straps around the client's body.
3 Moisten the pads evenly with saline solution.
4 Position pads securely over motor points.
5 Turn controls up slowly until client feels a tingling sensation.
6 Gradually increase intensity to obtain a contraction.
7 Cover client and leave for 15–20 minutes initially.

▸▸ **Practice point**:
  - Consecutive treatment times can be increased to a maximum of 30 minutes per session.
  - For maximum effect, EMS should be given 2–3 times per week for a course of 10–12 treatments.

Safe stopping

▸▸ Turn all dials to zero and switch off.
▸▸ **Practice point**: remove pads in reverse order to prevent tangling.

▸▸ Wash pads with hot soapy water.
▸▸ Wipe down machine and return to storage.
▸▸ Wipe over the treated area with cologne and continue with body therapy.

Assessment task 10.13

Describe, with attention to detail, pre-treatment preparation procedures related to EMS with due regard to health and safety. Describe the contra-indications and indications of EMS. (M)

Mrs Braithwaite comes to the salon for body EMS. Figure analysis highlights poor muscle tone in the abdominal and pectoral muscles following a recent pregnancy. The client also has heavy thighs and buttocks due to lack of exercise. Describe the method of padding up, timing, frequency and machine settings which would be appropriate for this client. (M)

Galvanism

You should revisit Unit 8: Facial therapy where the principles of galvanism are explored in detail (pages 109–204). Body galvanism involves the application of a direct current via electrodes which produces polar and interpolar effects. Body galvanism is used for the treatment of cellulite, hence its alternative name of **cellulite polarity**. As with all galvanic treatments, cellulite polarity uses paired sets of electrodes which 'push' and 'pull' electrically-charged cellulite products into the skin. Current flows from the active pad to the passive or indifferent pad, carrying the active product with it. Most cellulite products are negatively charged and therefore the negative electrode (black lead) is active and the positive electrode (red lead) is passive at the start of treatment. The active pad is placed on the affected area and the indifferent pad is placed underneath, to act like a magnet drawing the product into the skin. When used in conjunction with diet and exercise as part of a full body therapy programme, galvanism can be extremely effective for the reduction of cellulite.

Contra-indications to body galvanism:
- hypersensitive areas, e.g. inner thigh
- sensitive skin or sunburn
- lack of skin sensation, neuralgia
- circulatory disorders
- diabetes
- undiagnosed oedema
- metal pins or plates
- abdomen if IUD coil fitted
- low blood pressure
- pregnancy
- recent or extensive scar tissue
- skin diseases and disorders.

Indications for use:
- to disperse areas of cellulite and aid its absorption
- to disperse stubborn deposits of fatty tissue and aid its absorption
- to disperse non-medical fluid retention
- to stimulate blood and lymph circulation
- to improve the general condition of the skin.

Interpolar effects:
- stimulates blood circulation
- stimulates lymphatic circulation and lymph drainage
- increases metabolism and cell renewal
- lowers blood pressure.

Polar effects at the (-) cathode:
- localised heat
- vasodilation brings increased nutrients and oxygen and aids the removal of waste
- production of sodium hydroxide which softens skin and underlying tissues
- release of hydrogen which stimulate tissues
- tissue fluid is attracted away from the (+) anode towards the (-) cathode, which has a softening effect
- active anti-cellulite preparations are repelled into the skin by the (-) cathode and attracted into the skin by the (+) anode, thereby enhancing their effects, i.e. aiding the dispersal of cellulite.

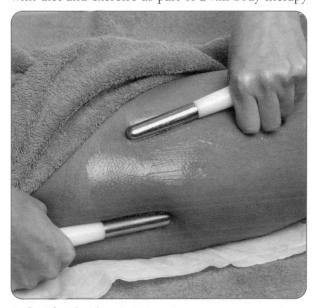
Body galvanism in progress.

Describe the contra-indications/indications to body galvanism. (M)

Body galvanism technique

Sensitivity testing:

Skin sensitivity test	Method
Hot and cold test	Fill one test tube with hot water and one with cold. Ask client to look away. Randomly touch different test tubes against the skin and ask the client to identify hot and cold.
Sharp and blunt test	Use an orange wood stick and a cotton bud. Ask the client to look away. Randomly stroke the items on the skin and ask the client to identify sharp and blunt.

Safe starting

- ▸ Prepare and sanitise equipment and work area.
- ▸ **Practice point:** carry out sharp/blunt and hot/cold skin sensitivity tests.
- ▸ Place machine on a stable base with no trailing wires.
- ▸ Turn all dials to zero before switching on.
- ▸ Test the machine on yourself.
- ▸ Prepare client and check for contra-indications to treatment.
- ▸ Cleanse the area thoroughly.

Safe working

- ▸ **Practice point:** if products are not used, dampen pads with saline solution.
1. Explain the treatment effects and sensation to the client.
2. If products are used, apply evenly to area/via gauze.
3. Place the active electrode over the pad on the treatment area.
4. Place the inactive electrode parallel to the active electrode.
5. Secure the pads with body straps.
6. Turn controls up slowly until client feels a slight tingling sensation.
7. Gradually increase intensity until a mild warmth is apparent (about 0.05 mA).

8. Cover the client and leave him or her for 15–20 minutes.

- ▸ **Practice point:** for maximum effect, body galvanism should be given 2–3 times per week for a course of 10–12 treatments in conjunction with a diet and exercise programme.

Safe stopping

- ▸ Slowly turn all dials to zero and switch off.
- ▸ Remove saline solution with warm soapy water.
- ▸ Do not remove anti-cellulite products.
- ▸ Wash pads with hot soapy water.
- ▸ Wipe down machine and return to storage.
- ▸ Continue with body therapy.

Assessment task 10.16

Describe, with attention to detail, pre-treatment preparation procedures related to body galvanism with due regard to health and safety. (M)

Assessment task 10.17

Discuss the benefits and uses of body galvanism techniques and equipment, showing their various applications. (M)

General electrical procedures

As with all treatments, it is necessary to record the details of electrical body therapy applications. Make a note of the intensity, duration and frequency of any equipment used as well as observations on skin reaction and client sensation. This will help you to plan consecutive treatments as part of a body therapy programme. It is also important to provide home care advice to the client to support the effects of the treatment and you should be fully aware of retail opportunities. Refer to the practical skills chapter and Unit 9: Body massage for further guidance, as well as the home care and retail recommendations for mechanical treatments.

Assessment task 10.18

Provide detailed home care advice and show an awareness of retail opportunities appropriate to body therapy. (D)

Assessment task 10.19

Explain the functions of the products used in body treatments. (M)

Light irradiation, sun tanning and self-tanning treatments

Light irradiation

As you have learnt from the previous sections, there are many treatments in body therapy which benefit from pre-heating the tissues. It is possible to apply general heat to the body by using saunas, steam baths, showers and jacuzzis, which are popular in health hydros and spas. Body therapists can also apply local heat to the body through the use of heat lamps or **light irradiation**.

Theory into practice

List the body treatments that benefit from pre-heating the body and explain the benefits.

General effects of heat on the body

The main effect of pre-heating the body in beauty therapy treatments is to make the tissues more receptive to other manual, mechanical or electrical treatments which follow. These effects include the following:

» increases cell metabolism
» increases circulation, higher pulse rate
» lowers blood pressure
» creates erythema
» promotes relaxation
» stimulates sweat glands
» stimulates sebaceous glands
» lowers the appetite
» soothes sensory nerves
» soothes muscular tension.

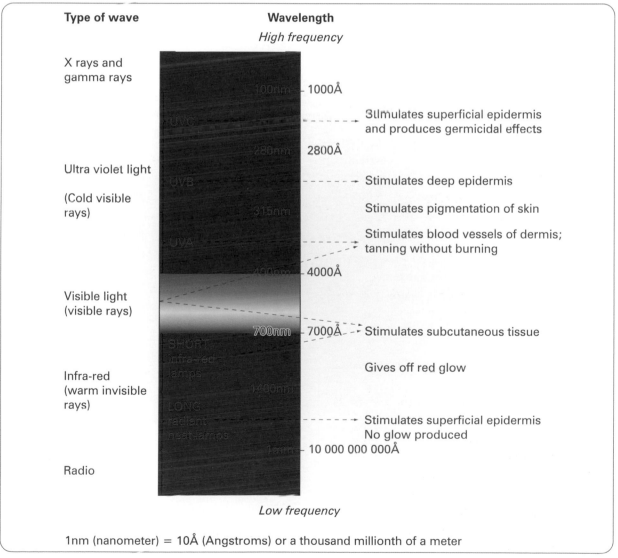

Type of wave	Wavelength
	High frequency
X rays and gamma rays	100nm — 1000Å
	UVC ‑ ‑ ‑ → Stimulates superficial epidermis and produces germicidal effects
	280nm 2800Å
Ultra violet light (Cold visible rays)	UVB ‑ ‑ ‑ → Stimulates deep epidermis
	Stimulates pigmentation of skin
	315nm
	UVA ‑ ‑ ‑ → Stimulates blood vessels of dermis; tanning without burning
	400nm — 4000Å
Visible light (visible rays)	
	700nm — 7000Å ‑ ‑ Stimulates subcutaneous tissue
	SHORT infra-red lamps
	Gives off red glow
	1400nm
Infra-red (warm invisible rays)	LONG radiant heat lamps
	‑ ‑ ‑ → Stimulates superficial epidermis No glow produced
	1mm — 10 000 000 000Å
Radio	
	Low frequency

1nm (nanometer) = 10Å (Angstroms) or a thousand millionth of a meter

The electromagnetic spectrum.

Explain how the application of heat can simultaneously lower blood pressure and increase heart/pulse rate.

Electromagnetic spectrum

The electromagnetic spectrum is explored in Unit 1: Scientific principles (pages 21–4). It consists of different types of rays, such as visible light and infra-red, which have different effects on the body because of their varying wavelengths (see the chart on page 243). Wavelengths were traditionally measured in **Angstrom** units (A) but it is becoming more usual to use **nanometres** (nm).

➡ **Practice point:** A nanometre is a minute measurement:
  10A (Angstroms) = 1 nm (nanometre)
  = 1 thousand millionth of a metre =
  1 millionth of a millimetre.

Inverse square law

The inverse square law applies to visible light, infra-red and ultraviolet rays, and governs intensity in relation to distance. It states that the intensity of radiation varies inversely with the square of the distance from the source. A client at point X, 1m from the source, will receive a particular treatment dose. If the distance is increased to 2m at point Y (Y is 2 times X) the intensity is reduced to one-quarter that of X (2 squared = 4).

Note:

➡ if the distance is increased, the intensity decreases by the square of the distance
➡ if the distance is reduced, the intensity increases by the square of the distance
➡ double the distance and the intensity is one quarter

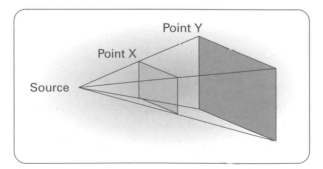

Illustration of the inverse square law.

➡ half the distance and the intensity is quadrupled.

Thus, intensity of radiation at 30 cm (1 ft) is four times that at 60 cm (2 ft) and nine times that at 1m (3 ft); this means that four minutes at 60 cm will produce the same effects as 1 minute at 30 cm or 9 minutes at 1m. Spend a few minutes thinking this through until you fully comprehend the scientific law of inverse squares.

Cosine law

The cosine law applies to visible light, infra-red and ultraviolet, and governs intensity in relation to the angle a ray strikes a surface. The cosine law states that the intensity of radiation at a surface varies according to the cosine of the angle of incidence (the angle between the ray and the surface). Maximum intensity, absorption and effect are ensured when rays strike the surface at an angle of 90°; greater angles produce lesser intensities. The amount of decrease can be calculated by measuring the angle between the incident ray and 90° and looking up its cosine in a book of cosine tables.

➡ There is maximum intensity and absorption when rays strike the body at 90°.
➡ As the rays move down towards the surface, the angle of incidence increases.
➡ The greater the angle of incidence, the lower the intensity.
➡ The cosine of 0° is 1; the cosine of 60° is 0.5.
➡ A 60° angle of incidence creates half the intensity of a 0° angle.
➡ **Practice point:** a good illustration of the cosine law is the fact that the midday sun, high in the sky, is more likely to cause sunburn than the late afternoon sun, which is low in the sky.

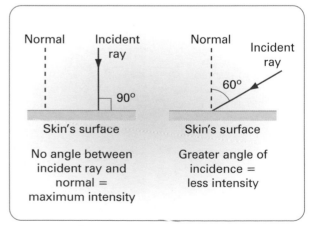

Illustration of the cosine law.

Infra-red and radiant heat

Infra-red and radiant heat lamps produce electromagnetic rays with wavelengths which are longer than visible light (see illustration on page 243). Infra-red rays are emitted by any hot object, such as the sun and electric and natural fires. There are two types of infra-red lamps used in body therapy: true infra-red or **non-luminous** lamps, and radiant heat or **luminous** types.

Infra-red (non-luminous)

These lamps consist of a wire coil which heats up in a bed of clay. The source is non-glowing, so it is not always apparent that the lamp is switched on and care should be taken to avoid burns. Infra-red lamps emit rays of about 4000nm, much longer than luminous types. They penetrate less deeply, only into the epidermis, and are therefore less irritating and have a more sedative effect. However, because of the increased superficial absorption, non-luminous rays can feel hotter than luminous rays at equal distance from the body.

Radiant heat (luminous)

These lamps consist of a glass bulb, often coloured red, surrounded by a reflector. They heat up instantly and it is obvious when the lamp is switched on because of the glow. Radiant heat lamps emit rays of about 1000nm as well as some visible rays. They penetrate more deeply, down into the subcutaneous layer, and are therefore more irritating than non-luminous types.

Infra-red and radiant heat lamps:

Infra-red (non-luminous)	Radiant heat (luminous)
▸ wire coil	▸ bulb
▸ takes 10 minutes to heat up	▸ heats up within 2 minutes
▸ no visible rays	▸ has some visible rays
▸ not obvious when it is switched on	▸ glows when switched on
▸ longer wavelength @ 4000nm	▸ shorter wavelength @ 1000nm
▸ penetrates epidermis.	▸ penetrates subcutaneous layer.

Contra-indications to infra red and radiant heat application:
- ▸ high or low blood pressure
- ▸ circulatory disorders
- ▸ thrombosis or phlebitis
- ▸ acute eczema and dermatitis
- ▸ hypersensitive skin
- ▸ previous burns or sunburn
- ▸ headache or migraine
- ▸ diabetes
- ▸ recent scar tissue
- ▸ later stages of pregnancy
- ▸ swelling or fluid retention
- ▸ menstruation.

Indications for use:
- ▸ for general pre-heating of the body
- ▸ to relieve aches and pains
- ▸ to relieve muscular tension
- ▸ to aid absorption of products
- ▸ to promote relaxation.

Benefits and effects:
- ▸ heating of body tissues directly or by conduction through the tissues
- ▸ increase in body temperature as local heat spreads to surrounding tissues
- ▸ increased circulation causing vasodilation, hyperaemia and erythema
- ▸ lower blood pressure due to vasodilation
- ▸ increased cell metabolism in local area.

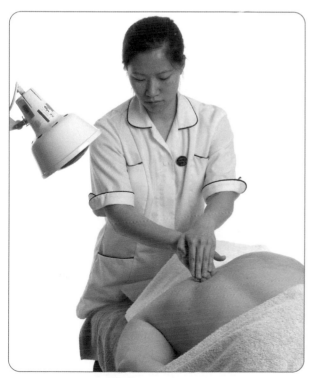

Infra-red heat lamp in use.

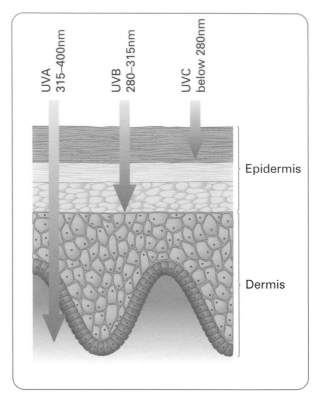

Assessment task 10.20

Discuss the indications and contra-indications to radiant heat and infra-red applications. (M)

Technique

Safe starting

▸▸ Prepare equipment and work area.

▸▸ Place machine on a stable base with no trailing wires.

▸▸ Check plugs, bulbs, leads and reflector.

▸▸ Prepare client and remove all jewellery.

▸▸ Check for contra-indications and cover any small abrasions.

▸▸ Cleanse the area thoroughly to remove any oils.

▸▸ **Practice point:** carry out a hot/cold skin sensitivity test.

Safe working

▸▸ **Practice point:** cover areas not being treated and protect the client's eyes with eye pads.

1 Explain the treatment effects and sensation to the client.

2 Direct lamp away from client and switch on.

3 When lamp is ready, position parallel to area being treated at a distance of about 60 cm.

4 Stay near to the client for the duration of the treatment (20 minutes).

Safe stopping

▸▸ **Practice point:** handle with care to avoid burns.

▸▸ Turn the lamp away, switch off and return to storage.

▸▸ Continue with massage or electrotherapy (not UV).

▸▸ As blood pressure is lowered, client should take care when rising.

Assessment task 10.21

Discuss the benefits and hazards of infra-red and radiant heat applications, describing timing, frequency and health and safety procedures. (M)

Ultraviolet radiation

Ultraviolet light consists of electro-magnetic rays which are invisible to the human eye. They have wavelengths of 100–400 nm and lie between x-rays

Penetration of UV rays into the skin.

and visible light on the electromagnetic spectrum (see illustration on page 243). Ultraviolet light is divided into three types according to wavelength: UVA, UVB and UVC.

UVA

UVA has the longest wavelengths at 315–400 nm. They penetrate deep into the dermis and cause tanning without burning. Because UVA rays penetrate deeply, they cause damage to collagen and elastin fibres and speed the skin's ageing process causing lines, wrinkles and dehydration. Sunbeds emit mostly UVA rays.

UVB

UVB is the middle band with wavelengths of 280–315 nm. They penetrate to the stratum germinativum or basal cell layer of the epidermis. UVB rays trigger tanning and also burning; over-exposure can contribute to the onset of skin cancer. The majority of UVB rays are filtered out of sunbeds but some sun lamps used for medical purposes do contain UVB rays.

UVC

UVC rays have the shortest wavelengths at 100–280 nm. They penetrate only as far as the stratum corneum, the uppermost layer of the epidermis. Exposure to UVC causes superficial skin damage and the destruction of bacteria. UVC rays are filtered out of sunbeds and the ozone layer serves to filter UVC out of natural sunlight. Depletion of the ozone layer has led to concerns that more harmful UVC will reach the earth's surface and cause damage to human skin.

Sources of UVA, UVB and UVC:

Natural sunlight	Artificial sunlight
Emits all ultraviolet rays	High and low pressure medical sunlamps emit UVA, UVB and UVC
Intensity varies according to the time of year, time of day, latitude, altitude and cloud cover	All harmful UVC is filtered out of sunbeds
Harmful UVC is absorbed by the ozone layer	Most UVB is filtered out of sunbeds
Effects of sunlight are caused by UVA and UVB rays	UVA rays are emitted by sunbeds to promote tanning

Sunbeds

There has been much debate between medical professionals and the leisure and beauty industry about the use of sunbeds, with the result that many local authorities have banned their use. It was widely reported when the Sanctuary day spa in London removed all sunbeds on the advice that they were a potential health hazard, and many other health and beauty establishments followed suit. However, those businesses which continue to offer tanning facilities are thriving and the demand for sunbeds remains high. There is no doubt that, for some people, the desire to look tanned outweighs the possible hazards. Some sunbeds emit only UVA and the manufacturers of these claim that they will tan without any harmful effects (i.e. from UVB or UVC). Dermatologists disagree and suggest instead that exposure to UVA is just as harmful as prolonged exposure to natural sunlight, causing degenerative skin changes and the development of skin cancer. Manufacturers believe that there is insufficient

evidence to support such claims and, indeed, most tests have been performed on animals rather than humans. As a beauty therapist, you need to be fully aware of the potential risk factors associated with the use of sunbeds and make up your own mind in order to ensure the safety of your clients.

Contra-indications to sunbeds:

» children under 16 years
» fair-skinned clients
» clients who do not tan easily in the sun
» high number of moles or freckles
» pigmented or inflamed naevi
» previously sun damaged skin
» previous heat treatment
» sunburn
» sensitive skin
» diabetes
» history of skin cancer
» pregnancy
» chloasma or vitiligo
» headaches, migraine
» certain medication (listed on page 249)
» high or low blood pressure
» fever, flu, high temperature
» skin diseases and disorders.

Assessment task 10.22

Discuss the indications and contra-indications to sun tanning applications. (M)

Equipment

Sunbeds come in various forms. The most popular are double canopy beds which tan both sides at once, and stand-up beds which tan all around the body simultaneously. Both types consist of fluorescent tubes lined with phosphorus which are designed to absorb UVC and most UVB rays. Sunbeds which only emit UVA are safer but tan slowly. So-called 'fast tanning' beds, which are currently very popular, emit about 96–98 per cent UVA as well as 2–4 per cent UVB. They produce a tan more quickly which lasts for longer, but they may also present greater risks.

(Skin cancer is discussed in Unit 6: Dermatology and microbiology, pages 114–117.)

Maintenance

» Sunbeds should be used in a well-ventilated room.
» Sunbeds should be wiped over before and after use with an appropriate sterilising solution.
» Sunbeds should be inspected annually by a qualified electrician.
» Sunbed use should be recorded and tubes changed as necessary.
» The intensity of sunbed tubes diminishes with use; refer to manufacturer's instructions.

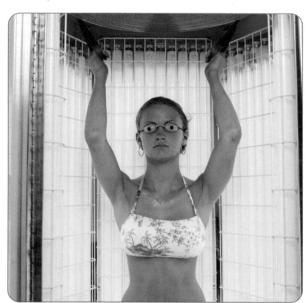

Upright tanning booth.

Ultraviolet lamps

High pressure mercury vapour lamps contain argon gas and mercury in small quantities, which ionises to give off ultraviolet light. This type of equipment emits UVA, UVB and some UVC as well as visible light and infra-red. The lamps are used in hospitals for the treatment of acne vulgaris, psoriasis, alopecia and other skin disorders. They are not used in beauty salons.

Potential hazards:

» uneven pigmentation and colouration of skin
» premature lines and wrinkles
» skin dehydration
» photosensitisation
» thickening of skin ('leathery' texture)
» changes to existing moles
» malignant melanoma and other forms of skin cancer
» cataracts, conjunctivitis
» can be addictive.

Consultation for UV treatment

The use of sunbeds can be made as safe as possible by following stringent guidelines and carrying out a full consultation with clients before use. You should check for contra-indications and examine the client's skin type, taking into account the presence of moles and freckles and his or her tanning history. Dermatologists suggest there are six skin types, which react differently to natural sunlight. You should assess the client, visually and verbally, and make a decision about exposure time based on this diagnosis:

» Type 1: never tans, always burns
» Type 2: tans with difficulty, burns often
» Type 3: tans easily, burns rarely
» Type 4: always tans, never burns
» Type 5: genetically brown skin
» Type 6: genetically black skin.

Indications for use of UV:

Indications for salon use of UV:	Indications for medical use of UV:
» to create a healthy glow	» as treatment for acne vulgaris
» to camouflage stretch marks and cellulite	» as treatment for psoriasis
» to improve skin blemishes	» as treatment for eczema
» to create a slimmer looking figure	» as treatment for alopecia
» to prepare skin for holidays in the sun	» as a general tonic
» to improve appearance for a special occasion	» as treatment for seasonal affective disorder (SAD).
» for relaxation.	

Assess your own, or a friend's, skin based on these six skin types and decide what advice you would offer for safe tanning and safe use of sunbeds.

Medical history, including current and previous medication, should be noted and, if you are in doubt, medical advice should be sought. Topical preparations, antibiotics, the contraceptive pill and hormone treatment can all make the skin photosensitive and prone to burning or pigmentation disorders (see below). You should also inform your clients of the potential dangers of use and over-use of sunbeds and ask them to sign a consent form (or the record card) as an acknowledgement that you have done so. You should provide goggles specifically designed for sunbed users and preferably each client will buy a pair for their individual use, to avoid cross-infection. Clients should not use sunbeds for more than 10 hours per year. Keep a tight record of their visits to maintain their safety as well as your professional reputation. You should also display a visible notice that warns clients of the potential risks of sunbed use and lists the precautions necessary prior to treatment.

Procedure

Safe starting
» Wipe over the bed with a recommended sterilising solution.
» Check for contra-indications and cover minor abrasions.

Recommendations for sunbed users:

» Remove make-up, perfume and body lotions.
» Remove all jewellery.
» Remove contact lenses.
» Check client's skin type.
» **Practice point:**
  - Provide clean goggles for each client.
  - Explain the potential hazards of sunbed use.

Safe working
» Set the timer switch according to skin type.
» Explain how to operate the 'stop' button.
» Start with the minimum dose.
» **Practice point:** clients should be able to stop the sunbed at any time if it becomes uncomfortable.

Safe stopping
» Client should rise slowly.
» Apply suitable face and body moisturiser.
» Record skin reaction.
» Record date, time and duration of treatment.
» Wipe over the bed with a recommended sterilising solution.
» **Practice point:** do not have a follow-up tanning session until the skin has calmed from the previous session.

Home care advice
» Avoid exposure to natural sunlight or other heat treatments such as waxing and electrolysis.
» Skin may be more sensitive for 6–8 hours after treatment, therefore avoid perfumed products.
» Monitor skin's reaction to treatment and contact the therapist if you notice any adverse reactions.

Doctor's permission is required if you are taking any of the following medication:
» antibiotics
» tranquillisers
» diuretics
» steroids
» contraceptive pill
» acne treatment, roacutane
» hormone replacement theory
» medication to control blood pressure
» medication for diabetes, insulin
» medication for thyroid treatment.

Pre-treatment precautions:
» remove all make-up, perfume and lotions
» remove all jewellery
» do not use suntan preparations
» remove contact lenses
» cover hair, especially if tinted
» wear protective goggles.

Maximum sunbed use = 10 hours per year

Retail recommendations

→ Sunbed goggles.
→ Facial moisturiser.
→ Body moisturiser.
→ Sunbed accelerator products.
→ SPF suntanning products and after-sun, if treatment is given prior to a holiday.

Assessment task 10.23

Discuss the benefits and hazards of sun tanning applications, describing timing, frequency, health and safety procedures. (M)

Assessment task 10.24

Design an after care leaflet for distribution to sunbed clients. Pay particular attention to potential hazards, frequency, timing, health and safety, after care and retail recommendations. (D)

Self-tanning application

The growth in popularity of self tanning has a direct correlation with the health scares associated with natural sun tanning and sunbeds, and the products available have advanced a long way since the streaky, orange creams of the past. Most cosmetic manufacturers have a range of sun care products which includes self-tan, as do chemist and supermarket chains. The choice of products is vast and the types available include creams, lotions, sprays and mousses. Some individuals are able to master the technique of self-application, but the best results by far are gained from the professional application of self-tanning products.

Product knowledge

Self-tanning products contain either chemical or vegetable pigments which tint the upper layers of the epidermis. Some products have an immediate effect but these tend to have more temporary results. The majority of formulations take about 4 hours to develop. They are applied as colourless lotions and tend to be quite sticky. As they dry, the tan develops and lasts for up to a week. More advanced formulas, such as St Tropez, Fantasy Tan or Sun FX, are applied as a tinted product which can be adapted to suit the individual skin tone. This is washed off after a longer period, 8 hours or more, looks most natural and lasts for longer – about 10–14 days. Modern self-tanning products are

safe to use, have no side effects and very few contra-indications, which make them a popular choice for a healthy, risk-free suntan and especially for clients who are contra-indicated to use sunbeds.

Contra-indications:
→ contagious skin diseases
→ skin inflammations
→ hypersensitive skin.

Indications for use:
→ to improve appearance
→ for fair skin which never tans
→ for sensitive skin that burns easily
→ during pregnancy
→ suitable for all age groups
→ for special occasions
→ to create a tan before holidays
→ to create a feeling of well-being.

Assessment task 10.25

Discuss the indications and contra-indications of self-tanning. (M)

Theory into practice

Consider the information you would need to record during a self-tan application.

Procedure
Safe starting
→ **Practice point:** make sure the treatment room is warm and well-ventilated.

→ Prepare the work area with regards to health and safety.
→ Check for contra-indications.
→ Protect the couch and floor with couch roll.
→ Protect the client's hair.
→ Provide disposable pants.
→ Choose a suitable method of application for the client's skin type and colour.
→ Agree colour choice with the client.

Safe working
→ **Practice point:** skin must be clean of oil and products, exfoliated and dried thoroughly before application.

→ Remove make-up, cleanse, tone and exfoliate.
→ Thoroughly exfoliate the body.
→ Ask the client to shower but refrain from using any products.
→ Apply face and body moisturiser.

- Apply product in a methodical sequence according to manufacturer's instructions.
- Wear disposable gloves or wash hands immediately.
- Leave the client to dry for up to 10 minutes, according to manufacturer's instructions.

Safe stopping

- **Practice point:** check that the application is even before the client departs.

- Buff the product according to manufacturer's instructions.
- Ask the client to dress in loose, dark clothing.
- Tidy the treatment area.

Home care advice

- Wear loose, dark clothes.
- Refrain from washing hands.
- Do not shower for the period instructed.
- Moisturise daily to maintain tan.
- Exfoliate after 5–7 days.
- Have re-application as required.

Retail recommendations

- Body scrub.
- Body lotion.
- Self-tanning product for top-up applications between treatments.
- Sun tanning products and after-sun if prior to a holiday.

Assessment task 10.26

Discuss the benefits and hazards of self-tanning applications, describing timing, and frequency, health and safety procedures. (M)

Assessment task 10.27

Provide detailed home care advice and show an awareness of retail opportunities following self-tanning application. (D)

Knowledge check

1. Compare and contrast the characteristics of an endomorph, ectomorph and mesomorph.
2. Describe various types of adipose tissue.
3. How can you ensure the accurate recording of body weight and measurements?
4. Describe the three main spinal deviations.
5. Explain the use of a plumb line.
6. Evaluate the use of audio sonic equipment in body therapy.
7. Describe the benefits of combining vacuum suction with gyratory massage.
8. What is the difference between mechanical and electrical equipment?
9. Give reasons for poor contractions in body EMS treatment.
10. Explain monophasic and biphasic current.
11. Explain longitudinal, duplicate and split padding.
12. What is a motor point?
13. Why is galvanism sometimes called cellulite polarity?
14. What is the purpose of pre-heating tissues in body therapy?
15. Explain the differences between infra-red and radiant heat.
16. Why do infra-red and radiant heat lamps not produce a tanning effect?
17. What is the inverse square law?
18. What is the cosine law?
19. Explain the different effects of UVA, UVB and UVC.
20. Are sunbeds safe?

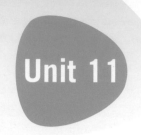

Permanent and long-term hair removal is now a multi-million pound business. A knowledge and understanding of the principles and application of electrical epilation is a valuable addition to your CV when you are looking for employment. Intense pulsed light systems and laser equipment are growing in popularity and are a good source of income. To be able to understand and use IPL systems in order to gain the best results for your clients, it is advisable to have trained in electrical epilation techniques.

This unit introduces you to the skills and knowledge you will need in order to practise electrical epilation. You will gain an insight into the structure and growth cycle of the hair and factors that influence the development of unwanted hair. In addition you will be introduced to the psychological effect that unwanted hair growth has on different people.

You will learn about the different methods of electrical epilation and techniques, as well as the benefits and drawbacks of each. You will gain the knowledge and understanding to diagnose and evaluate the client's problem and prescribe an appropriate treatment plan. You will also be given the opportunity to learn about and evaluate different equipment.

In order to achieve Unit 11 in Electrical epilation you must complete the following learning outcomes:

Learning Outcomes

1 Review the structure and growth cycle of the hair with regard to hair removal using electrical epilation.

2 Determine the type of hair and cause of hair growth and evaluate client suitability for treatment.

3 Explain types of current and their uses in electrical epilation.

4 Perform safe and effective treatment of electrical epilation.

Structure and growth cycle of the hair

To review the structure and growth cycle of hair, revisit Unit 6 pages 109–112.

Electrical epilation

You will find that when you apply electrical epilation correctly you should be able to destroy the lower third of the hair follicle. The way in which you achieve this depends on the method of epilation you use, i.e. blend, diathermy or galvanic. The most effective time to apply treatment is during anagen, when the follicle is at its deepest level in the skin and where the concentration of moisture is highest.

Shortwave diathermy coagulates the lower third of the follicle, changing the structure of the protein and destroying the cellular structure, including the germinal hair cells and dermal papilla. To achieve this you must apply the current through the needle to the base of the follicle and allow the current to flow for a sufficient period of time.

Blend destroys the follicle as a result of a chemical reaction which is achieved by the simultaneous application of high frequency current (to warm the sodium hydroxide) and galvanic, to produce sodium hydroxide (lye). Sodium hydroxide is caustic, causing the lower follicle to liquefy. You will only achieve the desired result when the blend of the two currents is correct. Blend is far more effective on curved or distorted follicles than shortwave diathermy. This is because sodium hydroxide is able to fill the follicle, whereas the high frequency heating pattern requires the needle to be placed accurately at the base of the follicle. You will find that it is not possible to place the tip of the needle accurately at the base of a distorted or curved follicle.

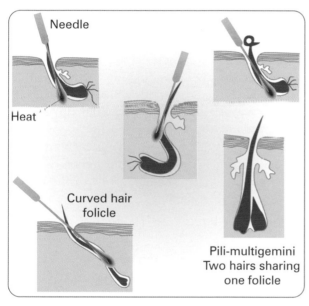

Heating pattern for high frequency and needle placement for distorted follicles.

Type of hair and causes of hair growth

Hair type

Hair can be grouped into specific types and each has a bearing on the treatment that you will give. You will find that most of the epilation treatments that you carry out will involve terminal hair. However, you must also be familiar with the structure and location of lanugo and vellus hair, both of which are entirely different in structure to terminal hair.

Lanugo hair

Lanugo is usually found in foetal life and is normally shed around the seventh to eighth month of pregnancy, to be replaced by vellus or terminal hair. This type of hair is long, fine, downy and soft in texture, without a medulla and usually does not contain pigment.

Vellus

Vellus hair is short, fine, downy hair and soft and does not contain pigment. It is found on the body generally and rarely exceeds 2 cm in length. These hairs do not contain a medulla. The base of the vellus hair lies very close to the skin's surface. Vellus hairs do not become terminal hair unless stimulated by topical or systemic conditions.

Vellus hair is the fine downy growth, often on the sides of the face, that some clients will become obsessed with. They are often the hairs that clients see but that you as the electrolysist cannot see – even with the aid of good light and a magnifying lamp moved in all angles and directions! The additional problem you will find when epilating vellus hair is that it lies very close to the skin's surface, so the insertions are very shallow. With blend application no moisture is present, therefore galvanic action for the production of sodium hydroxide (lye) will not occur. With shortwave diathermy, the current is applied too close to the surface, thereby risking burns through too much heat at the epidermis instead of in the dermis. You must observe the skin carefully during treatment to ensure that over-heating does not occur.

Terminal hair

Terminal hair is stronger than both lanugo and vellus hair, and has a defined structure. Located on the head, arms, legs, bikini area, under arms and face, this type of hair grows from a follicle and goes through a complete growth cycle.

Terminal hair is composed of three layers known as the cuticle, medulla and cortex, and grows to different lengths in different parts of the body (see page 208). This type of hair can be grouped into asexual, ambisexual and sexual.

1   **Asexual** – genetic hair present at birth.
    Asexual hair refers to hair found on the scalp, eyebrows and eyelashes, and to a lesser extent on the forearms and legs, in both sexes of all ages. Although this hair type is influenced by

hormone production, steroids do not influence growth.

2 **Ambisexual** – develops in both sexes at puberty. This type of hair growth is influenced by the increased gonadal and androgen

production. Areas where ambisexual hair growth occurs are the axilla, pubis, lower limbs and abdomen in both sexes. Growth on the forearms and legs becomes more profuse at this stage of life. The density and rate of growth differs widely between sexes, individuals of the same sex and various body sites.

3 **Sexual hair** – includes the beard, moustache, nasal passages, ears and external body hair, e.g. back and chest. Sexual hair is influenced by increased androgen hormone production by the gonads. Testosterone levels in men are 15–30 per cent higher than in women. Sexual hair is more pronounced in men due to the higher levels of progesterone production by the testes.

Needle size

You will discover that the needle size you use has an influence on the success or failure of epilation. A general guideline is that the diameter of the needle should match the diameter of the hair. The needle size varies slightly depending on whether you are using a one-piece or a two-piece needle. A one piece needle may be tapered between the tip and the shank whereas the diameter of a two piece needle does not alter. With practice and careful observation of skin reaction and ease of insertion into the follicle, you will soon be able to make the correct choice without hesitation.

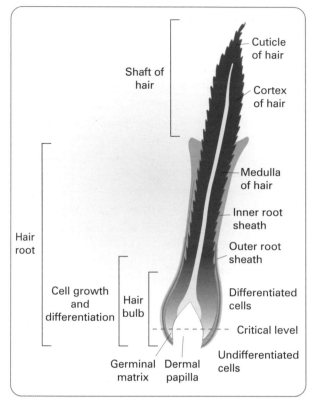

Longitudinal diagram of terminal hair.

Location of hair type:

Hair type	Location	Characteristics
Lanugo	Foetal	Shed around 7th and 8th months of pregnancy
Vellus	Generally on body and face	▸▸ Downy ▸▸ Rarely exceeds 2 cm in length ▸▸ Does not contain a medulla ▸▸ Clients often concerned about vellus hair ▸▸ cheeks, upper lip and sides of face
Terminal		▸▸ Pigmented ▸▸ Contains cortex, cuticle and medulla
▸▸ **Asexual**	Scalp, eyebrows, eyelashes	Genetic – present at birth
▸▸ **Ambisexual**	Axilla, pubis, lower limbs and abdomen in both sexes	Develops in both sexes at puberty
▸▸ **Sexual**	Beard, moustache, nasal passages, ears and external body hair, e.g. back and chest	Influenced by increased androgen production

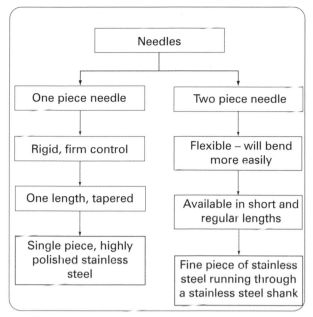

Needle types.

The needle diameter influences the result and comfort of treatment in a number of ways:

» *When the needle is too large:*
  a the follicle wall is stretched during insertion
  b the high frequency current may be applied at the skin's surface where the needle has made contact with the skin
  c you will find it difficult to insert the needle to the base of the follicle.

» *When the needle is too small:*
  a the needle will not encompass the base of the follicle
  b you will need to increase the current intensity to create sufficient heat in the follicle
  c the treatment will be painful for the client due to the high amount of current needed to epilate the hair.

» *When you use a needle that matches the diameter of the hair:*
  a the needle should slide easily into the follicle without touching the opening of the follicle
  b you will be able to apply sufficient current to encompass the base of the follicle thereby epilating the hair without causing unnecessary pain to your client.

Current timing and adjustment

When the current is set to the correct intensity the hair will slide out of the follicle easily, complete with bulb, depending on the stage of the hair growth cycle. Dark, terminal hairs on the chin will require a higher current intensity than fine terminal or vellus hairs on the upper lip. The client's pain threshold is much lower on the upper lip, particularly in the centre where the nerve endings are more numerous. A fine, sensitive skin will tolerate less current than a coarse or oily skin.

Incorrect adjustment of current causes a number of problems. If you set the current at too low an intensity there will not be enough heat produced (or galvanic lye in the case of blend) to successfully epilate the hair and destroy the follicle; you will find that there will be an unacceptable percentage of re-growth. On the other hand, if you use too much current you will create too much heat with high frequency or galvanic lye with blend. This will result in over-treatment of the skin, causing excess swelling, erythema, blanching and surface burns; too much current when using direct current (galvanic) may result in weeping follicles.

Cause of hair growth

In order to achieve a successful result with electro-epilation it is necessary to understand the causes of hair growth. This cannot be fully achieved without having first studied the endocrine system. Consideration should be given to genetic/heredity tendencies, topical causes and sensitivity of follicles to circulating androgens in the bloodstream.

A high percentage of hirsute women have either a hereditary predisposition or some subtle change in their androgen production. Hair distribution, type of hair and rate of growth varies from one race to another and from one person to another. For example, Caucasians have a higher number of hair follicles than the Japanese and Chinese. Some nationalities and individuals find the presence of hair both desirable and acceptable, whereas others prefer a complete absence of hair.

Sensitivity of follicle end receptors to circulating androgens encompasses a number of factors, from topical friction to endocrine influences. You will find that the degree of hormone sensitivity can vary from one area to another and between different individuals. Increased sensitivity of androgen receptors in the pilo-sebaceous unit may be a dominant or recessive hereditary trait.

There are a number of topical causes, including sustained friction, e.g. a plaster cast. Friction causes an increase in local blood circulation to the skin. This type of hair growth is temporary and usually returns to normal shortly after the plaster cast has been removed.

The tweezing of individual hairs tears out the lower follicle. The reconstructed follicle is usually stronger, with a better blood supply. Vellus and fine hairs are frequently removed at the same time, so aggravating the condition. Waxing of facial and vellus hair will have the same effect as tweezing. Hairs that have been waxed or tweezed invariably leave behind distorted follicles, so hindering electro-epilation unless blend or galvanic electrolysis is used.

Primary causes of hair growth

Hormones are responsible for influencing and stimulating growth of the follicle cells, which in turn determines the pattern, quantity, texture and distribution of body hair. It is important for clients to understand that both primary and secondary hirsutism can be managed successfully with medical treatment, which will correct or control endocrine disorders, thereby preventing the development of new growth.

Endocrine influences can be divided into **normal systemic** and **abnormal systemic** conditions. Normal systemic conditions include: puberty; pregnancy; menopause; stress; and sensitivity of follicle end organ receptors to androgens. Abnormal endocrine conditions include: Stein Leventhal syndrome, more commonly referred to as polycystic ovary syndrome; Cushings syndrome; adrenal tumours; ovarian tumours; diabetes mellitus; and anorexia nervosa.

Androgens and growth hormones increase the size and diameter of hair follicle. Cortisols, oestrogens and thyroid hormones alter and influence without increasing hair growth. Although oestrogens do not initiate growth they can prolong an existing hair growth cycle (see *The Cause and Management of Hirsutism*, Greenblatt et al).

Surgery can also contribute towards the development of unwanted hair, e.g. total hysterectomy, which involves the removal of the ovaries and therefore alters the hormone balance.

Puberty

The anterior pituitary gland secretes gonadotrophic hormones, which influence the target organs. These are ovaries in the female and testes in the male. At puberty, the adrenal cortex becomes active. Between them, the adrenal cortex and the gonads secrete large quantities of steroid hormones into the circulatory system.

The appearance of both pubic and axillary hair is due to the increased level of adrenocortical androgens. Hereditary sensitivity in combination with the amount of hormone produced is responsible for the appearance of hair in other areas. Androgen levels increase in women during puberty, pregnancy and menopause; however, women produce smaller quantities of androgen than men.

Pregnancy

During pregnancy there is an increase in hormone activity. On occasions, excess androgens are produced, with the result that fine hair growth may appear on the lip, chin and sides of the face. Quite often this is a temporary growth that disappears shortly after the end of pregnancy, without treatment.

Menopause

The menopause marks the end of a woman's reproductive life. Between the ages of 40 and 50 years there is a gradual decline in the oestrogen and progesterone levels. This is because ovarian tissue slowly ceases to respond to stimulation by the gonadotrophic hormones of the anterior pituitary gland. Facial hair often develops because of the increased level of circulating androgens.

Assessment task information

Mrs Sutherland is a 47-year-old woman who is embarrassed by the presence of hair growth on her chin, sides of face and upper lip. During the consultation you discover that she is diabetic, has started the menopause and that her hair growth has increased during the past five years. This lady has previously received epilation in another establishment, which has unfortunately left her with scars around the chin and upper lip. You will be asked to complete Assessment tasks 11.1–11.6 based on this information.

Assessment task 11.1

Describe the manner in which you would conduct the consultation with Mrs Sutherland. Produce evidence to show what information you would gather from the consultation and the bearing of this information on future treatment. List the methods of communication that you would employ. (M)

Secondary causes of hair growth

Endocrine disorders which affect hair growth

Endocrine disorders result from a glandular defect, which may be inherited from either parent (or their predecessors) or may be an acquired disease. Disorders that affect hair growth are: Cushings syndrome, Stein-Levethal syndrome and adrenal neoplasms.

Adrenal influences in hirsute women

People vary greatly in their skin sensitivity to androgens owing to their genetic background: a high level of circulating androgens may have no effect on one individual, whereas a low level may induce hair growth in another.

Adrenogenital syndrome

Adrenogenital syndrome fortunately is a rare condition and very unlikely to be seen by the practising electrolysist. The effect of androgen disorder is more noticeable in girls who show an abnormal development of the external genitalia. In extreme cases, the clitoris protrudes and may be mistaken for a penis. The adult female will eventually have a male build and develop a deep voice, as well as having a male distribution of hair growth.

When a boy is affected, he will reach puberty between the ages of 3 and 5 years, with secondary sex characteristics becoming noticeable. High androgen levels in both sexes cause rapid body growth that stops early. The epiphyses in the bone fuse at an earlier age than normal.

Symptoms which may be present in the adult woman are due to over-secretion of androgens. These include: receding hairline; the appearance of bald patches; increased hair growth in a masculine pattern on the face and limbs; breasts becoming atrophied; and the menstrual cycle may be absent or become irregular. Feminine fat is replaced by masculine muscle.

Adrenal tumours

These are small, non-encapsulated masses and are usually single, solitary nodules. Adrenal tumours (also known as neoplasms) can occur at any age, although they are more common around the age of 30 to 40 years. Their presence is indicated by a sudden onset of virilisation, or Cushings syndrome. This type of tumour may be masculinising, causing hirsutism, increased muscle mass and deepening of the voice in women.

Virilising congenital adrenal hyperplasias

Virilising congenital adrenal hyperplasias are the result of enzyme deficiency that affects the production and levels of adrenal hormones. Partial or total enzyme deficiency results in decreased cortisol levels. At the same time, production of androgen is increased by the adrenal cortex, leading to excess production and thereby causing hirsutism.

Cushings syndrome

Cushings syndrome is brought on by an excess of glucocorticoids as a result of a tumour or excessive adrenal cortex function. Pituitary tumours and certain cancers, such as lung and pancreatic cancers, result in over-production and aldosterone production.

There are a number of symptoms associated with Cushings syndrome which include: osteoporosis owing to decreased calcium absorption; obesity of the trunk with purple stretch marks on the abdomen; muscular weakness and wasting of the limbs; thinning of the skin plus a tendency to bruise easily; rounding of the face due to fat deposits in the cheeks; diabetes could occur due to increased steroid production; salt retention leading to high blood pressure and oedema; vellus hair growth due to increased cortisol levels; and excess androgens possibly leading to hirsutism.

Stein-Leventhal syndrome

This condition is more commonly referred to as polycystic ovary syndrome. You, the electrolysist, may be the first person to observe the signs that indicate a client may be suffering from this condition. Referral of the client back to her doctor for further investigation is advisable. Symptoms associated with polycystic ovary syndrome include: enlarged ovaries with numerous follicular cysts; irregular menstrual cycle; weight gain; and the development of excess hair growth. The onset of hirsutism is gradual, occurring from puberty onwards. Polycystic ovaries are capable of secreting large quantities of androgens. Epilation may not eliminate the excess hair growth due to the underlying cause; however, you will find that it is possible to reduce the growth considerably especially when combined with medical treatment.

Masculinising ovarian tumours

This type of tumour is rare, but when present it may cause an excess production of androgen. Hirsutism caused by masculinising ovarian tumours has a rapid onset, usually but not always later in life. Menstruation may stop and will only start again after surgery.

Archard-Thiers syndrome

This is another relatively rare endocrine disorder. The characteristics include: generalised obesity; diabetes mellitus; hypertension; and hirsutism. Hair growth is most noticeable on the face, with emphasis on the moustache and beard. Menstrual disorders may occur.

Anorexia nervosa

Anorexia nervosa is a condition that usually affects adolescent girls. It is a condition that involves the nervous, digestive and endocrine systems.

Anorexia nervosa exhibits a number of characteristics which include: increased growth of vellus hair on the face, trunk and arms; persistent refusal to eat food; absence of menstrual periods; weight loss and wasting muscles; emotional stress or disturbance.

Definition of hirsutism

Hirsutism refers to a masculine pattern of hair growth in women – one that is normal in men. There is an increase in cyclic growth, diameter of the hair and rate of growth. Hirsutism is considered a disease by many medical authorities and may arise from a serious underlying disorder that can often be diagnosed by some simple blood test and detailed notes of medical history.

Hirsutism is caused by the following two factors:

1 Increased follicle sensitivity to normal levels of circulating androgens in the blood. This is referred to as **primary hirsutism**. The onset of primary hirsutism occurs at puberty, increasing until the thirties when it stabilises. Secondary hirsutism begins just before or just after puberty.

2 Increased androgen production by the adrenal glands and ovaries. This is referred to as **secondary** or **true hirsutism**. Secondary hirsutism is due to an endocrine disorder that causes increased hormonal secretion by the glands.

▶▶ **Practice point:** The total number of hair follicles for an adult human is estimated at 5 million, with 1 million on the head of which 10,000 alone cover the scalp (Szabo 1958).

Definition of hypertrichosis

Hypertrichosis refers to a generalised over-growth of vellus and terminal hair in either sex. Hairs grow faster than normal, although there is no increase in diameter size. This type of growth is not due to a systemic disorder; causes are genetic and racial tendencies or constitutional variations in follicle sensitivity.

Definition of superfluous hair

Superfluous hair can be defined as hair growth that is not wanted; in other words, it is surplus to requirements. It may be an excess amount of hair growing in a natural pattern with no underlying causes, or it may be due to hypertrichosis of hirsuitism.

Client suitability for treatment

Preliminary consultation

What are clients looking for during the initial contact with the electrolysist? Usually they are seeking a professional approach which is warm and welcoming – one that is not patronising or flippant, or which makes them feel abnormal or inferior. Questions may arise relating to: the professional qualifications of the electrolysist; knowledge of the subject; frequency and length of treatments; time taken to clear the problem permanently; methods of dealing with the hair growth between treatments; cost involved; approach to hygiene; and the use of sterile disposable needles.

Having considered the advantages to the client, some thought should be given to the benefits of the consultation to the electrolysist. Valuable information can be obtained at this stage that will help the electrolysist plan an effective course of treatment. Several factors need to be considered before a decision on treatment is reached.

During the initial consultation you should assess the client's suitability for epilation treatment, having determined the cause of hair growth. You should explain in detail the process and the time commitment to ascertain whether or not the client is prepared to make the commitment to attend for treatment on a regular basis. You will need to be sure that there are no contra-indications that will prevent treatment. You should also check by means of a medical questionnaire whether you client has a condition which will need her or his doctor's consent before treatment can be started, e.g. pace maker, epilepsy. You must also establish that your client's expectations of time involved and anticipated results are realistic!

During the menopause it is possible that hair growth will increase due to the change in the hormone balance. Some follicles become sensitive to these circulating hormones in the blood and hair growth is stimulated. This can and does cause embarrassment.

A woman can become more sensitive with a lowered pain threshold immediately before and during menstruation, therefore the treatment will often be painful at this time. The healing rate of the skin may also be slower.

During pregnancy there is an alteration in hormone levels and sometimes hair growth increases. This growth is often temporary and disappears after the birth of the baby, without any treatment. There is no known reason why treatment of an existing problem should stop during the pregnancy but it is advisable to notify the client's GP of the treatment details. Blend should not be given during pregnancy.

Certain medications stimulate hair growth, e.g. steroids and some forms of hormone replacement, whereas others increase the risk of pigmentation, e.g. the contraceptive pill and those hormones used in large doses for transsexual clients.

Diabetic conditions require liaison with the GP and consideration should be given to the fact that skin is slower to heal, therefore treatment sessions should be spaced further apart. The pain threshold is also lower, particularly before a meal when the blood sugar levels will be low, therefore the timing of appointments needs to be carefully considered.

You should give a short explanation of the hair growth cycle to help your client understand what is happening below the skin's surface and the importance of attending for treatment on a regular basis. The removal of a few hairs will enable the client to see how treatment feels, while giving you the opportunity to assess the skin's reaction. A simple description of how electrical epilation works will give your client an insight as to why it is not possible to guarantee the destruction of any one hair permanently after a single treatment.

No consultation would be complete without an examination of the skin, preferably with the aid of a magnifying lamp. The condition and colour of the skin often gives an indication as to the health of the client.

Establishing the cause of hair growth

This can be achieved by observation of:

1 **The skin** – presence of acne; oily, dry, sensitive; thin, moist, general condition, texture and health of the skin; allergies, presence of infection in the treatment site, eczema, psoriasis, epilation scars from previous treatment by another electrolysist.

2 **Area to be treated** – face, sides of face, chin, upper lip, bikini, legs, etc.

3 **Type and distribution of hair growth** – coarse, fine, vellus.

You should ask questions relating to:

▸ age – puberty, menopause
▸ family history
▸ medication, e.g. steroids, HRT, insulin, etc.
▸ previous methods of hair removal
▸ the length of time that the hair growth has been present.

▸ **Practice point:** If scars are present from previous electrical epilation treatment, it is essential that these be pointed out to the client as tactfully as possible during the consultation. This will prevent any confusion at a later date as to the length of time the scars have been evident and will protect the electrolysist who gives further treatment.

Medical history

At this stage a detailed medical history should be taken which must include the following:

▸ possible contra-indications, such as asthma and emphysema (see overleaf)
▸ prescribed medications, to include: steroids, anti-depressants, hormones, hormone replacement therapy, contraceptive pill, drugs for the control of epilepsy
▸ pregnancy: stage and any complications that may have arisen during the pregnancy
▸ hepatitis B: date of illness, prescribed drugs (notification of the proposed treatment to the general practitioner)

- hepatitis C
- diabetes: whether it is controlled by diet, tablets or insulin injections; healing rate, tendency to bruise and sensitivity of skin
- epilepsy: severity and frequency of fits; medication used; ascertain whether the condition is controlled
- endocrine and gynaecological problems: polycystic ovary syndrome, menstrual irregularities, menopause, endometriosis
- organ transplant, i.e. lungs, kidney; nature; date; and medication
- surgery: date and nature.

Why is it necessary to obtain the above information, and how can it be of use in treatment planning? Most importantly, it enables you to assess whether the treatment is right for the client. Conditions such as diabetes require liaison with the client's GP before starting treatment. Medical treatment is required for conditions such as polycystic ovary syndrome, since without this complete elimination of the hair growth is not possible.

Contra-indications to electrical epilation

There are a number of conditions that are either contra-indicative (showing that treatment is inadvisable or should not be given) or require advice from the client's doctor before beginning electro-epilation. These include:

- **Asthma** – defined as 'a condition characterised by transient narrowing of the smaller airways'. During an asthmatic attack the patient experiences great difficulty in breathing. An attack may be triggered by anxiety or stress. Should the client's GP agree to electro-epilation treatment, particular attention should be given to positioning during the session.
- **Dermagraphic skin condition** – congenital sensitivity to any form of friction on the skin. Swelling appears shortly after treatment and may last up to 24 hours. There are no long-term adverse effects, but the decision concerning continuation of treatment should be the client's.
- **Dermatitis/eczema in area** – increased sensitivity, skin irritation and often a build-up of dry skin blocks the opening to the hair follicle, thereby hindering insertion.
- **Fungal infections** – e.g. tinea: risk of transmitting infection.
- **Bacterial infections** – e.g. impetigo: risk of transmitting infection.

- **Viral infections** – e.g. herpes simplex, herpes zoster: risk of cross-infection.
- **Heart problems/circulatory disorders requiring medical treatment** – advisable to consult with GP.
- **Haemorrhage/bruising** – disturbed blood supply interferes with healing process. Heating effect of short-wave diathermy causes blood vessels to dilate.
- **Hypertension/anxiety, stress** – nerve endings highly sensitive, client unable to relax therefore treatment more painful. Insertion to follicle hindered. Risk of scarring due to client pulling away during current application.
- **Loss of skin sensation** – inability to sense when current is too high, which could result in over-treatment of area.
- **Metal plate** – concentration of high-frequency field causes overheating in tissues.
- **Pre-malignant/malignant lesions** – possible stimulation of metabolism due to increase in temperature could accelerate growth.
- **Hepatitis B and C** – can be transmitted through needle stick injury and contact with infected blood.

An additional consideration when using galvanic or blend treatments is the presence of excessive fillings, which often give rise to a metallic taste in the mouth that may be unacceptable to the client.

Doctor's referral

There are times when it is advisable to write to your client's GP before starting any treatment. However, it is important to keep correspondence short and to the point, detailing the relevant information and including a tear-off slip or duplicate letter that the doctor can sign, to save time.

Conditions which need to be referred to the GP are:

- **Epilepsy** – electrical impulses to the brain may be disturbed, which could result in a fit. Only shortwave diathermy should be given, particularly if anxiety is present.
- **Vascular disorders requiring anti-coagulant drugs** – the coagulation of the blood supply at the base of the follicle will be impaired.
- **Hepatitis B** – strict attention to hygiene and the use of disposable sterile needles is essential. The clotting mechanism is often affected and the healing rate of the skin is inhibited. The client bruises easily.

- **Naevi/moles** – hairs growing out of moles must be referred to a GP for checks on possible malignancy.
- **Diabetes** – slow to heal; low pain threshold; shorter treatments; longer healing gaps; increased length of time between treatment sessions.
- **Endocrine disorders** – several endocrine disorders, such as polycystic ovary syndrome, result in increased hair growth in a male pattern. It is essential that correct medical treatment is carried out, which may help in the reduction of unwanted hair. However, it is worth remembering that electrical epilation in conjunction with medical treatment will speed up the final result.
- **Emphysema** – some drugs used in the control of emphysema can lead to increased hair growth. In extreme cases it may only be possible to keep the hair growth under control rather than eliminate it. However, it must be remembered that, psychologically, electrical epilation will be of great value to the client. Extra care and a detailed explanation of the cause of hair growth in this situation must be given at the time of the consultation. The client must be fully aware of the process involved, to avoid unrealistic hopes with regard to length of time and degree of hair removal. Consideration must be given to the positioning of the client during treatment due to breathing difficulties.
- **Steroids** – can often be instrumental in encouraging hair growth.
- **Hiatus hernia** – positioning of the client during treatment is of the utmost importance. The client should be raised into a sitting or semi-sitting position to avoid discomfort.

Assessment task 11.2

Continuing with your consultation, evaluate the cause of the hair growth, describe in detail the most suitable method of treatment and formulate a detailed treatment plan. Provide evidence of the information you have gathered. (M)

Professional ethics

Professional ethics refer to the code of conduct or standards of behaviour practised by the professional electrolysist in relation to:

- clients
- colleagues
- the medical profession.

Courtesy, honesty and integrity are all essential qualities for caring professionals.

Ethics towards clients

Clients should receive caring, professional treatment at all times. Honest information should be given in relation to the duration and progress of treatment. False promises or prolonged treatment for financial gain are not beneficial to the electrolysist's long-term reputation.

Clients should be able to expect and receive total confidentiality at all times. Information relating to one client should not be discussed with another. Conversations relating to controversial subjects such as politics, religion and racial matters are best avoided.

Clients' appointments, once made, should not be cancelled or altered by the electrolysist without good reason. There are times when an event such as illness, a death in the family, failure of the electricity supply or a major crisis may prevent the electrolysist from keeping an appointment. In such instances the clients should be notified in advance, so avoiding wasted journeys and possible ill feeling. Most clients are very understanding in such circumstances.

The appointment book should be organised to allow for accurate time keeping so that clients are not kept waiting. Running late occasionally is acceptable; to do so on a regular basis shows inefficient organisation together with lack of courtesy towards the client.

Many clients are inclined to talk about their personal problems during treatment. The electrolysist may often be the only person they can talk to about such matters. It is essential that conversations remain totally confidential and are *never* discussed with anyone else. In these circumstances you should not offer personal advice, but simply be a sympathetic listener.

The client's best interests should always be of prime consideration.

Ethics concerning colleagues

A true professional does not attempt to poach clients from colleagues, and does not speak disparagingly about another electrolysist's standard of work.

Psychological considerations

Never under-estimate the psychological effect that unwanted hair growth has on your client. It is not unusual for clients to take several *years* to work up the courage to telephone for an appointment for a consultation, and it takes yet further courage to walk through the door. The way in which he or she is greeted in reception, and your approach and manner throughout the consultation, will determine whether or not the client will come back for further treatment.

Watch your client's body language very carefully. Is the client anxious, nervous or argumentative? Is he or she hiding behind his or her hand when he or she speaks to you? Is the client's hair long and covering the sides of his or her face? Is the client extrovert or introvert? Non-verbal communication can tell you much about your prospective client.

It is not uncommon for clients to burst into tears once they start discussing the problem – usually as a result of the sheer relief of talking to someone who understands their problem, and who can provide a solution.

Record keeping

Completion and storage of record cards

Record cards should contain details of treatments; for example, date of treatment, length of treatment, treatment site, needle size, current intensity, machine used, skin reaction. You should update these at the completion of every treatment and add your signature. Accurate and well-maintained records enable you to keep track of treatment, noting progress or any changes in hair growth patterns that occur.

When records have been updated after treatment they should be filed in alphabetical order and kept in a locked fireproof filing cabinet, cupboard or similar. Where records are kept on computer the salon should register with the Data Protection Registrar and take every precaution to ensure that a client's records cannot be seen by unauthorised persons.

▶▶ **Practice point:** Clients' records contain sensitive and confidential information. These records should only be seen by authorised personnel.

Alternative methods of hair removal

Methods suitable and unsuitable for use in conjunction with electrical epilation

Depilatory wax is a temporary method of hair removal that lasts between 4–6 weeks. Hair is allowed to grow until it is approx 3–5 mm in length. Warm wax is applied to the area, then a paper or fabric strip is pressed firmly onto the wax and ripped off very quickly against the hair growth. In this way, the hair is torn out of the follicle. This is acceptable for the legs and areas such as the bikini line, but not for the face. It must be remembered that facial hair is under hormonal control. When hair is torn out of the follicle the follicle may become distorted, so encouraging ingrown hairs. Blood goes to injured or damaged skin tissue and, bearing in mind that blood carries oxygen, nutrients and circulating hormones, it is inevitable that the follicle will regenerate to produce a stronger and healthier hair. Fine, downy hairs are also removed; if these follicles are sensitive to circulating hormones they may be stimulated into producing terminal hairs.

Sugaring dates back hundreds of years. Sugar, lemon juice and water is combined to form a sticky paste. This is warmed to a temperature of 55–60°C for strip sugar and 50–55°C for non-strip sugar, then applied to the skin firmly with the fingers and worked onto the hair (so gripping it). The hair is then ripped out of the follicle with a lifting motion. The effects are similar to those of depilatory wax.

Shaving removes the hair level with the skin's surface. The end will be blunt, therefore re-growth will feel bristly and rough to the touch.

Re-growth occurs within 2–3 days (most men need to shave on a daily basis). Shaving can cause skin irritation so should not be carried out immediately after epilation treatment, but left for 24–48 hours. Shaving can be used as a management method between epilation treatments.

Plucking/tweezing has exactly the same effect as waxing on the hair follicle. When clients have been plucking hairs on the chin area for some time they are often left with a dark shadow and/or bruising in the area. The skin also becomes desensitised and rough to the touch, with a coarse appearance.

Depilatory creams are effective for 4–5 days. The cream is applied in a thick layer where the active ingredients (which are alkaline) dissolve the hair, level with the follicle opening. Due to the alkaline nature of the creams, there is a risk of an allergic reaction occurring in the skin. When this happens the skin becomes inflamed, red and itchy and it may take several days to return to normal. It is essential that a patch test is carried out on the area before applying depilatory creams. Depilatory creams may be used to manage hair growth in between epilation treatments. However, they should not be used within 48 hours of treatment – when the skin is sensitive or tender – and a patch test must be carried out on each occasion.

Mechanical epilators: these electric, hand-held devices work by grasping the hair and tearing it out of the follicle by means of a metal coil. The side effects associated with this method of hair removal are ingrown hairs, inflammation and folliculitis. As with waxing, tweezing and threading, mechanical epilators can be painful to use.

Threading: the skillful application of cotton sewing thread held between the thumb and forefinger of each hand achieves hair removal. The thread is then moved backwards and forwards, in a rhythmic motion, with the cotton closing over the hair, which is then pulled out of the follicle. This method is effective when treating eyebrows but, as with waxing and tweezing, is not recommended for the rest of the face. Threading is practised extensively among the Asian community. This method is not suitable for use in conjunction with epilation. The results will be the same as for plucking, i.e. distorted follicles and stronger regrowth.

Lasers and intense pulsed light (IPL):
In comparison to electrical epilation, lasers and intense pulsed light (IPL) systems are relatively new treatments for the removal of unwanted hair. Both systems target the pigment contained within the hair and follicle. As yet it is too early to claim permanent hair removal but long-term removal can be guaranteed. Intense pulsed light works by raising the temperature within the follicle to destroy the lower follicle by the application of selective photo-thermolysis (the production of heat by the application of light). Lasers disable the follicle either by selective photothermolysis or photo-mechanical effects.

The colour of the hair must be darker than that of the skin. Hair also needs to be long enough to absorb the light into the follicle, but not so long that the light will be absorbed by the hair on the skin's surface (which will result in surface burns). Both systems are ideal for treating large areas such as full face, arms, legs or bikini.

Your client may wish to follow the quicker but not so thorough route of hair removal by IPL or laser, yet have a percentage of blond or white hairs that will not respond due to lack of pigment. In this instance the two treatments can be combined. Allow at least two weeks before and after IPL or laser treatment before applying electrical epilation. This will give the skin a period of time to recover from the build up of heat in the tissues.

Assessment task 11.3

Identify the procedures you must follow before Mrs Sutherland is able to start treatment with electrical epilation. Justify your answers. (M)

Types of current

Types of current used in electrical epilation

True electrolysis using galvanic current was discovered by Dr Charles Michel in 1875. Galvanic application was used until the early 1900s when this method was superseded by the faster but less thorough application of high frequency. During the 1940s, shortwave diathermy treatment, also known as high frequency and thermolysis, superseded galvanic electrolysis. Initially, shortwave diathermy appeared to be a much faster and more effective method. However, the main disadvantage is the higher percentage of re-growth. In 1949 Arthur Hinkle and Henrie St Pierre were granted a patent for the 'new' **blend** method of electrolysis which combines both methods.

The different types of electrolysis – galvanic, high frequency and blend – are described overleaf. Each method has advantages and disadvantages, therefore you should use the method that is most suited to your client's needs.

Types of electrolysis:

Galvanic electrolysis	Brings about the permanent destruction of a hair follicle by the chemical action that occurs in the follicle .
High frequency	Causes destruction by the production of heat within the tissues follicle.
Blend	Combines the benefits of both by achieving the thoroughness of galvanic application with the speed of high frequency.

High frequency

High frequency is often referred to as **shortwave diathermy, RF** (radio frequency) or **thermolysis**. Why are these terms used? The answer is simple – epilation equipment uses the shortwave band of radio frequency. Thermolysis occurs when the high frequency is applied to the follicle. Tissue is destroyed as a result of the heat (therm) produced by the agitation of molecules in the surrounding tissue.

High frequency is an oscillating alternating current of very high frequency and low voltage. This ranges from 3–30 MHz or 3–30 million cycles per second.

The high frequency value describes the number of times the current completes a cycle every second. Each frequency has a fixed wavelength. As the frequency increases, the wavelength decreases. Thus the wavelength of a 13.56 MHz machine is twice that of a 27.11.062 MHz machine.

Production of heat by high frequency

During the application of high frequency to the follicle, the electrovalency of molecules within the

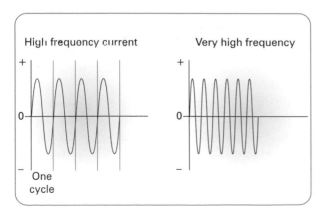

High and very high frequency pattern.

tissues is altered. The rapid agitation of atoms causes the atoms to vibrate against each other, which results in friction. This in turn causes a temporary release of energy in the form of heat. It is the moisture within the tissues that is heated – not the needle.

The heating pattern commences at the sharpest point of the needle (which should be the tip) where the high frequency energy is most intense, gradually building up around the needle. The term 'high frequency field' is used to describe the heating pattern radiating from an epilation needle, connected by a wire to a high frequency oscillator. The high frequency field is strongest close to the needle, and in practice will concentrate around the needle tip.

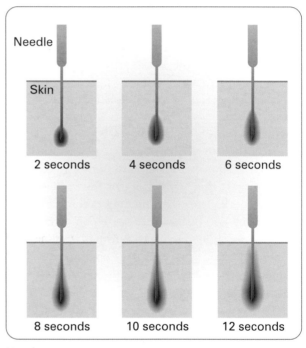

Heating patterns.

Effect of heat on tissue

Heat destroys tissue either by cauterisation or by coagulation.

When a high intensity of high frequency is passed into the tissue, moisture vaporises, the tissue becomes dry and cauterisation occurs. In comparison, by using a lower intensity of high frequency, the cellular structure in the tissue breaks down, protein is congealed and coagulation occurs. Your aim when applying high frequency is to achieve coagulation rather than cauterisation of the lower follicle, to bring about destruction without damaging the surrounding tissue.

You should remember that the successful application of high frequency in the follicle relies on a number of factors.

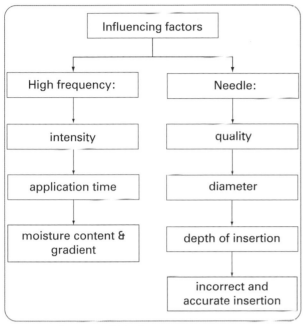

Factors influencing high frequency.

The galvanic current

The galvanic current, discovered by Luigi Galvani, is a direct current. It is a flow of electrons along a conductor in an electric circuit. When a direct current passes through an electrolyte, which contains ions, the ions move in opposite directions. The ions carry the current.

▸▸ **Practice point:** High frequency alternates between positive and negative whereas galvanic or direct current flows in one direction only, i.e. negative to positive, or positive to negative.

Electrolysis can be defined as a chemical process that occurs when a direct current is applied to tissue salts and moisture or salt-water solution.

The direct current causes the salts and water to split into their chemical elements, which then rearrange themselves to form entirely new substances. During the passage of direct current through salt-water solution, the negative chloride ions (anions) are attracted to the positive anode, and the positive sodium ions (cations) are attracted to the negative cathode. When the chloride ions reach the anode they lose an extra electron to become chlorine atoms. Sodium ions arriving at the cathode gain an electron and become sodium atoms. The sodium atoms react with water to form sodium hydroxide, while the chloride ions form hydrochloric acid.

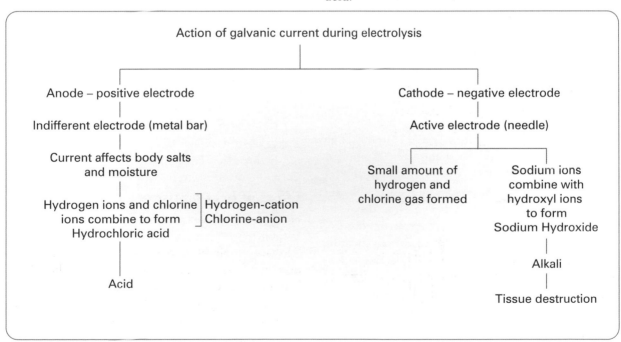

Action of galvanic current during electrolysis.

Galvanic electrolysis is very rarely used today without the addition of high frequency. The reasons for this are:

▸ the procedure is too slow, taking about 60 seconds to successfully destroy the follicle;

▸ an excessive build-up of sodium hydroxide in the follicle, causing scarring and weeping follicles.

Blend

The blend technique is an exciting development that enables you to treat superfluous hair more effectively. The high percentage of re-growth experienced with high frequency (shortwave diathermy) is reduced; the length of time taken to clear an area is reduced; and subsequent scarring, which often results when using galvanic alone, should be eliminated.

The principle of blend is to enhance the chemical action of galvanic electrolysis with the simultaneous application of high frequency. The blend is a versatile epilation method that can be adapted to treat most hairs effectively, including curved or distorted follicles and deep bulbous hairs. Blend requires approximately 75 per cent less time to provide the same degree of destruction as galvanic electrolysis alone. It is faster than galvanic electrolysis but slower than shortwave diathermy.

How does blend work?

The application of the two currents works in the following way: both currents are present at the needle – either separately or together – with each retaining its own characteristics and identity. The dual or blended action takes place within the follicle. The galvanic current brings about tissue destruction by chemical action, whereas high frequency produces heat to speed up the chemical action brought about by the galvanic current. (High frequency when used in shortwave diathermy destroys tissue by heat.)

Curved or distorted follicles are unsuitable for treatment by high frequency because the tip of the needle cannot be placed accurately at the base of the follicle, therefore the high frequency heating pattern cannot reach the base of the dermal papilla and base of the lower follicle. The sodium hydroxide produced during blend, being fluid, can easily move into any open space that will accommodate a liquid.

The successful application of the blend technique relies on the correct balance between the two currents. When used together, galvanic and high frequency currents are superimposed, with both currents being available at the needle either separately or together, as required. Each current retains its own true form and is not changed by the presence of the other current. The tissue is affected by each current in the following way:

▸ *Galvanic current:* electrons flow along the needle into the follicle. When making contact with tissue and moisture within the follicle a chemical reaction takes place. Sodium hydroxide is produced and, being highly caustic, destroys the surrounding tissue.

▸ *High-frequency current:* the rapid oscillations of the high-frequency current cause vibrations of water molecules within the tissue. This results in friction, which in turn causes heat. The action of sodium hydroxide is accelerated by heat.

The action of the two currents is blended in the tissue. The combination of the action from both currents is more effective than the 'sum' of the separate actions.

Action of high frequency during blend application

The action of high frequency current in the follicle enhances that of galvanic electrolysis in three ways:

1 Heat produced by high frequency breaks down the cellular structure of the follicle, causing the protein to congeal. The congealed tissue becomes porous allowing the passage of sodium hydroxide into the tissue.

2 The turbulence created by high frequency forces galvanically-produced sodium hydroxide into the porous tissue.

3 The action of sodium hydroxide is increased by the heat, thereby shortening the time needed to destroy the lower follicle. Heated sodium hydroxide is between two and sixteen times more effective in destroying tissue.

You will only achieve good results when the balance of the two currents is correct during treatment. When too much galvanic current is used, the advantages of high frequency speed are lost: this is due to there being less causticity, porosity and turbulence owing to the decreased heat production. Over-treatment of skin will result in weeping follicles. Should too much high frequency be used, the effect would be to evaporate moisture in the tissue thereby reducing galvanic action and production of sodium hydroxide, resulting in cauterisation of the lower follicle. Over-treating will result in blanched skin.

The combined currents can reduce the application time of galvanic to between 6 and 15 seconds, with the average being 10–12 seconds on most machines. With a number of modern machines the time is reduced to between 6 and 8 seconds. A minimum of 6 seconds is necessary to achieve the blended action of the two currents in the follicle. Less than 6 seconds does not allow sufficient production of sodium hydroxide.

Much depends on the client's pain tolerance. The treatment appears to be less painful than either current used individually: the combined currents seem to have a numbing effect on the nerve endings.

Before you apply the current you should cover the indifferent electrode (which your client holds) with damp cotton wool or sponge. This prevents irritation to the skin caused by the build up of hydrochloric acid that forms at the anode.

▸▸ **Practice point:** Using a thin indifferent electrode can cause a higher build up of hydrochloric acid (produced by the positive pole) and consequently result in irritation of your client's skin.

Setting blend currents and intensity

To achieve the required results it is necessary to ensure that sufficient **sodium hydroxide** is produced in the follicle. The amount of sodium hydroxide is directly related to the degree of moisture in the tissues, plus the current intensity and the length of time the current is applied to the follicle.

Sodium hydroxide is not produced instantaneously (unlike the heat produced by high frequency/shortwave diathermy). Arthur Hinkle (the inventor of blend), devised a system called 'Units of Lye' to help the electrolysist. The amount of 'lye' needed will differ according to the type of hair, the depth and the moisture content.

▸▸ **Practice point:** 1/10th of a milliamp of galvanic current flowing for 1 second equals one unit of lye, e.g. 0.5 milliamps dc × 3 seconds = 15 units of lye.

Setting the current intensity for blend application

The aim of blend is to achieve the complete destruction of the lower follicle and dermal papilla in the shortest possible time without damaging the skin or causing unnecessary discomfort to your client. To set blend currents:

1 Apply high frequency to the follicle and establish the number of seconds taken to loosen the hair.

2 Divide the number of seconds needed to loosen the hair by the number of units of lye to determine the galvanic setting in milliamp tenths. (See the chart at the top of page 268.)

Guide to units of lye:

▸▸ Fine soft pigmented hair	10–20 units
▸▸ Medium/shallow pigmented terminal hair	15–30 units
▸▸ Deep terminal hair	35–40 units
▸▸ Very deep terminal hair	45–60 units

During blend application you will find that it is the high frequency that influences the length of application in the follicle.

In summary, two currents are used for the application of electrical epilation:

▸▸ galvanic, which is a direct current and the original current used to apply true electrolysis, bringing about a chemical action within the follicle;

▸▸ high frequency, which is an alternating current and breaks down the tissue by the production of heat.

The combined application of galvanic and high frequency is known as blend epilation. This application is used to gain the benefits of high frequency and galvanic treatment whilst minimising or eliminating the disadvantages.

Assessment task 11.4

Highlight any problems that may occur with Mrs Sutherland's treatment. Give clear and coherent information on how these problems may be overcome. (D)

Relationship between high frequency and galvanic settings:

Seconds of h.f	Divided into	Units of lye	Milliamp tenths DC	Milliamps
5	divided into	15	3 tenths	0.3
15	divided into	30	2 tenths	0.2
6	divided into	30	5 tenths	0.5
5	divided into	30	6 tenths	0.6
9	divided into	45	5 tenths	0.5
5	divided into	45	9 tenths	0.9
10	divided into	60	6 tenths	0.6
6	divided into	60	10 tenths	1.0

Assessment task 11.5

Compare and contrast alternative methods of long-term hair removal with electrical epilation. Analyse the benefits and identify the drawbacks of each method from your client's point of view. (M)

Safe and effective treatment

The aim of electrical epilation is to remove unwanted hair without leaving visible signs that your client has received treatment. No one should be able to tell that your client has undergone epilation and it is one of the few treatments where you eventually lose your client because the hair has disappeared!

There are several areas to be considered in order to give safe and effective epilation treatment. These include:

- needle selection
- techniques of probing (correct and incorrect) and angle and depth of insertion
- skin sensitivity
- manipulation of the skin
- operator position during treatment
- preparation of the skin
  - before treatment
  - aftercare immediately following treatment
  - home care advice
  - management of growth in-between treatments

- treatment procedure
- timing of treatment
- application of high frequency (shortwave diathermy)
- application of blend (galvanic and high frequency combined)
- duration and frequency of treatment
- equipment
- preparation of the treatment room
- working environment
- sterilisation and hygiene.

When your client has attended for the initial consultation, you will have considered his or her skin type, contra-indications, causes of hair growth, most suitable method of treatment, and the length and frequency of treatments that will be needed to achieve the desired result.

Assessment task 11.6

During your consultation with Mrs Sutherland you noticed that she had scars from previous epilation. Describe how you would raise this point with her, and how you would approach the subject of evidencing this fact with 'before' and 'after' photographs. Explain why it is important to do this. (D)

With regard to the practical application, you must consider the way in which you manipulate, stretch or hold the skin in order to open the follicle and facilitate needle insertion without causing undue pressure or discomfort to your client; neither should your insertion distort the follicle in any way. The needle holder should be held very lightly and without tension: you will lose the sensitivity in your fingers if you hold the needle holder too tightly. The hand holding the needle holder should rest very gently on the skin, with the fingers of the opposite hand positioned in a way that will not interfere with the correct insertion of the needle. The way in which you handle the needle holder, needle and tweezers during treatment will also contribute to the efficiency of the treatment.

Needle selection

Never be tempted to economise on needles – always buy the best that you can afford. For your peace of mind and that of your clients, you should only use pre-sterilised disposable needles. You should look for a manufacturer who supplies a choice of needle sizes with a good quality finish to the surface, so there is no risk of scratching the skin or uneven current distribution. (This subject has been covered in depth on pages 254–5.)

Technique of probing (correct and incorrect)

Accurate probing has a crucial influence on a successful end result. The needle should slide into the follicle easily, in line with the direction of the hair growth. When your needle reaches the base of the follicle you should feel a slight resistance, as you would if you accidentally make contact with the follicle wall. You should not obstruct the entry of the needle into the follicle with the fingers that are lightly holding the follicle open (skin stretch). Neither should you be able to see a depression or puckering of the skin.

Never be tempted to rotate the needle in the follicle because this will reduce your sensitivity in the fingers whilst increasing the risk of piercing the follicle wall. Double depression of the finger switch on the needle holder is also another bad habit to fall into. The need for double depressions indicates that you are not using sufficient current to epilate the hair – there is also a risk of forcing the needle through the base of the follicle with the second depression.

The finger switch should be depressed gently and smoothly. A heavy depression may cause the needle to move in the follicle, causing the needle to make contact with the follicle wall and/or pierce the base.

Insertions which are not deep enough (too close to the skin's surface) do not reach the base of the follicle, therefore preventing the current from reaching the target area. The current could also be applied too near to the epidermis, causing surface burns. On the other hand, insertions that are too deep place the current below the base of the follicle, causing destruction of the deeper tissue. In time, this will show as pit marks in the skin where the tissue has collapsed.

Angle and direction of insertion

The angle and direction of insertion are also important. The angle of hair growth differs depending on the area being treated and whether your client has been shaving, plucking or waxing. The latter two methods of hair removal are known to cause distorted follicles, which will interfere with the accuracy of insertions.

The angle of insertion should follow the direction of hair growth, with the needle raised slightly from the skin's surface. You should not be able to see loss of colour or a depression in the skin as a result of leaning the needle on the surface.

The incorrect angle of insertion could also cause the needle tip to pierce the follicle wall or enter the sebaceous gland, thereby releasing the current in the wrong area.

Causes of scarring

There are several ways in which you could leave your client with scars; however, when you probe correctly with the right amount of current, you will find that your clients will lose their hair without any obvious sign that they have received epilation treatment! Avoid the following bad practices and you will not have cause for concern:

1 Enter the follicle with the high frequency current flowing.

2 Keep the high frequency flowing when the needle is removed from the follicle.

3 Probing through the follicle base with the current on will cause a depression or pit mark to form in the skin, due to destruction of the lower dermal tissue.

4 Probing through the side of the follicle wall with the current on will give the same results as above.

5 Shallow insertion will concentrate the current at the epidermis. Probing in this manner will

lead to surface burns or the development of pigmentation marks, particularly in dark and Asian skin types.

6   Insertions which are too deep result in destruction of the deeper tissue, eventually leaving pit marks in the skin where the tissue has collapsed.

7   If the position or angle of magnifying lamp casts a shadow over the area, this may result in difficulty in seeing the follicle opening, giving rise to incorrect insertion.

Assessment task 11.7

Describe correct and incorrect probing techniques. Illustrate your answers. (M)

Assessment task 11.8

Identify the problems that occur as a result of incorrect probing techniques. Discuss the solutions. (D)

Skin types and their influence on treatment

Your client's skin type does have an influence on treatment application, therefore you should practise recognising and analysing different skin types and conditions.

Dry skin

Dry and/or dehydrated skin will be lacking in moisture or sebum and at times both. When moisture is lacking the skin will be dehydrated, and as both high frequency and galvanic currents need moisture to be present, treatment will not be so successful. With dry skin there is often a build-up of dead cells on the epidermis, which block the follicle opening and hinder needle insertion.

Oily skin

Oily skin can be identified by the presence of open pores and a shiny appearance due to a surface covering of sebum. The texture is often thick and coarse. The benefit of an oily skin is that sebum is an excellent insulator. This will prevent the current reaching the surface and confine the effects to the lower third of the follicle. The moisture content of the lower follicle is usually good. The presence of open pores helps with needle insertions. Comedones, papules and pustules may be present, however, and,

due to the fact that the pH balance may be disturbed, there is an increased risk of infection.

Moist skin

Moist skin has a high content of moisture in both the epidermis and dermis. You must be very careful when applying current to make sure that the needle is placed away from the surface and that the current is not too high. (See moisture gradient on page 110.) There is a risk of the high frequency action rising up the follicle too quickly and reaching the surface before the lower follicle has been successfully treated. Blend is most suitable for skin containing a high percentage of moisture because a lower intensity of high frequency is used and, in addition, galvanic action will occur more quickly.

Sensitive skin

Sensitive skin often has a fine texture and is generally fair in colour with flushing present. Telangiectasia (dilated capillaries) are often visible on the cheeks and across the nose. The skin will react quickly to heat and stimulants such as alcohol, aggressive skin care products and touch. Blend is usually more suitable due to the lower intensity of high frequency used during treatment. Phoresis applied after blend treatment will help to reduce the erythema and restore the natural pH balance.

Operator's position during treatment

Your position during treatment should at all times be relaxed and free from muscular tension. You should be able to maintain the correct posture for several hours at a time. You should be sitting at the correct side of the treatment couch, with your stool or chair at the height that is right for you – this is where an adjustable stool is a real asset. You should be able to reach your client easily during treatment.

Incorrect working posture over a period of time will lead to the following problems:

▸▸ fatigue
▸▸ tense, painful muscles in the neck and shoulders
▸▸ backache
▸▸ headaches
▸▸ frozen shoulder.

The correct working position during treatment should enable you to:

▸▸ align the probe to the direction of the hair growth, making it easier to slide the needle into the follicle without obstruction

- reach the area requiring treatment easily
- keep levels of fatigue to a minimum
- reach the foot pedal easily.

The correct working position if you are right-handed is the left-hand side of the couch; if you are left-handed it will be the right-hand side of the couch.

Preparation of the skin before treatment

You should inspect the skin carefully to ensure that there are no abrasions, cuts, infections or contra-indications present. Make-up or lipstick in the immediate area should be removed thoroughly with a suitable cleanser, then wipe the area with a swab of cotton wool and antiseptic solution. Surgical spirit is flammable and has a drying effect on the skin so it should be avoided, particularly on sensitive skin.

Post treatment and home care recommendations

When you have finished the treatment, apply suitable soothing and antiseptic aftercare in the form of witch hazel gel, aloe vera, lacto calamine or similar. Tinted lotions – formulated specifically for use after electrical epilation – are also available: the advantage of these is that post-treatment erythema is camouflaged. At this stage you should remind your client verbally of home care procedures that must be followed. Written home care instructions should always be given to your clients during their initial consultation.

- **Practice point:** You will find that many of your clients have a short memory span and will soon forget aftercare advice and recommendations that have been given to them verbally!

You should include the following points in your homecare advice:

- make-up should not be applied to the treatment site for at least 24 hours
- a suitable aftercare cream or lotion should be applied to the skin under make-up; this will help to form a protective barrier
- soaps and perfumed products should be avoided for 24 hours
- no swimming for 24 hours – there is the risk of picking up an infection and chlorine in the water may irritate the skin
- heat exposure, either to sunlight or sun beds, could result in slower healing and/or pigmentation marks

- loose, non-restrictive clothing that does not cause friction should be worn after epilation to the bikini line.

Remember: the above list contains guidelines and is not exhaustive.

Management of hair growth in-between treatments

A percentage of your clients will get very distressed when they have a heavy growth which cannot be removed completely during a treatment. Such clients will worry about how to manage the growth in-between treatment sessions; therefore, you should be sure that the necessary information is given with regard to the correct management of growth in-between appointments.

The method that you recommend to your client will depend on the size of the area involved. For small areas with just a few hairs, the preferred method is to cut the hair close to the skin with a small pair of scissors. For larger areas, shaving may be the answer. Contrary to some beliefs, shaving does not interfere with the growth cycle; neither does it increase growth. What does happen is that the pointed end is removed, leaving a blunt bristle. However, shaving does not distort the follicle and shaving regularly can cause skin irritation.

- **Practice point:** You should advise clients who shave or cut between treatments that the hair should be long enough for you to be able to grasp it with the tweezers when they come in for treatment.

Plucking and waxing will distort the hair follicles and encourage in-grown hairs. Depilatory creams may cause allergic reactions in some people, therefore a patch test must be carried out before use.

Treatment procedure

- **Practice point:** The needle should slide smoothly into the follicle followed by application of current, withdrawal of needle and removal of hair. A correctly epilated hair should slide out of the follicle easily, without signs of traction or resistance. The sequence should be smooth, rhythmic and unhurried. Unnecessary hesitation during treatment wastes time and does not fill the client with confidence.

Regardless of whether you are giving high frequency (shortwave diathermy) or blend, the treatment will start in the same way:

1 A thorough examination of the skin and removal of make-up from the area.

2 Question your client as to which hairs are causing most distress (treat these first).

3 Insert sterile, disposable needle into the needle holder, remembering to choose the needle size according to the diameter of the hair.

4 Turn the epilation unit on. It is at this stage that the application of high frequency and blend differ. See the chart opposite.

5 When you have completed the treatment, dispose of the needle into the 'sharps' container and apply suitable aftercare.

Factors which influence length of treatment and current intensity

Your client's tolerance and reaction to treatment is influenced by a number of factors, which will vary from one day to another and from one treatment to the next. Therefore, you should not assume that the settings that were suitable for the last treatment will be suitable for the next one.

As mentioned before, sufficient current should be used to destroy the hair follicle permanently without causing unnecessary discomfort to the client or adverse skin reaction. You must always remember that the following conditions have an influencing effect:

▸ Type and diameter of hair.
▸ Skin sensitivity.
▸ Treatment site.
▸ Pain threshold.
▸ Weather and temperature, e.g. humidity and hot weather, both of which bring about increased circulation and a higher moisture content in the skin; hairs usually epilate more easily with a lower current setting. During cold weather the follicles close and the nerve endings become more sensitive; the pain threshold is often higher.
▸ Premenstrual tension and stress can both affect the pain threshold.

Differences in application between high frequency and blend epilation:

High frequency (shortwave diathermy)	Blend application
1 Your client does not hold an electrode.	1 Give the sponge-covered positive electrode to the client to hold firmly. The grip on the electrode should remain constant, to prevent fluctuating current intensity to the follicle.
2 Probe the follicle, treating the darker, coarser or more noticeable hairs first.	2 Apply anaphoresis if required.
3 Apply sufficient high frequency to remove hair easily without causing adverse skin reaction. The current intensity should be set within the client's pain threshold. Stop the flow of current and remove hair with sterile tweezers. The hair should slide out of the follicle easily, without traction or resistance.	3 Find the balanced combination of high frequency and galvanic currents to epilate the hairs without causing adverse skin reaction or the production of too much 'lye'. Stop the flow of current and remove hair with sterile tweezers. The hair should slide out of the follicle easily, without traction or resistance.
	4 At the end of treatment cataphoresis may be applied. This has a number of advantages: use of the positive electrode has a germicidal effect by producing hydrochloride acid and restoring the skin's pH balance; nerve endings are soothed, which gives a feeling of well-being to the client; erythema is reduced.

When the current is set to the correct intensity the hair will slide out of the follicle easily, complete with bulb (depending on the stage of the hair growth cycle). Dark, terminal hairs on the chin will require a higher current intensity than fine terminal or vellus hairs on the upper lip. The client's pain threshold is much lower on the upper lip, particularly in the centre where the nerve endings are more numerous. A fine, sensitive skin will tolerate less current than a coarse or oily skin.

Application time of high frequency

You will find that the application time of high frequency in the follicle has a direct effect on the heating pattern. When the high frequency application time is too short, insufficient heat will be generated. When the application time is too long, the heating pattern will eventually reach the surface of the skin, resulting in scars.

Application time of blend

The application of blend is slower to achieve a result in the follicle. This is due to the length of time needed for galvanic action to occur and produce the necessary amount of sodium hydroxide in the follicle. You will find that you need a minimum of 6 seconds to achieve the desired result, in comparison to the 1–2 seconds required with high frequency (see the table on page 268).

Duration and frequency of treatments

You will need to consider a number of points when recommending a treatment plan to your client. These include:

- the density and texture of hair growth
- client's pain threshold
- skin sensitivity
- size of the area to be treated
- the hair growth cycle
- method of treatment, i.e. blend or high frequency
- the time that the client can commit to appointments.

You should allow a minimum of 7 days between treatments to the same area, to allow the skin time to heal and to ensure that there is sufficient hair present to treat at the next session. Explain the hair growth cycle to the client so that he or she fully understands the importance of attending regularly for treatment. The effect on your client's psychology can also play a part in determining the frequency of treatments. When a large area such as the legs needs treatment, your client may prefer longer treatments to clear as much hair as possible in any one session. On the other hand, where an area such as the lip, chin and sides of the face need attention, the areas can be worked in rotation so that your client can attend for several shorter treatments. Psychologically your client often feels better when attending more frequently.

Treatment area
Equipment

There are certain items of equipment that are essential when you are setting up an epilation practice: the epilation unit, autoclave, treatment couch, operator's stool, trolley and magnifying lamp.

The **treatment couch** needs to be comfortable for the client, well-padded and preferably with an adjustable lifting head. Other considerations include easy access, so that you can work comfortably with your knees under the couch, while an electronic or hydraulic facility for height adjustment will help you to give a more efficient treatment whilst making your working position far more comfortable and less tiring.

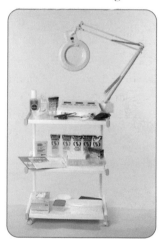

A trolley set up for epilation.

There is a wide selection of **trolleys** available. The trolley should be chosen to suit the size of the treatment room and the size of the epilation unit that it is going to hold. Some trolleys have an electric side panel, some have lower drawers and others have a facility for attaching the magnifying lamp. Castors, to allow easy movement, are an advantage for all trolleys.

A **magnifying lamp** can often seem to have a mind of its own during treatment: just as you get the lamp in the right position and you are about to insert the needle, the lamp drifts off, as if by magic!

You want the lamp to provide good light and magnification, with the head of the lamp remaining perfectly still. The whole unit should be well balanced so that it does not over-balance during treatment.

A good **operator's chair/stool** makes all the difference to the efficiency and your comfort during treatment. The ideal is a chair that has castors to enable you to move around the treatment couch with ease, with a back support and an adjustable height facility.

The **epilation unit** must be reliable and enable you to give a comfortable and effective treatment. There is a wide selection of machines available, from the very basic shortwave diathermy units through to the sophisticated computerised blend units. You will find that a good blend machine, which gives a choice of three methods of treatment – shortwave diathermy, galvanic electrolysis and blend – would be an excellent investment that should serve you well for many years. These units offer flexibility according to the client's needs.

Preparation of the treatment room

The treatment room should be checked on a daily basis before the clients arrive. You should make sure that the room is clean, with clean covers and linen on the couch. The couch should also be covered with a fresh sheet of paper (this should be changed after every client).

Consumables, such as needles, tissues, cotton wool, medi-wipes, cleansers, skin prep solution and aftercare products, should be stocked up at the beginning of the day. By making this part of your daily routine you will not need to interrupt your client's treatment because you are missing an item, for example, needles or forceps, etc.

Washable surfaces, such as the trolley, wash basin and floor, should be cleaned on a daily basis, preferably at the end of the day to give the floor time to dry before clients arrive. Waste bins should be emptied and washed at the end of the day.

Always check that equipment is in good working order, without broken cables or trailing flexes.

Keep your clients' records within easy access so that you have an opportunity to read them before you start treatment. This will refresh your memory with regard to contra-indications and treatment progress.

Sterilisation and hygiene

Sterilisation and hygiene are covered in Section 1. However, because of the invasive nature of electrical epilation there are a few additional procedures that should be followed for the protection of both you and your clients. You should take extra measures to avoid cross-infection from one client to another, or from your client to you and vice versa. Prevention of cross infection can be achieved easily by:

- ⇥ carrying out thorough cleaning of treatment rooms
- ⇥ cleaning and sterilisation of all equipment, forceps and needles
- ⇥ attention to personal hygiene
- ⇥ keeping cuts and abrasions covered
- ⇥ hand washing after client contact
- ⇥ correct disposal of clinic waste.

In addition to the above you can protect yourself from Hepatitis B by having a course of vaccinations from your GP. This course consists of three vaccinations: the first and second spaced one month apart with the third six months later. Contaminated needles and blood may easily transmit the Hepatitis B virus. It has been found that the virus can remain inactive on hard surfaces for several years; therefore, high standards of hygiene in the clinic are imperative.

- ⇥ **Practice point:** Hepatitis B can be transmitted through: needle stick injury; contact with infected blood; an open wound; blood transfusion; drug users sharing needles.

Preparation of hands before treatment

Your hands should be washed both before and after treatment, preferably with liquid soap or bactericidal preparations. You should cover cuts and abrasions or open wounds with a waterproof dressing. Wear a fresh pair of disposable gloves to treat each client, changing these if you have to interrupt a treatment or if they become damaged.

Hygiene within the salon is easily achieved and the procedure should be a routine matter. All equipment, hard work surfaces and washable floors should be wiped over daily with a hospital-grade disinfectant. There are many of these available on the market, a number of which are environmentally friendly. Hand-wash basins should be cleaned regularly. Soap bars should be placed in a soap rack in-between use; soap pump dispensers are more hygienic. Hands should be dried on disposable paper towels.

Although it is possible to sterilise needles with an autoclave, the use of pre-sterilised, disposable needles rules out the possibility of cross-infection from one client to another, particularly as far as HIV and hepatitis are concerned. Disposable needles are sterilised by one of two methods:

1   Needles are packed in hospital-grade blister packs and sterilised with ethylene oxide gas.

2   Individually-packed needles are sterilised by gamma-irradiation. These packs have a red dot on the outside of the packet to indicate that sterilisation has taken place.

You should dispose of used needles by placing them in the 'sharps' box as soon as you have finished the treatment. Never leave the needle in the needle holder after it has been used.

Needle holders, caps, chucks and forceps

You should ensure that needle holders are wiped over with a detergent solution (germicide/disinfectant) after each treatment. Plastic or metal caps, chucks and forceps should be immersed in a disinfectant solution for at least one hour, then rinsed in water and dried with tissue or paper towel, then rinsed and immersed in 70 per cent isopropyl alcohol for at least 10 minutes. Empty the covered container used to hold the alcohol, either daily or whenever visibly contaminated. Forceps, metal caps and chucks are all suitable for sterilisation in an autoclave.

When you practise electrical epilation you are legally required to register with the Environmental Health department at your local council under the **Local Government (Miscellaneous Provisions) Act 1982**. The registration fee varies from one council to another. When you apply for registration the Environmental Health Officer will come to inspect your premises and check your qualifications, paying particular attention to your health and safety procedures, including hygiene and sterilisation provisions.

Knowledge check

1   Explain why an understanding of the hair growth cycle has a bearing on the application and results of epilation treatment.

2   Give a detailed description of the structure of a terminal hair in the anagen stage of growth.

3   Explain how high frequency and galvanic currents bring about the destruction of the hair follicle.

4   Give six examples of scars caused by incorrect epilation and explain how they are caused.

5   Compare and contrast the following:
    a   hypertrichosis
    b   hirsutism
    c   superfluous hair.

6   Describe Stein Leventhal's syndrome (P.C.O.S.) and discuss its effect on hair growth.

7   Explain the differences between normal systemic and abnormal systemic endocrine influences on hair growth.

8   Demonstrate an understanding of how the shape and size of the follicle influences:
    a   the application of epilation
    b   needle selection.

9   Identify the problems that can arise due to curved and distorted follicles.

10 Evaluate the benefits of blend epilation over high frequency (shortwave diathermy) and galvanic electrolysis.

References and bibliography for Unit 11: Electrical epilation

Greenblatt, R.B, Mahesh, V.B. and Don Gambrell, R.(1987) *The cause and management of Hirsutism: A Practical Approach to the Control of Unwanted Hair*, CRC Pr I Llc

Small, J.C.& Clarke-Williams, M.J. (1972)*Endocrinology*, Heinemann

Godfrey, S. (2001) *Principles and Practice of Electrical Epilation*, Butterworth Heinemann

Stretch, B. et al (2002) *BTEC National Health Studies*, Heinemann

Aromatherapy

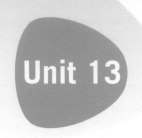

Unit 13

This unit will enable you to use and adapt your massage techniques from body massage as the medium to deliver the healing properties of carrier and essential oils. This will mean using a lighter pressure and removing some of the more stimulating moves associated with body massage. Massage is the way you will engage and interact with your clients.

It is important to be aware that some of your future clients may be vulnerable both physically and emotionally. Massage and the use of essential oils will enable you to help resolve many of these situations.

The word aromatherapy can be translated as 'smell therapy'. Your sense of smell can exercise powerful influences over your body via the olfactory nerve, which connects directly with the limbic portion of the brain. This part of the brain is the earliest to develop in the womb and acts as a 'guardian', controlling emotion, memory and behaviour.

This unit will introduce you to a selection of essential and carrier oils; the benefits of each oil; their therapeutic properties and the potential hazards of these concentrated essences. The consultation process will give you an understanding of contra-indications and contra-actions for this approach to complementary care.

You will be assessed via an assignment, which may be made up of written or other elements and will be assessed by your tutors internally. The following is a suggested scenario that can be used to cover all your assessment criteria:

'Mr Vitak arrives for an aromatherapy treatment and during the consultation he tells you that he suffers from high blood pressure, which is controlled by medication. He also tells you that he has recently experienced a major trauma relating to his business, which is causing high levels of stress both at home and work'.

In order to achieve Unit 13 Aromatherapy you must complete the following learning outcomes:

LEARNING OUTCOMES

1 Explain the legal requirements and codes of conduct.

2 Prescribe and apply aromatherapy treatments.

3 Research the extraction and chemistry of essential oils.

4 Examine the therapeutic uses of essential oils and carrier oils.

Background

Smell can trigger emotional responses to memory; a perfume worn by someone we are or were close to is a good example. The perfume of flowers can evoke memories of holidays or places.

It helps to remember the effects and outcomes when using essential oils.

The three P's of aromatherapy

- ▸ **P**harmalogical – the chemical interaction between the enzymes, hormones and the essential oils in the bloodstream.
- ▸ **P**hysiological – how essential oils can stimulate, for example, to help counteract lethargy or to sedate and deal with anxiety.
- ▸ **P**sychological – how essential oils can enhance mood.

The sense of smell can be used for neuro-associative conditioning and has proved successful in controlling epileptic fits and painful spasms. Therefore, it will be part of your training to learn how to use this remarkable ability of smell to tailor the outcomes of physical responses.

As with all holistic approaches, the blending of essential oils will be unique for each client. Their needs will be different as will their responses to each individual oil. As the therapist you will use your knowledge of the curative properties of these beautiful oils, but it will be the client's sense of smell which decides which oil best suits their needs. It is the client that defines the choice of oil and the final blend.

A brief history of aromatherapy

Many ancient cultures have a history of herbal medicine. The Egyptians are renowned for their use of herbs and spices for embalming the dead, but they also perfected the art of making pills, powders, ointments and pastes using a variety of trees and plants. Numerous jars and oil bottles have been found during excavations of Egyptian tombs: frankincense and myrrh were found when Tutankhamun's tomb was opened in 1922, and the Ebers Papyrus, which dates back to 1500BC, lists some 800 herbal remedies.

The ancient Greeks, expanding the knowledge gained from the Egyptians, discovered that certain aromas could be either stimulating or sedating. They used olive oil to macerate petals and herbs, which would then be used for the treatment of wounds.

Dioscorides was a Greek surgeon employed by the Roman army and, as he travelled around the Mediterranean, he was able to compile his 'Materia Medica'. We owe the discovery of aspirin to this amazing ancient healer; he used a decoction of willow to ease the pain of gout, and some two thousand years later we are still using information he recorded on the best time for harvesting plants and herbs for medicinal purposes. Hippocrates, known as the father of medicine, recommended a daily aromatic bath and massage using scented oils.

Traditional Chinese Medicine also has a rich history of using herbs and spices, with records dating back to 2000 BC.

Manuscripts from the Middle Ages contained recipes to make scented oils and lavender water, and it became common place to make lavender bags and other herbal sachets to use around the home. The spoils of war from the Crusades included exotic herbs, spices and rose water.

However, once chemists in the nineteenth century were able to imitate the medicinal properties of plants, herbal medicine began to lose its popularity.

Modern aromatherapy

Most practising aromatherapists will know that a chemist called Gattefosse discovered the amazing healing properties of lavender after an accident in his laboratory. After badly burning his hand, he plunged it into a vat of lavender oil and discovered that it healed with little scarring in a very short time. This discovery encouraged further experiments in the healing properties of essential oils during the First World War, with remarkable outcomes. These experiments were continued by another French physician, Dr Jean Valnet, during the Second World War, for the treatment of burns, to sterilise surgical instruments and to disinfect hospital wards. However, it was the discovery of penicillin that replaced the use of essential oils for treating bacterial infections.

Madam Maury, with her interest in beauty therapy, set up her first clinic in London. Applying the accumulated knowledge of Dr Valnet, she would create a personal blend for each of her clients, taking into account health issues and temperament. Her work with beauty therapists, herbalists and medical practitioners has encouraged the practise of aromatherapy worldwide.

Using essential oils

You will need to understand how the body interacts with essential oils in order to draw up your treatment plans.

Olfaction

The nose does not enable us to smell but it does perform some very useful functions. It modifies the humidity and temperature of the air we breathe and acts as a filter for any debris in the air, such as pollen and dust, thereby preventing access to the nasal passages. The olfactory bulb or nerve is responsible for our sense of smell. It is the first of the cranial nerves, with nerve fibres, that track upwards from the cell receptors through microscopic holes in the skull, joining together to form the olfactory track.

Theory into practice

As a group, discuss why, during the evolutionary process of man, the nerves associated with our ability to smell are situated at the front of the brain (at the top of the nose) whereas the sight cells are positioned at the back of the brain. Does this mean smell is more important than sight? List some reasons why smell might offer greater protection from harm.

There are two groups of smell receptor cells positioned at the top of the nostrils. When inhaling an essential oil, the molecules lock onto hairs protruding from the receptor cells at the top of the nose and an electro-chemical message is sent via the olfactory tract to the limbic system, triggering emotional and memory responses. These responses are then sent via the hypothalamus to other parts of the brain and body, and it is the reaction to these messages that result in the release of other neuro-chemicals; these can be euphoric, relaxing, sedative or stimulating.

How does this happen?

The nerve impulses from the olfactory bulb interact with two important centres in the brain. One is the locus caeruleus, which is responsible for triggering the production of nor-adrenaline, thereby controlling the non-voluntary functions of the sympathetic nervous system. The second is the raphe nucleus, responsible for triggering the production of serotonin. This neuropeptide has been called the 'happy hormone' because of its ability to influence mood and emotion.

The act of breathing enables the body to absorb the tiny oil molecules via the small air sacs in the lungs, or alveoli. This happens if you use oils when bathing and they interact with the steam. The most relaxing and enjoyable way to introduce the curative properties of essential oils is by massage. The oils diluted by carrier oil readily penetrate the skin through the deep tissue layers to the capillaries, where they pass into the bloodstream to be transported around the body.

Legal requirements and codes of conduct

All salons and clinics operate under approved guidelines for health and safety and COSHH. All students must be able to identify and control exposure to hazardous oils and understand the potential for harm in using essential oils that are toxic.

The following are toxic oils that are **never** used in aromatherapy.

▶ Aniseed	▶ Bitter Almond
▶ Arnica	▶ Broom
▶ Bitter Fennel	▶ Camphor (brown and yellow)
▶ Cassia	▶ Chervil
▶ Horseradish	▶ Cinnamon Bark
▶ Mugwort	▶ Deertongue
▶ Pennyroyal	▶ Mustard
▶ Sassafras	▶ Oregano
▶ Rue	▶ Pine (Dwarf)
▶ Savin	▶ Thyme (Red)
▶ Thuja	▶ Wormwood
▶ Tansy	▶ Wintergreen

A toxic reaction can be classified as acute or chronic. The oils gain access to the body by the mouth or through the skin. An acute reaction by mouth means the person has been poisoned, which may result in death. An acute reaction via the skin could lead to liver or kidney damage, as these organs process and filter all the substances before they gain access to the bloodstream. A chronic reaction takes longer to produce symptoms.

Controlling exposure to the hazards of certain oils requires the student to be aware of the contra-indications of certain oils and medical conditions. This means that you must be aware of which oils can cause irritation and which oils clients may become sensitised to.

Professional ethics

In any professional discipline, it is important to have a standard of acceptable behaviour. Once qualified, it is advisable to become a member of a professional

Explain how you would comply with the necessary legal requirements. Explain what is meant by potential hazards, which justify safety procedures and meet with the necessary codes of conduct. (M)

Show a comprehensive knowledge of the need to comply with the necessary legal requirements. Identify potential treatment hazards and offer a solution that complies with safety procedures and codes of conduct. (D)

Working together in a group:

1 List the situations that might make it necessary for you to disclose information about a client to someone in authority.

2 What other disciplines would you consider studying to continue your professional development?

GP referrals

Always work within the guidelines of any referrals you receive from a doctor, consultant or other health professional.

Aromatherapy treatments

Preparation

Treatment area

The way in which you decorate and set out the treatment area is a very important aspect when planning your room/clinic, ranking alongside considerations of hygiene.

▸ **Accessibility:** think about the type of clients you are hoping to attract and consider their ability to access your room/clinic.

▸ **Position in the building:** how will the room feel when in the full heat of the sun? If you have a choice of rooms, try to choose a room or position in the building that gives you some control over sun and shade. Remember that a room which adjoins a busy road would mean noise pollution.

▸ **Choice of colour and accessories:** this is very important; the choice of both should reflect what you are trying to achieve. Colours in themselves are healing.

▸ **Ventilation:** it is essential that you are able to ventilate the room between treatments to avoid the build-up of aromas becoming overpowering. Remember that as a therapist you need fresh air as well: you are breathing in all the different oils you choose for client treatments.

▸ **Lighting:** overhead lights are very disturbing when lying on your back; make sure you can adjust the glare or use lamps.

▸ **Shower facilities:** these may be a luxury but if you have clients with stressful lifestyles and you

association or governing body that has a code of ethics to which members are expected to adhere. The following is what is expected of a student during training and will form the basic guidelines for acceptable professional standards once qualified.

▸ Therapists must conduct themselves in a professional manner at all times.

▸ Respect the religious, spiritual, social and political views of your clients irrespective of creed, race, colour or sex.

▸ Never abuse the relationship between yourself and your client.

▸ Always co-operate with other health care professionals, referring cases outside your skill range or therapeutic knowledge to those with the relevant qualifications.

▸ Always explain the services you offered and discuss fees with your client before any treatment starts.

▸ Keep accurate, up-to-date, confidential records of treatment.

▸ Never disclose client information without the prior written permission of the client, except when required to do so by law.

▸ Never claim to cure, diagnose a medical condition, or give unqualified advice.

▸ Ensure that all marketing material represents your practice professionally.

▸ Ensure that your working environment complies with all current health, safety and hygiene legislation.

▸ Ensure that you have insurance from a recognised professional body.

▸ Endeavour to become a member of a professional association which sets high standards for the industry.

▸ Continue with your professional development.

▸ Keep personal and professional life separate.

do not want the oils removed by bathing for 24 hours, offering a pre-treatment shower is a must.

▸ **Privacy:** guaranteeing privacy is very important. Not only will it ensure client relaxation, but the more vulnerable clients will feel comfortable.

Theory into practice

Working in a group, design your own treatment room, taking into account the recommendations for health and safety.

Health, safety and hygiene for the therapeutic space

To avoid cross-infection you must consider the following:

▸ the treatment area
▸ the equipment
▸ the client
▸ the therapist.

Health, safety and hygiene for the treatment area

▸ Keep this area hygienically clean at all times; never leave it 'to do' later.
▸ Make sure that all fire exits are clearly marked.
▸ Arrange for the checking of fire extinguishers according to manufacturer's recommendations. Know where they are and how they should be used.
▸ Check all equipment used for both health and safety; for example, tears in couch coverings can harbour germs.
▸ All items used for treatment should be disinfected at the end of each working day, e.g. couch, stool, trolley, storage boxes and bins.
▸ All floors should by non-slip and washable.
▸ Keep client and staff towels in separate linen bins.
▸ For disposable wipes make sure that all bins are lined with a disposable bag. If using wipes to remove spillage of essential oils, make sure that these are disposed of in an outside bin.
▸ Ensure hand-washing facilities are available in the vicinity of the treatment area.
▸ Check all equipment used and make sure that it is maintained regularly.
▸ Maintain a first aid box.

Client considerations

Clients will come into a clinic or salon with certain expectations. Your business will grow if you are able to meet these expectations. Safe working practice is also essential.

▸ The consultation ensures that the client is suitable for treatment. This will cover any possible contra-indications.
▸ Clean towels and couch roll – should be provided for each client. To avoid any cross-infection via the feet, use a replaceable mat or couch roll on the floor.
▸ Wash your hands before and after each treatment.
▸ Remove all jewellery, allowing the client to place his or hers in a container.
▸ If possible, a pre-treatment shower will remove old perfume and perspiration and slightly open the pores before treatment.
▸ Help the client on and off the couch.
▸ Check for any infectious conditions, open wounds or sores.
▸ Patch test for the oils to avoid skin reactions.

Therapist considerations

You will attract and retain clients by being professional in all circumstances. Massage means being in very close proximity to your clients and personal hygiene is therefore very important.

▸ Cover any cuts or abrasions with a waterproof plaster.
▸ Protect your back when lifting or moving objects and use the correct posture when carrying out a massage routine.
▸ Renew your first aid experience every 3 years.
▸ Know where the first aid box is kept.
▸ Know where the fire extinguishers are kept and how to use them.
▸ Check the stock dates of products used on your clients.
▸ Maintain hygiene at all times by washing your hands thoroughly between client treatments

Theory into practice

Working in a group:
1 How would you deal with a client who had several warts on his or her feet? Would you be able to massage them safely?
2 Why is it important to rotate stock? Devise a system that would help you to do this.

Procedures

Consultation

Consultation is about communication, which involves talking and listening. The information given during this process is designed to keep both the client and the therapist 'safe'.

It is important to engage with your clients by listening to them. The consultation will require you to ask a series of questions and complete a consultation form. It will be especially important to consider the effects of the essential oils as well as the contra-indications to certain oils in relation to physical or medical conditions, e.g. pregnancy as a physical consideration or high/low blood pressure as a medical consideration. Information about lifestyle and personality will help also to give you an overall picture of the person and will guide you on oil choice.

During the consultation be aware of the non-verbal messages (body language) that your clients send. Together with the questions you ask, those will help you to build a complete picture of your client and draw up a treatment plan.

Consultation aims for a massage include:
- evaluating client expectations
- ensuring the client's suitability for treatment
- establishing a good rapport
- answering client queries
- agreeing a treatment plan.

Theory into practice

How do you think the consultation form, on page 282, can be improved? Design your own consultation form including your logo and company name.

Contra-indications

Contra-indications are about safe practice. There are times when the body would find it hard to deal with the extra stimulation of touch; for example, when the person has a fever. However, a client would benefit from this approach when he or she has a terminal or chronic illness. Contra-indications to any massage are:
- When the client is feverish, has an acute infectious disease or is generally unwell.
- When the client is being treated for cancer, unless the treatment is being carried out under medical supervision.
- When the client is under the influence of drugs or drink.

Contra-indications to **localised massage** include:
- A history of thrombosis or phlebitis in the blood vessels of any limb.
- An area of the body with a skin infection.
- An area of inflammation, e.g. a rash or boil.
- Sunburn.
- Areas of bruising; cuts, recent scars or abrasions.
- Sprains, fractures or surgical procedures.
- Hot or swollen joints.
- Undiagnosed swellings or lumps.
- Tender or painful muscles.
- Severe varicose veins.
- Moles and warts.
- The first three months of pregnancy (avoid the abdomen).

Conditions where special care should be exercised include: diabetes, epilepsy, heart disease, high or low blood pressure.

Record keeping

An in-depth consultation will require the use of a confidential record system, whether using record card or a computer database. You must comply with the laws on data protection and always protect your client's privacy.

Assessment task 13.2

Incorporating the known facts, describe, with attention to detail, how you would proceed with a consultation. (M)

Illustrate a comprehensive knowledge of consultation techniques, showing an understanding of the use of 'non-verbal communication' during the consultation process and how this information affects any decisions relating to the treatment process. (D)

Aftercare

Absorption rates vary with different oils and you will need to advise your clients not to shower immediately after a massage to gain the full benefit of the blend of oils. Advise your client to:
- arrange all appointments which will enable them to continue the enjoyment of a relaxed state
- avoid stressful situations
- drink plenty of water or herbal teas
- avoid tea, coffee and alcohol

- ⇥ eat light meals
- ⇥ make a note of any outcomes which he or she would like to discuss with you.
- ⇥ **Practice point:** Always give your client an aftercare leaflet confirming what you have said. It is safe practice to confirm verbal instructions in writing.

Theory into practice

Design your own aftercare leaflet incorporating your own logo and company name.

Oil knowledge

Aroma families

Smells are identified by the different families they come from, e.g. lemons will fit in the fruit family.

- ⇥ **Fruit:** Lemon, Grapefruit, Orange, Tangerine.
- ⇥ **Flower:** Geranium, Rose, Roman Chamomile, German Chamomile, Lavender, Patchouli, Jasmine, Melissa, Neroli, Ylang Ylang.
- ⇥ **Herb:** Peppermint, Rosemary, Clary Sage, Marjoram (Sweet).
- ⇥ **Resin:** Frankincense, Myrrh.

Diploma in Aromatherapy Massage Record Card

For Massage

PERSONAL DETAILS

Name:

Address:

Tel. No:	Date of Birth:
Doctor's Name:	Tel. No:

Address:

Reasons for coming:

Any previous treatment:

GENERAL HEALTH *please tick*

Allergies/skin problems ☐	Lumps/swellings ☐
Menstruation pattern ☐	Digestive/bowel disorders ☐
Epilepsy ☐	Operations ☐
Blood pressure ☐	Hepatitis/HIV ☐
Fluid retention ☐	Headaches/migraine ☐
Respiratory problems ☐	Diabetes ☐
Medication ☐	Metal plates/pacemaker ☐
Pregnancy ☐	Circulatory disorders ☐
Throat/sinus ☐	Bladder/kidney disorders ☐
Back problems ☐	Liver disorders ☐
Nervous conditions ☐	Injuries ☐
Heart conditions ☐	

Details of above:

Are you currently being treated by a Doctor, Chiropractor or other practitioner?

LIFE STYLE

Home involvement:

Work involvement:

Active/Sedentary:

Eating habits:

Drinking/Alcohol/Other:

Smoking:

Sleeping pattern:

Interests:

Stress levels:

Personality:

OBSERVATIONAL

Skin:

Hair:

Body shape/Type:

Expressions/Body language:

Posture:

RELEVANT CASE HISTORY NOTES/CLIENT ASSESSMENT

RECOMMENDED TREATMENT PLAN/TREATMENT OBJECTIVES

I confirm that I understand fully the consultation and treatment proposed and that all the information I have forwarded is accurate. As a trainee giving treatment he/she cannot be held wholly responsible for possible outcomes.

Client's signature			Date

RECORD OF TREATMENTS

Date	Treatment given	Medium	Home advice

Aromatherapy consultation form.

- **Wood:** Sandalwood, Juniper, Cypress, Tea Tree, Eucalyptus, Nauoili, Petitgrain, Pine.
- **Spice:** Black Pepper, Ginger.

Extraction and chemistry of essential oils

Steam distillation

This method, thought to have originated in Persia, has been used for obtaining essential oils since the tenth century. The plant material is heated by placing it in water, which is then brought to the boil; this is called direct distillation. This method can cause 'burning' of sensitive plant material. An alternative is to place the plant material on a rack or grid and heat the water beneath, allowing the steam to pass through the racks; this is called steam distillation. Vulnerable plants, such as rose, need to be treated immediately. Other plants are dried, crushed or grated before undergoing the distillation process.

The heat and steam cause the walls of the plant cells to break down, releasing the plant essence in the form of vapour. This is gathered into a pipe and passed through cooling tanks or jackets; the vapour returns to a liquid and is collected in vats at the end of the process. The steam condenses into a watery distillate, which is sold as flower water, e.g. lavender or rose water, while the essence of the plant has become essential oil.

Enfleurage

This method, used for the extraction of essential oils from delicate flowers such as jasmine and rose, was once the favoured method of the perfume industry to avoid spoilage by steam distillation. Purified cold fat is spread over sheets of glass mounted in wooden frames. The flowers are placed on the fat, which absorbs the essential oils. The flowers are continually replaced until the fat is saturated with essential oils. At this stage the fat is cleaned of plant debris and is called, a 'pomade'; this is then diluted in alcohol to separate the fat from the essential oil. The solution is gently heated to evaporate the alcohol leaving behind the essential oil. Because the process is very labour intensive it is no longer commercially viable.

Solvent extraction

This method is favoured by the perfume industry since the fragrance return is much higher than by steam distillation. The flowers are mixed with a volatile solvent, such as petrol ether, benzene and hexane, to extract the essential oil. The solvent is then distilled off, leaving a semi-solid perfume called a 'concrete'. The concrete is repeatedly treated with alcohol; this is then evaporated off leaving behind the oil, known as an absolute.

Oils produced by this method are not recommended for therapy because of solvent residues, which may produce reactions on sensitive skins.

- **Practice point:** Always check the process used to obtain essential oils from resins such as frankincense, myrrh and benzoin. Benzene, which is sometimes used in the extraction process, is potentially carcinogenic.

Expression

The essential oils of citrus fruits are obtained by this method. The rinds are pressed or grated and the oil collected in a sponge and squeezed out. At one time this was all done by hand, but today machines are mostly used. However, the best quality oils are still extracted by hand.

Liquid carbon dioxide extraction

Because of the equipment cost, the financial expenditure on this form of extraction remains extremely high, but it does have the ability to produce oils that remain closer to their original format. Oils produced by this process have more esters and less terpenes.

Hydrofission

This process is similar to steam distillation but instead of the steam being introduced from below the plant material, it is used in the form of a steam spray from above. Oils produced by this method have a richer colour and aroma.

Aroma chemistry

Knowledge of the chemical qualities in essential oils is important; it is the starting point of understanding how the various oils can heal. Plants have the ability to synthesise chemical substances and the oils extracted from the various plant materials may contain several hundred different chemicals.

Carbon (C), hydrogen (H) and oxygen (O) are the building blocks of essential oils and of life itself. Essential oils are organic compounds, which means they will contain the element carbon (C). Carbon, hydrogen and oxygen are made up of elements. Atoms are the smallest unit of an element, and bond together to form a compound. Molecules are the smallest unit of a compound.

Using the first letter of the Latin name identifies atoms, which are molecular building blocks:

- Carbon (C)
- Nitrogen (N)
- Oxygen (O)
- Sulphur (S).
- Hydrogen (H)

Hydrocarbons contain the molecules of hydrogen and carbon and are classified as terpenes.

When the compound contains oxygen as well, they are classified as:

- acids
- ketones
- alcohols
- lactones
- aldehydes
- oxides
- esters
- phenols.

One of the chemical structures of an essential oil is the **isoprene unit**, which is a branched chain containing five carbon compounds:

$$CH_2 = \overset{\overset{\displaystyle CH_3}{|}}{C} - CH_2 - CH_2$$

Bonds between atoms are always shown as a dash.

The second chemical structure is when six carbon atoms join together to form a ring. The potential for an aromatic ring to form becomes more probable as the length of the chain increases, but some rings will form with less than six carbon atoms.

Chemical compounds containing carbon will also use nitrogen (N) and sulphur (S) as well as oxygen (O) as basic molecular building blocks.

Terpenes

Terpenes are based on the isoprene unit, the five-carbon compound, and the two terpenes of most interest to aromatherapists are sesquiterpenes and monoterpenes.

- Sesquiterpenes has 15 carbon atoms = 3 isoprene units.
- Monoterpenes has 10 carbon atoms = 2 isoprene units (common to most essential oils).

In a few oils, diterpenes, which contains 20 carbon atoms, is found in very small quantities; Clary sage is one example.

High monoterpene content can often be recognised by looking at the oil. The oil is clear, has low viscosity and is volatile. This reflects the small molecular size of a terpene molecule.

Oils with a high sesquiterpene content have a higher viscosity, are darker in colour, are much less volatile and because of the lingering aroma and low volatility are used as a fixative in a blend.

Alcohols

Monoterpenic alcohol is based on monoterpene and has 10 carbon atoms. They are classified on which terpene is involved in their production and are known as terpene derivatives. They belong to the most gentle and useful terpene molecules, being non-toxic to humans and extremely effective against micro-organisms.

Sesquiterpenic alcohols are not so common, but the interplay between effect and the chemical structure is more varied than with the monoterpenic alcohol.

Esters

Esters are one of the most important constituents of essential oils.

Alcohols, including terpene alcohols, react with acid to form a new chemical compound, which is based on the carboxyl group (COOH). Oils with a high ester content are antispasmodic and balancing. The strength of the antispasmodic effect is dependent on the chain length of the acid content of the molecule.

- Esters of formic acid – one carbon atom. This is the main component of geranium oil.
- Esters of acetic acid (acetates) – two carbon atoms. This is a component of rosemary oil.
- Esters of acids with five carbon atoms are the main components of Roman chamomile. Its antispasmodic properties can be used for skin and joints when there is inflammation.
- The strongest antispasmodic effect is achieved with oils that have esters of acids with seven carbon atoms, for example, Ylang Ylang.
- Esters are also fungicides.

Aldehydes

Aldehyde is a common component of an essential oil, based on the carbonyl group (C=O). Oils with high aldehyde content are both anti-inflammatory and sedative. A low concentration of this type of oil, which is diluted by air or liquid, will produce the best effect – a real case of 'less is best'.

Ketones

These oils can be potentially toxic, although they have a similar structure to aldehydes and are based on the carbonyl group. Oils that contain ketones have a stimulating effect on tissue regeneration.

Oxides

These compounds are quite rare in essential oils but high levels are found in eucalyptus and melalenca oils. They have strong anti-viral effects, as in Tea Tree, and expectorant effects, as in Naiouli. The oxygen atom is situated between two carbon atoms (C-O-C).

Lactones

These compounds usually occur in expressed oils (citrus) and some absolutes, e.g. jasmine. They have expectorant effects and have the ability to regulate temperature. They also have anti-viral and anti-fungal properties. Care must be taken because they can be phototoxic.

Phenols

Phenols are similar to alcohols because they have (-OH) group, which attaches itself to carbon in a aromatic group; this makes the phenol molecule very reactive. Oils with a high phenol content can severely irritate the skin and are not used in aromatherapy.

Therapeutic uses of essential oils and carrier oils

Essential oils can be used in numerous ways. It is too easy to become focused on using these beneficial oils for massage only. Smell therapy is a clue as to how you can introduce home care and advise your clients on alternative uses.

Throughout history, herbs, oils and resins have been used in religious ceremonies. Frankincense is still used in the Roman Catholic Church in the form of incense because of its ability to lower the rate of breathing, thereby preparing churchgoers for the act of prayer and worship.

Candles are used more and more in the home in an effort to enhance the atmosphere. Be wary of aroma-candles as they often contain aroma-smells, not aroma-oils. Use candles by all means, but blend your own unique aromas to both set and lift the mood.

Theory into practice

Remembering that skin is semi-permeable, what other ways can you use essential oils for home care?

Essential oil profiles

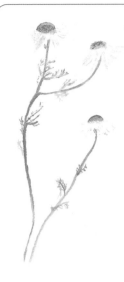

Roman Chamomile – Chamaemelum nobile

Family: Asteraceae (Compositae).

Country of origin: Hungary, England and Belgium.

Volatility: Middle note.

Method of extraction: Steam distillation of flower heads.

Principal constituents: Esters (75–80%). Monoterpenes – pinene, camphene, myrcene. Sesquiterpenes – sabinene, chamazulene. Alcohols – farnesol, nerolidol. Aldehydes – myrtenal.

Properties: Anti-inflammatory, antiseptic, antispasmodic, analgesic, bactericidal, carminative, digestive, emmenagogue, febrifuge, hepatic, hypnotic, nerve sedative, stomachic, tonic, vulnerary.

Common uses: Aches and pain, acne, anxiety, arthritis, depression, dry skin, eczema, heavy painful periods, headaches, hysteria, irritability, insomnia, minor wounds, nappy rash, PMT and menopausal symptoms, reduces inflammation, rheumatism, stress.

Safety: Non-toxic, non-irritant, can cause dermatitis and wheezing in hyper-sensitive people. Avoid during the first three months of pregnancy.

N.B. Be aware of substitutes, e.g. Moroccan Chamomile.

Herbal traditions: For two thousand years this herb has been used in medicine and is still widely used today. It is also known as the 'plant's physician' since it promotes the health of adjacent plants. For several hundred years chamomile has been used to lighten hair colour for fair-haired people.

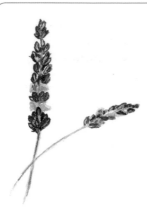

Lavender – Lavandula Officinalis

Family: Lamiaceae (Labitatae)

Country of origin: Native of the Mediterranean, now grown commercially in France, Spain and England.

Method of extraction: Steam distillation of flowering tops.

Volatility: Middle note.

Principal constituents: Monoterpenes – pinene, limonene, camphene. Alcohols – linalool, kerpineol, borneol, geraniol, lavandulol. Esters (40–45%) linalyl acetate, lavandulyl acetate, terpenyl acetate, geronyl acetate.

Properties: Probably the most versatile of all the essential oils. Balancing, calming, uplifting, antiseptic, anti-inflammatory and healing are among its many properties.

Common uses: Athlete's foot, anxiety, burns, colds, depression, dermatitis, diarrhoea, eczema, flu, headaches and migraine, insomnia, muscular aches and pains, nausea and vomiting, rheumatism and arthritis, reduces fever and stimulates the immune system, sinusitis, sprains, stress, throat infections, wounds and sores.

Safety: Non-toxic, non-irritant, non-sensitising. Possible dermatitis through overuse. This form of skin reaction can become a problem for aromatherapists.

Do not use if any form of haemorrhage has occurred.

Avoid during pregnancy, especially if there is a history of miscarriage. Do not use if low blood pressure is the problem.

Spike lavender: Do not use on small children as it can cause palpitations.

Herbal traditions: Lavender is well established as a folk remedy and almost everyone is familiar with its scent. It has been used for years to protect against moths by placing lavender bags in drawers and chests. Used as an insect repellent and in water to relieve tired feet and to alleviate the pain of toothache.

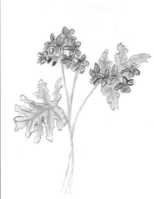

Geranium – Pelargonium Graveolens

Family: Geraniaceae

Country of origin: Native of Africa, now grown in France, Italy, Spain and Corsica. Main regions for essential oil production – Egypt, Russia, China and Reunion.

Method of extraction: Steam distillation of leaves, stalks and flowers.

Volatility: Middle note.

Principal constituents: Monoterpenes – pinene, myrcene, limonene, phellandrene. Alcohols (55–60%) citronellol, geroniol, linalool, nerol.

Properties: Analgesic, anti-depressant, anti-inflammatory, antiseptic, astringent, cicatrisant, deodorant, diuretic, fungicidial, haemostatic, stimulant of adrenal cortex, tonic, vulnerary.

Common uses: Acne, anxiety states, depression, dry eczema, gentle diuretic, PMT and menopause, sore throats and mouth infections, skin problems, uterine cancer, ulcers (internal and external).

Safety: Non-toxic, non-irritant, generally non-sensitising. Possible dermatitis in hyper-sensitive people.

The Bourbon type can cause reaction on a sensitive skin. Avoid during pregnancy.

Herbal traditions: Used for healing wounds, tumours and fractures.

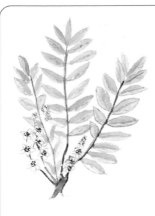

Frankincense – Boswellia Carteri

Family: Burseraceae

Country of origin: North Africa and the Middle East.

Method of extraction: Steam distillation of bark resin (often described as 'tears').

Volatility: Base note.

Principal constituents: Monoterpenes (40%) – pinene, limonene, sabinene, myrcene, phellandrene. Alcohol – borneol, farnesol. Esters – octyl acetate.

Properties: Anti-inflammatory, antiseptic, antistringent, carminative, cicatrisant, cytophylactic, digestive, diuretic, emmenagogue, expectorant, sedative, tonic, uterine, vulnerary.

Common uses: All respiratory complaints, physical or emotional, asthma, cystitis, psychological conditions like obsession and fear – helps to let go of the past and move on, skin care for ageing skin, slows and deepens breathing, ulcers, wounds.

Safety: Non-toxic, non-irritant, non-sensitising. Avoid during the first three months of pregnancy.

Herbal traditions: Used as incense in India, China and in the West by the Roman Catholic Church. In Egypt it was used in cosmetics, such as facial masks and perfumes. It was also used in the mummification process. Frankincense has been used medicinally to treat syphilis, rheumatism and urinary tract infections.

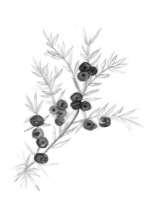

Juniper Berry – Juniperis Communis

Family: Cupressaccae

Country of origin: France, North America, Canada and Eastern Europe.

Method of extraction: Steam distillation of ripe berries.

Volatility: Middle note.

Principal constituents: Monoterpenes (60–80%) – pinene, limonene, camphene, thujene, sabnene, myrcene, phellandrene. Alcohols – terpeol, borneol, geraniol. Esters – bornyl acetate, terpinyl acetate.

Properties: Anti-rheumatic, antiseptic, antispasmodic, antitoxic, aphrodisiac, astringent, carminative, diuretic, emmenagogue, nervine, parasiticide, rubefacient, sedative, tonic, vulnerary.

Common uses: Aches and pains, acne, anxiety, cellutitis, cramps, cystitis, flu, gout, kidney stones, loss of appetite, mental fatigue, oily skin and hair, rheumatism, scanty periods, weeping eczema, wounds.

Safety: Non-sensitising, may be slightly irritating but generally non-toxic.

Do not use if kidney problems or urinary tract infections are present. Avoid during pregnancy. Always use in moderation.

Herbal traditions: The needles and berries have a long tradition of being used for chest problems, bronchitis and troublesome coughs. The berries can be used to help expel the build up of uric acid in the joints and help to eliminate the pains of rheumatism and arthritis. They have also been used to treat cystitis.

Juniper berries are used to give gin its flavour.

Vets use products with juniper berries to prevent ticks and fleas.

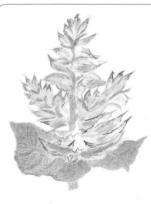

Clary Sage – Salvia Sclarea

Family: Lamiaceae (Labiatae)

Country of origin: Native of Southern Europe. Cultivated in Russia and USA. The main producers of oils are France and Britain.

Method of extraction: Steam distillation of leaves and flowering tops.

Volatility: Top/middle note.

Principal constituents: Monoterpenes – pinene, camphene, myrcene. Alcohols (15%) – linalool, citronellol, geraniol. Esters (50–75%) – linalyl acetate, geranyl acetate, neryl acetate. *Constituents vary depending on geographical area.*

Properties: Anticonvulsive, anti-depressant, antiseptic, antispasmodic, aphrodisiac, astringent, bactericidal, carminative, deodorant, digestive, emmenagogue.

Common uses: Acne, anxiety, asthma, boils and skin inflammation, depression, digestive problems (colic, flatulence), frigidity, impotence, insomnia, lower blood pressure, menopausal problems, menstrual stimulant, muscular problems.

Safety: Non-toxic, non-irritant, non-sensitising. Should not be used if your client has cancer. Avoid during pregnancy and if you suspect your client may be the 'worse for alcohol': this oil will make the side effects of drinking much worse. It can exaggerate drunkenness and induce a narcotic effect.

Clary sage is used in aromatherapy in place of sage, because it has a lower toxicity level.

Herbal traditions: During the Middle Ages, this herb was used for digestive disorders, kidney disease, uterine and menstrual complaints, for treating ulcers and as a nerve tonic.

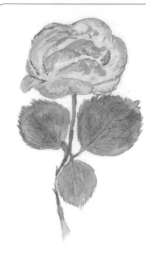

Rose – Rosa Damascena

Family: Rosaceae

Country of origin: Morocco, Turkey, France, Bulgaria.

Method of extraction: Steam distillation of flower petals (Rose Otto). Solvent extraction of petals (Rose Absolute).

Volatility: Base note.

Principal constituents: Monoterpenes (30–37%) – pinene, camphene, myrcene, phellandrene. Alcohols – linalool, borneol. Oxides (30–55%) – 1,8 cineole.

Properties: Antidepressant, antiseptic, antispasmodic, antiviral, anti-tubercular agent, astringent, aphrodisiac, bactericidal, choleretic, cicatrisant, detoxifying, sedative, emmenagogue, haemostatic, heptatic, laxative, tonic for heart, liver, stomach and uterus.

Common uses: Asthma, depression, dry or sensitive skin, frigidity, good for all female problems, grief and sadness, hay fever, herpes, impotence, insomnia, nausea, palpitations, poor circulation.

Safety: Non-toxic, non-irritant, non-sensitising. This oil can promote menstruation and should be avoided during pregnancy. Rose Absolute may cause skin irritation in hyper-sensitive clients.

Herbal traditions: The rose has been used for healing since antiquity. During the Middle Ages it was used for digestive and menstrual problems, headaches, poor circulation, the plague, eye and skin infections.

French and Moroccan roses possess narcotic properties; hence their reputation as aphrodisiacs.

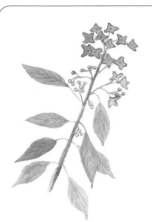

Sandalwood – Santalum Album

Family: Santalaceae

Country of origin: East India.

Method of extraction: Steam distillation of the wood and roots.

Volatility: Base note.

Principal constituents: Sesquiterpenes – santalene, farnesene. Alcohols (40–60%) – santalol.

Properties: Anti-depressant, antiseptic, antispasmodic, aphrodisiac, bactericidal, carminative, cicatrisant, diuretic, expectorant, fungicidal, insecticidal, sedative, tonic.

Common uses: All skin care, anxiety, bronchitis, cystitis, depression, diarrhoea, insomnia, menopausal symptoms, morning sickness, nausea, PMT, rashes, sore throats, tension, urinary infections.

Safety: Non-toxic, non-irritant, non-sensitising. Avoid if severe clinical depression is the problem. Neat application may cause contact dermatitis.

Herbal traditions: Sandalwood has been used in perfume for over 4000 years. In India it is combined with Rose to produce the famous scent 'Aytar'. It is used as incense, to embalm and as a cosmetic. The wood is also used to build temples.

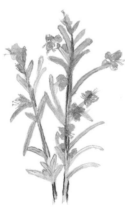

Rosemary – Rosmarinus Officinalis

Family: Lamiaceae (Labiatae)

Country of origin: Native of Mediterranean coasts. Main oil producing countries are France and Spain.

Method of extraction: Steam distillation of leaves and flowering tops.

Volatility: Middle note.

continued ▸▸

Principal constituents: Monoterpenes (15–30%) – pinene, camphene, myrcene, limonene. Alcohol – borneol. Oxides – 1,8 cineole trace 20%. Ketones (monoterpenones) – berbonene.

Properties: Analgesic, aphrodisiac, antiseptic, antispasmodic, carminative, digestive, diuretic, emmengogue, fungicidal, nervine, rubefacient, tonic, vulnerary.

Common uses: Aches and pains, arthritis and rheumatism, colds, flu, coughs, fluid retention, headaches, migraine, improving circulation, improving memory, helping with lymphatic congestion, lowering cholesterol.

Safety: Non-toxic, non-irritant (in dilution only), non-sensitising. Do not use if asthma or high blood pressure are the problems. Do not use in pregnancy or on a client with epilepsy.

Cautions: Different types may contain higher levels of ketones, check with your supplier. This oil is subject to adulteration. May antidote homeopathic remedies.

Herbal traditions: Rosemary was highly prized in many civilizations. During ancient times sprigs were burnt at shrines in Greece and used in the Middle Ages to drive away evil spirits, and to protect against the plague and infectious illness.

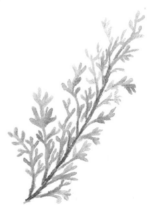

Cypress – Cupressus Sempervirens

Family: Cupressaceae

Country of origin: Cultivated in France, Germany and Spain.

Method of extraction: Steam distillation of twigs, needles and cones.

Volatility: Middle note.

Principal constituents: Monoterpenes (40–50%) – pinene, camphene, limonene. Sesquiterpenes – cadinene. Alcohols – terpineol, borneol, linalool, sabinol. Ester – terpenyl acetate.

continued ▸▸

Properties: Antirheumatic, antiseptic, antispasmodic, astringent, deodorant, diuretic, hepatic, styptic, sudorific, tonic, vaso-constrictive.

Common uses: Asthma, broken capillaries, bronchitis, cellulites, chilblains, cramps, dry cough, haemorrhoids, nose bleeds, reducing swelling, rheumatism, varicose veins.

Safety: Non-toxic, non-irritant, non-sensitising. Do not use with breast cancer, glaucoma, menstrual or prostate problems.

Herbal traditions: Highly valued as a medicine by ancient civilisations and still used in Tibet as incense.

Safety: Non-toxic, non-irritant, with possible sensitisation in some people. May cause irritation on sensitive skin areas.

N.B. This oil is subject to adulteration.

Herbal traditions: Tea Tree gets is name because the leaves are used to prepare a herbal tea. It has been used for hundreds of years by the Aboriginal people of Australia. Recent research has shown it to be a very powerful immuno-stimulant and it has been found to be active against infectious organisms, bacteria and viruses.

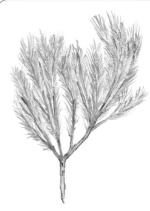

Tea Tree – Melaleuca Alternifolia

Family: Myrtaceae

Country of origin: New South Wales, Australia.

Method of Extraction: Steam distillation of leaves and twigs.

Volatility: Top note.

Principal constituents: Monoterpenes (25–40%) – pinene, terpinene, cymene, limonene, myrcene, phellandrene. Alcohols (25–57%) – terpene-4-ol. Oxide – cineole.

Properties: Anti-inflammatory, antiseptic, antiviral, bactericidal, balsamic, cicatriant, diaphoretic, expectorant, fungicidal, immuno-stimulant, parasiticide, vulnerary.

Common uses: Athlete's foot, abscess, acne, blisters, boils, bronchitis, chesty coughs, chickenpox, cold sores, colds, cuts and wounds, cystitis, flu, gum and mouth infections, insect bites, rashes including nappy rash, shingles, sinusitis, thrush, sunburn, warts, veruccae.

continued ▶▶

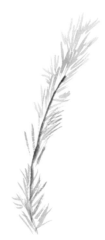

Naiouli – Melaleuca Viridiflora

Family: Myrtaceae

Country of origin: Australia.

Method of extraction: Steam distillation of the leaves and young twigs.

Volatility: Top note.

Principal constituents: Monoterpenes – pinene, limonene. Alcohols – linalool, viridflorol, nerolidol. Oxides (38–65%) – 1,8 cineole.

Properties: Analgesic, anticatarrhal, antirheumatic, antiseptic, antispasmodic, bactericidal, balsamic, cicatrisant, expectorant, stimulant, vermifuge.

Common uses: Acne, boils, burns, cuts, insect bites, oily skin, spots, ulcers, wounds, muscular aches and pains, poor circulation, rheumatism, asthma, bronchitis, catarrhal conditions, coughs, sinusitis, sore throats, whooping cough, cystitis, urinary infections, fever, flu.

Safety: Non-toxic, non-irritant, non-sensitising. No known contra-indications.

N.B. This oil is subject to adulteration.

Herbal traditions: It has been used in Australia for ailments such as general aches and pains, cuts and infections, and all types of respiratory conditions. It was also used to purify water.

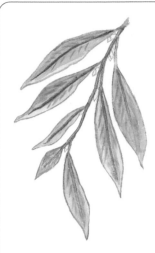

Eucalyptus – Eucalyptus Globulus

Family: Myrtaccae

Country of origin: Australia. Main oil-producing countries are Spain, Russia and China.

Method of extraction: Steam distillation of the leaves and young twigs.

Volatility: Top note.

Principal constituents: Monoterpenes – pinene, cymene, limonene, camphene. Alcohols – terpineol. Aldehydes – myrtenal, geranial. Oxides (60–85%) – cineole. Esters – terpenyl acetate.

Properties: Analgesic, antineuralgic, antirheumatic, antiseptic, antispasmodic, antiviral, balsamic, cicatrisant, decongestant, deodorant, diuretic, expectorant, febrifuge, parasiticide, rubefacient, stimulant, vermifuge, vulnerary.

Common uses: Arthritis (rheumatoid), asthma, blisters, boils and skin infections, bronchitis, burns, poor circulation, colds, flu, cold sores, dry coughs, headaches, insect bites, insect repellent, lice, muscular aches and pains, neuralgia, rheumatism, shingles, chicken pox, throat infections.

Safety: Externally non-toxic, non-irritant (in dilution), non-sensitising. Do not use with any form of urinary tract infection. Do not use if high blood pressure or epilepsy are the problem. Avoid using on sensitive skin.

Cautions: When taken internally, eucalyptus oil is very toxic: as little as 3.5 ml has been reported as fatal.

Herbal traditions: A traditional Australian household remedy. Used especially for bronchitis and croup with the dried leaves used like tobacco and smoked for asthmatic conditions. It is also used for feverish conditions such as malaria.

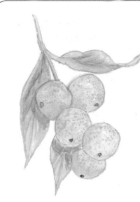

Petitgrain – Citrus Aurantium var. amara

Family: Rutaceae

Country of origin: France, Italy, Spain and North Africa. Main oil-producing countries are Italy and Eygpt.

Method of extraction: Distillation of leaves and twigs of the orange tree that produces bitter orange oil.

Volatility: Top note.

Principal constituents: Monoterpenes – myrcene, pinene, cymene, sabinene. Alcohols (30–40%) – linalool, terpineol, nerol, geraniol. Esters – linalyl acetate, neryl acetate, geranyl acetate.

Properties: Antiseptic, antispasmodic, deodorant, digestive, nervine, stimulant (digestive, nervous), stomachic, tonic.

Common uses: Acne, anti-depressant, dyspepsia, excessive perspiration, refreshing, relaxing, sedating for the nervous system, skin care – tonic for all skin types.

Safety: Non-toxic, non-irritant, non-sensitising and non-phototoxic. No known contra-indications.

Herbal traditions: The oil used to be extracted from unripe green oranges about the size of a cherry, hence the name 'little grains' (petitgrain). It is one of the main ingredients of eau-de-cologne.

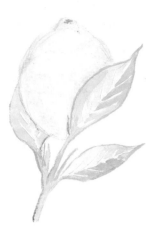

Lemon – Citrus Limon

Family: Rutaceae

Country of origin: Sicily, Italy, USA. (Grows wild in Spain and Portugal.) Main oil-producing countries are Italy, Israel and USA.

Method of extraction: Expression of the rind and fruit.

Volatility: Top note.

Principal constituents: Monoterpenes (90–95%) – limonene, pinene, terpinene, sabinene. Alcohols – hexanol, octanol. Aldehydes – geranial, neral, citronellal. Esters – neryl acetate, geranyl acetate.

Properties: Antiseptic, antianaemic, antimicrobial, antirheumatic, antisclerotic, antispasmodic, antitoxic, bactericidal, carminative, cicatrisant, diuretic, febrifuge, haemostatic, hypontensive, insecticidal, rubefacient, tonic, vermifuge.

Common uses: Asthma, arthritis, boils, bronchitis, chilblains, colds, cuts, dyspepsia, fever, flu, herpes, mouth ulcers, rheumatism, throat infections, varicose veins, warts.

Safety: Non-toxic; may cause dermal sensitisation or reaction to some people. Apply in moderation. Phototoxic – do not use on skin exposed to direct sunlight.

Calming despite high hydrocarbon content. Avoid if high blood pressure is the problem.

N.B. This oil has a short shelf life and should be used within six months.

Herbal traditions: In Europe, lemon is regarded as a 'cure all' for infectious illness. It has been used for such fevers as typhoid and malaria, for liver congestion, and for acidic orders such as arthritis and rheumatism.

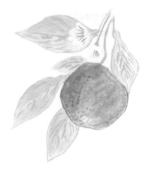

Orange – Citrus sinesis

Family: Rutaceae

Country of origin: Native to China. Extensively cultivated in America and the Mediterranean.

Method of extraction: Cold expression of the peel.

Volatility: Top note.

Principal constituents: Monoterpenes (80–98%) – limonene. Alcohols – linalool, nerol. Esters – linalyl acetate.

Properties: Antidepressant, anti-inflammatory, antiseptic, bactericidal, carminative, choleretic, digestive, fungicidal, hypotensive, sedative (nervous), stimulant (digestive and lymphatic), stomachic, tonic.

Common uses: Skin care, mouth ulcers, obesity, palpitations, water retention, bronchitis, constipation, colds, flu, nervous tension, stress-related conditions.

Safety: Generally non-toxic (although large amounts of orange peel eaten by children has been known to be fatal). Non-irritant, non-sensitising, but limonene can cause dermatitis in some people.

Distilled orange oil is known to be phototoxic but the oil of expressed sweet orange is not considered so; however, it would be wise to avoid strong sunlight after treatment.

Prolonged use as well as high dosage may cause irritation on sensitive skin areas.

N.B. This oil has a short shelf life and should be used within six months.

Herbal traditions: In Chinese medicine the dried peel of sweet oranges is used to treat coughs, colds, anorexia and malignant breast sores.

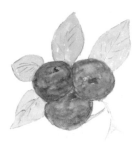

Tangerine – Citrus reticulata

Family: Rutaceae

Country of origin: A native of China, it has the same botanical source as the Mandarin. Most of the tangerine oil is produced in America.

Method of extraction: Cold expression from the outer peel.

Volatility: Top to middle.

Principal Constituents: Monoterpenes (75–80%) – limonene, myrcene, pinene, phellandrene. Alcohols – citronellol, linalool.

Properties: Antiseptic, antispasmodic, cytophylactic, sedative, stomachic, tonic.

Common uses: Stress – especially in young children, tension – especially in young children, digestive problems, flatulence, diarrhoea, constipation, vascular tonic, skin tonic – especially when blended with neroli and lavender for stretch marks.

Safety: Non-toxic, non-irritant, non-sensitising. Possibily phototoxic: do not expose the skin to strong sunlight after treatment.

N.B. This oil has a short shelf life and should be used within six months.

Herbal traditions: None for the tangerine, but the mandarin was given as a token of respect to the rulers of China, who were called Mandarins.

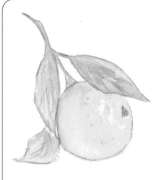

Grapefruit – Citrus x paradisi

Family: Rutaceae

Country of origin: Native of Asia. Cultivated in America, Israel and Brazil. The oil is produced mainly in California.

Method of extraction: Cold expression of the peel.

Volatility: Top note.

Principal constituents: Monoterpenes (90%) – limonene, pinene. Alcohols – linalool, geraniol.

Properties: Antiseptic, antitoxic, astringent, antidepressant, bactericidal, diuretic, stimulant (lymphatic and digestive), tonic.

Common uses: Acne, promotes hair growth, skin care, cellulite, obesity, stiffness, water retention, immune system, depression, headaches, nervous exhaustion.

Safety: Non-toxic, non-irritant, non-sensitising, non phototoxic. This oil has a very short shelf life as it oxidises very quickly. Although it is non phototoxic it is best to avoid strong sunlight after treatment.

Herbal traditions: It shares the history of other citrus fruits, being used for protection against infectious illness because of its high vitamin C content.

N.B. All citrus oils oxidise very quickly: use after six months may cause skin actions. Date all bottles and use stock rotation to avoid this problem.

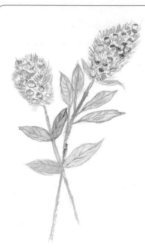

Peppermint – Mentha Piperita

Family: Lamiaceae (Labiatae)

Country of origin: Cultivated in Europe, USA and Japan.

Method of extraction: Steam distillation of leaves and flowering tops.

Volatility: Top/middle note.

Principal constituents: Monoterpenes – pinene, limonene, sabinene, phellandrene, myrcene. Alcohols (50%) – menthol, isomethol. Esters – menthyl acetate.

Properties: Analgesic, antimicrobial, anti-inflammatory, carminative, cephalic, emmenagogue, expectorant, febrifuge, hepatic, nervine, stomachic, vasconstrictor.

Common uses: Colds, colic, flatulence, flu, throat infections, headache, heartburn, hot flushes, indigestion, nausea, neuralgia, shock and hysteria, sinusitis, toothache, travel sickness.

Safety: Non-toxic, non-irritant (except in concentration). Possible sensitisation due to menthol. Always use in moderation and avoid during pregnancy. Do not use on nursing mothers and avoid use on sensitive skin. Do not use on children under 30 months old.

Caution: Avoid use on clients susceptible to cardiac fibrillation. Antidote to homeopathic remedies.

Herbal traditions: Mints have been in China and Japan for hundreds of years. A type of peppermint was found in Egyptian tombs dating from 1000BC. It has been used regularly to help indigestion, toothaches, headaches and sore throats.

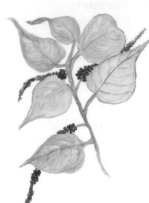

Black Pepper – Piper Nigrum

Family: Pipeaceae

Country of origin: Singapore, India, Malaysia. Main oil producing countries are USA and Europe

Method of extraction: Distillation of unripe berries.

Volatility: Middle note.

Principal constituents: Monoterpenes – limonene, pinene, thujene, sabinene, terpinene, myrcene, camphene. Sesquiterpenes – carophyllene, bisabolene, farnesene. Alcohols – terpineol, linalool.

Properties: Analgesic, antimicrobial, antiseptic, antispasmodic, antitoxic, aphrodisiac, bactericidal, carminitive, digestive, diuretic, laxative, rubefacient, stimulant (nervous, circulatory, digestive), stomach, tonic, warming prior to exercise.

Common uses: Arthritis, catarrh, chilblains, chills, colds, colic, constipation, diarrhoea, flatulence, flu, heartburn, loss of appetite, muscular aches and pains, nausea, poor circulation, poor muscle tone, sprains, stiffness.

Safety: Non-toxic, non-sensitising, irritant in high concentration. Can also be an irritant on sensitive skins because of its rubifacient properties. Always use in moderation as it can over-stimulate the kidneys.

Herbal traditions: Black and white pepper has been used for medicinal and culinary purposes in the East for over 4000 years. White pepper is used in Chinese medicine to treat fevers such as malaria and cholera. The Greeks used it for intermittent fevers and digestive problems.

German Chamomile – Matricaria recutica

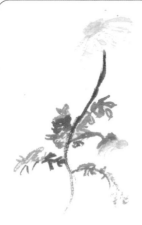

Family: Asteraceae (Compositae)

Country of origin: Native to Europe and cultivated for oil production in Hungary and Eastern Europe.

Method of extraction: Steam distillation of the flowers.

Volatility: Middle note.

Principal constituents: Chamazulene, farnesene.

Properties: Analgesic, anti-allergenic, anti-inflammatory, antispasmodic, bactericidal, emmenagogue, fungicidal, hepatic.

Common uses: Aches and pain, acne, anxiety, arthritis, depression, dry skin, eczema, heavy painful periods, headaches, hysteria, irritability, insomnia, minor wounds, nappy rash, PMT and menopausal symptoms, reduces inflammation, rheumatism, stress.

N.B. Because of its higher content of azulene it has excellent anti-inflammatory properties.

Safety: Should not be used in the early stages of pregnancy as it is an emmenagogue. Use in a lower concentration, 0.5%, because of possible allergic reactions on sensitive skin.

Herbal traditions: Has a long history of being used to deal with all situations of a nervous origin.

Neroli – Citrus aurantium

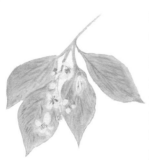

Family: Rutaceae

Country of origin: Major producers are Italy, Egypt, USA and France.

Method of extraction: Steam distillation of the flowers.

Volatility: Middle to base.

continued ▶▶

Principal constituents: Alcohol – linalool 34%, gerniol, nerol. Esters – linalyl acetate, neryl acetate. Ketone – jasmone.

Properties: Anti-depressant, antiseptic, antispasmodic, bactericidal, deodorant, fungicidal, hypnotic.

Common uses: Scar tissue, stretch marks, sensitive skin, palpitations, colic, anxiety, depression, PMT.

Safety: Non-irritant, non-sensitising, non-phototoxic. Can be quite hypnotic, use with care.

Herbal traditions: Orange petals symbolise innocence and were used in bridal bouquets.

Pine – Pinus sylvestris

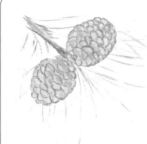

Family: Pinaceae

Country of origin: Northern Europe and Scandinavia.

Method of extraction: Steam distillation of needles (high grade oil). Steam distillation of cones and twigs (low grade oil, which is not suitable for aromatherapy).

Volatility: Middle note.

Principal constituents: Alcohol – borneol. Esters – bornyl acetate, terpinyl acetate. Monoterpenes – camphene, diphene, phellandrene, pinene, sylvestrene.

Properties: Antiseptic, decongestant, deodorant, disinfectant, expectorant, stimulant.

Common uses: Excessive perspiration, head lice, muscular pains, rheumatism, respiratory problems, neuralgia.

Safety: Other species can be toxic and should not be used for aromatherapy treatments.

Herbal traditions: Used by ancient civilisations for respiratory illnesses.

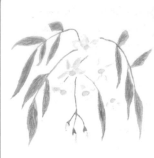

Jasmine – Jasminum officinale

Family: Oleaceae

Country of origin: Native to China. Main oil-producing countries are France and Egypt.

Method of extraction: Enfleurage/Solvent.

Volatility: Middle to base.

Principal constituents: Alcohols – farnesol, geraniol, nerol, terpincol. Esters – Linalyl acetate, Methyl anthralate.

Properties: Analgesic, anti-inflammatory, antiseptic, antispasmodic, aphrodisiac, sedative.

Common uses: Sensitive skin, sprains, spasms, frigidity, depression, stress.

Safety: Avoid during pregnancy. Very hypnotic: use with care. If adulterated may irritate sensitive skin.

N.B. Subject to adulteration.

Herbal traditions: Used in India for religious ceremonies.

Melissa – Melissa officinalis

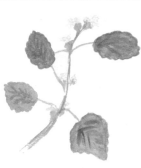

Family: Lamiaceae (Labiatae)

Country of origin: Oil production is mainly in France, Spain, Germany and Russia.

Method of extraction: Steam distillation of the leaves and flowers.

Volatility: Middle note.

Principal constituents: Acids – citronellic. Alcohols – citronellol, geraniol, linalool. Aldehydes – citral, citronellal. Ester – geranyl acetate.

continued ▶▶

Properties: Antidepressant, antispasmodic, bactericidal, emmenagogue, nervine, sedative.

Common uses: Allergies, respiratory problems, indigestion, nausea, insomnia, migraine, nervous conditions, stress, panic attacks.

Safety: This oil is often adulterated with other oils or synthetic chemicals. Always use in low doses to avoid sensitisation – 0.5%. Avoid during pregnancy.

Herbal traditions: Long history of medicinal use with a reputation as a 'cure all'.

Ginger – Zingiber officinale

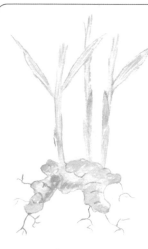

Family: Zingiberaceae

Country of origin: Oil mainly distilled in Britain, China and India.

Method of extraction: Steam distillation of dried ground roots.

Volatility: Top note.

Principal constituents: Alcohol – borneol. Aldehyde – citral. Monoterpenes – camphene, limonene, phellandrene.

Properties: Analgesic, antiseptic, anti-spasmodic, aphrodisiac, bactericidial, expectorant, laxative, stimulant.

Common uses: Arthritis, fatigue, poor circulation, rheumatism, sprains, coughs, sore throats, colic, nausea.

Safety: Can irritate sensitive skin; always use in low doses – 0.5%.

Herbal traditions: Used in ancient Greece for stomach problems. Chinese herbalists use it for respiratory problems.

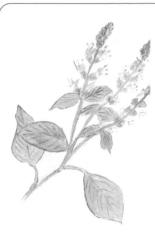

Patchouli – Pogostemon cablin

Family: Lamiaceae (Labiatae)

Country of origin: Native to Malaysia. Oil produced in Europe and the USA.

Method of extraction: Steam distillation of dried leaves.

Volatility: Base note.

Principal constituents: Alcohol – patchoulol. Aldehydes – cinnamic, benzoic. Sesquiterpene cadinene.

Properties: Antidepressant, anti-inflammatory, antiseptic, antiviral, bactericidal, deodorant, diuretic, fungicidal, nervine, stimulant.

Common uses: Skin conditions, hair problems, acne, athlete's foot, bed sores, insect repellent, depression, nervous disorders, stress.

Safety: Non-irritant, non-sensitising. Perfume can be overwhelming: use in low doses – 0.5%.

Herbal traditions: Used as an antidote for snake-bite and in herbal sachets to stop bed bugs.

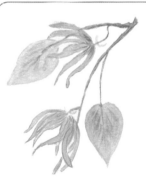

Ylang Ylang – Cananga odorata var. genuina

Family: Anonaceae

Country of origin: Native to tropical Asia. Oil produced mainly in Reunion and Madagascar.

Method of extraction: Steam distillation of the flowers. (This oil is available in several different grades – always check before purchase.)

Volatility: Middle to base note.

continued ▸▸

Principal constituents: Acid – benzoic. Alcohols – farnesol, geraniol, linalool. Ester – benzyl acetate. Phenols – eugenol, safrole. Sesquiterpene – cadinene.

Properties: Antidepressant, antiseptic, hypotensive, nervine, sedative, stimulant.

Common uses: High blood pressure, palpitations, depression, nervous conditions, stress.

Safety: Can cause sensitisation in some people: use in low doses: (0.5–1%). Overuse can cause nausea and headaches.

Herbal traditions: Used in the hair preparation known as Macassar oil, which was why anti-macassars were used to protect armchairs from the oil stains.

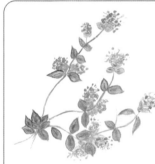

Sweet Marjoram – Origanum marjorana

Family: Lamiaceae (Labiatae)

Country of origin: Originates from Libya and Egypt. Main oil production is in France.

Method of extraction: Steam distillation of dried flowering herb.

Volatility: Middle note.

Principal constituents: Alcohols – borneol, terpineol. Monoterpenes – pinene, sabinene, terpinene. Sesquiterpene – caryophyllene.

Properties: Analgesic, antiseptic, antispasmodic, antiviral, bactericidal, emmenagogue, expectorant, hypotensive, laxative, nervine, sedative.

Common uses: Arthritis, muscular problems, sprains, rheumatism, respiratory problems, colic, PMT, high blood pressure, nervous disorders, stress.

Safety: Avoid during pregnancy. Do not use any other marjoram for aromatherapy use.

Herbal traditions: Used in Greece as an antidote for poison and for digestive problems.

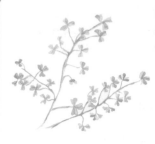

Myrrh – Commiphora myrrha

Family: Burseraceae

Country of origin: Native to the Middle East, North Africa and Northern India.

Method of extraction: Steam distillation of crude myrrh tears.

Volatility: Base note.

Principal constituents: Acid – myrrholic. Aldehydes – cinnamic, cuminic. Monoterpenes – pinene, dipentene, limonene. Sesquiterpene – cadinene.

Properties: Anti-inflammatory, antiseptic, stringent, carminative, emmenagogue, expectorant, fungicidal, sedative, uterine.

Common uses: Skin care and all forms of skin problems, respiratory problems, mouth infections, diarrhoea, thrush.

Safety: Non-irritant, non-sensitising. Avoid during pregnancy.

Herbal traditions: Myrrh was mixed with wine and offered up to Jesus on the cross. The Egyptians used it in both mummification and cosmetics.

Assessment task 13.3

Describe in detail the choice of essential oils, method of extraction, chemistry and the possible therapeutic outcomes of both the essential and carrier oils. (M)

Evaluate the choice of essential oils, using the Latin name; identify problems with possible contra-indications and justify the decision of oil choice because of the therapeutic outcome. Illustrate an in-depth understanding of the extraction process and chemical make-up of the choice of oils, including the carrier oil. (D)

Sources of oils

Essential oils, also known as essences, aromatic or volatile oils, are the basic materials of the aromatherapist. Plants make these aromatic substances in specialised tissues, distributed throughout the flowers, leaves, stems and bark.

Three separate oils are derived from the orange tree, all with different therapeutic properties:

- neroli comes from the flowers
- petitgrain from the leaves
- orange from the rind of the fruit.

Until they undergo extraction, they remain the essence of the plant.

Oils are usually secreted from glands or ducts. The more glands or ducts present in the plant, the cheaper the final cost of the oil.

Factors that influence the quality of the oil

These include:

- soil conditions – e.g. calcium-rich soils encourage a higher oil yield from German Chamomile
- variations in climate.

The plants and herbs used for oil extraction have to be gathered at precisely the right moment; the time of day and season of the year can change the chemical composition of an essential oil. Each plant has its own bio-rhythm.

- **Practice point:** Jasmine has a high concentration of oil at night. Damask Rose has a higher concentration before the heat of midday.

Oil purity

It is important to be able to guarantee the purity of the oils used during treatment. An essential oil may carry traces of chemical contaminates if the plants were grown with artificial pesticide or fertilisers. To avoid this problem, try to buy oils which have been grown organically in a controlled way. Some oils will be sold on the promise that they have been taken from the wild, but if they are growing 'wild' alongside a road they are unlikely to be of a good enough quality to be used therapeutically.

Try to ascertain which part of the plant the oil has been extracted from. Pure juniper oil should be extracted from the berries; a much lower grade oil can be obtained from the twigs.

It has been known for some producers to resort to adulterating oils for economic reasons. Rosemary oil can be adulterated by adding camphor oil, which would give a poor crop a better 'rosemary' aroma. Synthetic materials can be mixed with a pure oil, improving the aroma and decreasing the overall cost, but this would drastically alter any therapeutic qualities.

Buy oils from suppliers who know:

▸▸ the source of the oils they retail
▸▸ the country or region of origin
▸▸ the botanical name of the plant
▸▸ the part of the plant used
▸▸ the method of extraction used.

Oil safety

1 Essential oils must always be kept out of the reach of children.

2 Keep oils in a locked cabinet and store in date order.

3 Store oils in dark glass bottles in a controlled temperature. Oils stored in plastic bottles can either melt the plastic or draw impurities from the plastic container.

4 Do not stand oils on a window ledge in direct sunlight: heating and cooling the contents of the bottle may alter the chemical composition.

5 Essential oils should never be taken internally, unless prescribed by a medical practitioner. On the Continent, some doctors are also medically qualified aromatherapists.

6 Many beverages contain essential oils as approved flavour enhancers. These have undergone strict quality control before being selected for use.

7 If an essential oil accidentally enters the mouth, rinse thoroughly. If a quantity of oil is swallowed, medical attention must be sought. If an essential oil splashes into the eyes, rinse immediately and if any pain or inflammation is experienced, medical attention must be sought.

8 Essential oils are flammable; keep well away from naked flames.

9 If using a rag or paper to mop up spills, dispose of it in an external bin. Atmospheric oxidation of terpenes can cause a change in temperature, which may ignite the oils.

Assessment task 13.4

Explain the procedures you would use for the use of 'home care' information and products in this situation. (M)

Evaluate potential problems with 'home care' information and the storage of blended products and purchased oils. Describe, with attention to detail, the safety procedures required to achieve a solution. (D)

Classifying oils

It was a Frenchman called Piesse who classified odours with the musical scale. Oils are given 'notes' to denote their volatility rate, which means how quickly they evaporate once they are exposed to the air.

▸▸ 'Top notes' evaporate the fastest; they act quickly and are usually light and stimulating. Lemon and other citrus oils are good examples.

▸▸ 'Middle notes' evaporate more slowly and can form the heart of a blend; they are used to help the general metabolism. Floral and fruity oils are good examples, such as geranium.

▸▸ 'Base notes' evaporate very slowly and are used as a fixative for the blend. They are relaxing and sedating. Sandalwood is a good example of a base note.

A more complex way of categorising oils is by the chemical constitutes, but this will vary according to where the plant was grown and under what conditions. The predominant chemical classifies oils.

▸▸ **Aldehydes** are anti-inflammatory, antiseptic, anti-rheumatic, calming and soothing.

▸▸ **Ketones** are classified toxic in mugwort, pennyroyal and sage, which are not used in aromatherapy, and non-toxic in other oils including jasmine, which contains jasomone, and sweet fennel, which contains fenchone. Oils with a ketone content have excellent curative properties but they should always be used in moderation in a blend. They should not be used continuously over a long time span since clients and therapists may become sensitised to the oils.

▸▸ **Esters** are the most widespread group of chemical found in essential oils. They are anti-spasmodic, anti-inflammatory, anti-parasitic, cooling and soothing.

- **Ethers** are anti-inflammatory, anti-spasmodic and anti-stress.
- **Sesquiterpenes** are anti-inflammatory, anti-allergic and anti-parasitic.

The oils containing these chemical constituents are calming oils.

- **Sesquaialcohols** act as a general tonic.
- **Alcohols** are germicidal and some are very stimulating.
- **Terpenes** are antiseptic and anti-inflammatory. The component limonene is found in 90 per cent of citrus oils.
- **Oxides** are expectorant and decongestant. Some are anti-parasitic and anti-viral.
- **Phenols** are anti-bacterial, anti-viral, anti-fungal and anti-parasitic.

The oils containing these chemical constituents are stimulating oils.

Skin test

It is always advisable to carry out a skin test before using an essential oil. It is particularly important if your client suffers from hay fever or allergies of any kind. A skin test must always be done before using essential oils in the treatment of children and the elderly. The dilution percentages are different for these two categories of client.

Put one drop of the oil on a cotton bud and use it to lightly touch the inside of the elbow, the inside of the wrist or under the arm. Cover the area with a plaster and leave unwashed for 24 hours. If there is itching, redness or any other type of reaction, do not use that oil. Always check first that your client is not allergic to plasters.

Skin irritation

The majority of essential oils are safe when used on the skin with the correct dilutions. It is usually clients with ultra-sensitive skins, typically those with fair or red hair, who are more likely to experience a reaction to the oils.

Blending

For the trainee and newly-qualified practitioner this process can be the most daunting part of an aromatherapy treatment. All essential oils are diluted in a 'carrier oil' (see page 302).

- **Practice point:** Each person you blend for is unique. More surprisingly, your mood will leave its signature on blended oils. As with all complementary treatments that involve 'touch', your approach to your client will impact on the outcomes.

Theory into practice

Personality signatures
- Choose four or five students from your group, making sure that there is a mix of personalities.
- Using a 30 ml bottle containing carrier oil, add:
  - 5 drops of lavender
  - 2 drops of bergamot
  - 2 drops of cedarwood.
- Each student should mix up an identical blend. Make sure they keep the mixture about their person for about 15 minutes.

Smell test
The rest of the group then undertake a 'smell test', smelling each blend in turn, making sure that they do not handle the bottles.

Record the outcomes – it should prove very interesting.

How much to mix

A useful rule of thumb for a female client is the dress size, otherwise measure as follows:

- 10 ml for a small person
- 14 ml for a person of medium build
- 20 ml for the larger frame.

For body massage the essential oils are 2 per cent of the total blend; for facials it is 1 per cent. The simplest formula for working out the required number of drops is:

- For a 1 per cent blend divide the amount of carrier oil by 4, e.g. 20 ml divided by 4 = 5 drops.
- For a 2 per cent blend divide the amount of carrier oil by 2, e.g. 20 ml divided by 2 = 10 drops.

A 1 per cent blend is also used on children and older clients.

Factors to consider when blending for your clients

▸ The right choice of both carrier oil and essential oils.

▸ The fragrance of the individual oils must be acceptable to your client. Many oils have similar properties but the oil you may choose which smells right to you, may be unacceptable to your client. For this reason, when making a selection always have a replacement in mind. Studies at Warwick University have shown that if an aroma is intensely disliked this will block its effect on the central nervous system.

▸ The fragrance of the blend should be acceptable to your client. When offering each individual oil to your client, make a mental note of how he or she responds to each of the oils. If you have 8 drops to add to your blend, you will need a guide for the number of each oil you have decided to use; your client's reactions to the oils will be an excellent indicator for choice: the body knows its needs. To validate this, check if the 'client's choice' will respond to 'presenting symptoms'.

▸ If using a strong fragrance be aware that this may dominate the blend. Use oils that complement each other.

When understanding the function of the oils internally, two words seem to sum up the properties of essential oils:

adaptengonic = to normalise.

To emphasise the requirement of the blend to be unique and its ability to normalise an imbalance, French aromatherapy doctors use an 'aromatogram' to decide on the best oil/oils required for treatment. A swab is taken from an infected area; it is then cultured in a laboratory. The cultures are tested with up to 15 different oils before a decision is made on the 'oil' prescription.

▸ **Practice point:** No two patients with the same infection are given the same essential oil prescription.

Synergy (Greek – *syn* = together, *ergon* = work) = *working in harmony.*

When a blend is working in harmony, the combination or choice of oils is called a synergy. This is when you have taken into consideration the three P's (see page 277) and created a holistic blend aimed at treating any underlying causes.

Madame Maury would prescribe individual prescriptions for all of her clients, which always took into account temperament and circumstances alongside any physical symptoms. One oil that seems to enhance just about any blend is lavender; that is of course, if your client finds it acceptable.

There are no hard or fast rules for teaching you to blend. More than two oils can be used but no more than four, as they will 'fight' each other. Be wary of pre-blended oils that can be purchased, extolling the virtues of the numerous oils they contain – often they contain chemical substitutes with no therapeutic value.

Do not use a particular blend for a prolonged period or too frequently. Both you and your client can become sensitised to a particular blend or oil. Always respect the power of essential oils and use them with care.

As a safety net, you can use blend charts or work suggestions given by experienced writers in aromatherapy, but eventually you will be able to blend your own oils intuitively.

Oil contra-indications

Whenever you select an oil for a massage blend, always refer to the original consultation and check with your client that there has not been a change of circumstances.

Special note: Ravensara is becoming more popular for aromatherapy use. Always make sure you purchase Ravensara aromatica (leaves) and not Ravensara anisata (bark), which has a high estragole content.

Theory into practice

As you progress as a therapist and wish to add new oils to your repertoire, always investigate the outlines you will find under essential oils.

You will notice that the majority of oils should be avoided during pregnancy. There is growing concern at the high levels of essential oils being used on pregnant and nursing mothers and very young babies. The act of massage stimulates the body to use its own internal pharmacy without introducing very concentrated plant essences.

Carrier oils

Carrier oils are used to 'carry' or administer the essential oils. It is important to choose the carrier oil with as much care as you would an essential oil. Many of the carrier oils have their own therapeutic properties and can be chosen to complement the essential oil.

Cold pressed oils are superior because the process limits the damage to the natural characteristics of the oil.

The following are some of the processes undergone by refined oils, which generally makes them unsuitable for massage or as a carrier in aromatherapy.

- Removal of the basic colour by a bleaching process, which enables manufacturers to make the batches uniform in colour.
- Adding synthetic antioxides to improve the shelf life.
- The use of solvents, such as hexane and petroleum spirit, to increase the yield. Although they are removed, there will a residue left in the oil.

Sweet almond oil

Odour:	Sweet smell with a hint of marzipan.
Colour:	Pale yellow.
Skin types:	All skins.
	Helps to soothe inflammation, including sunburn. Relieves the itching caused by eczema, dry scaly skin, psoriasis and dermatitis.
Contains:	Vitamins A, B1, B2, B6 and E.
Cautions:	Because of an increase in nut allergy, check with your clients and do not use on babies for baby massage.

Grapeseed oil

This is a refined oil as it is a by-product of the wine-making industry. The seeds of the grape are washed, dried and ground before being pressed. It is not available cold pressed.

Odour:	Little or no smell.
Colour:	Pale green.
Skin Types:	All skins.
Contains:	Little nutrients.
Cautions:	This oil is non-toxic and hypoallergenic.

Sunflower oil

Organic sunflower oil is used as a macerating medium for calendula (pot marigold).

Odour:	None.
Colour:	Pale yellow.
Skin types:	All skins.
Contains:	Vitamins A, D and E. Minerals – calcium, potassium, zinc, phosphorus and iron.
Cautions:	None known.

Wheatgerm oil

A cereal grass native to West Asia. Wheatgerm is similar to grapeseed oil as it contains approximately. 13 per cent oil. The oil is extracted by hot pressing and also by a process similar to maceration. This oil is a natural antioxidant and is used as a preservative for other carrier oils.

Odour:	Can have a strong smell.
Colour:	Golden.
Contains:	Vitamins A, B1, B2, B3, B6, E, F.
Cautions:	This oil should not be used on clients with a wheat allergy.

1 How do aromatherapy oils trigger physical responses?

2 What are the three P's of aromatherapy?

3 Why is it important to understand the potential hazards of essential oils?

4 Explain the need for a Code of Ethics.

5 List four essential requirements to avoid cross-infection.

6 List the five aims of a consultation.

7 What is your understanding of contra-indication?

8 Why is it necessary to keep your records confidential?

9 List the recommendations for aftercare.

10 Give a brief description of steam distillation.

11 Why do you need a basic understanding of aroma chemistry?

12 Why is oil purity important?

13 List five questions you need to ask your supplier to guarantee oil purity.

14 What should you do if an essential oil accidentally enters the mouth?

15 How are oils classified?

16 Why do you need to do a patch test?

17 Who chooses the final blend?

18 What do you use a carrier oil for?

References and bibliography for Unit 13: Aromatherapy

Lawless, J. (1995) *Complete Essential Oils*, Element Books.

McGuiness, H. (1997) *Aromatherapy Basics*, Hodder Stoughton

Montagu, A. (1986) *Touching:The Human Significance of Skin*, Harper & Row

Price, L. (1990) *Carrier Oils*, Riverhead.

Price, S & Price, L. (1995) *Aromatherapy for Health Professionals*, Churchill Livingstone.

Schnaubelt, K. (1995) *Advanced Aromatherapy, The Science of Essential Oil Therapy*, Healing Arts Press.

Tisserand, R. & Balacs, T. (1995) *Essential Oil Safety*, Churchill Livingstone

Wildwood, C. (1996) *Encyclopaedia of Aromatherapy*, Grange Books.

Wildwood, C. (1998) *Encyclopaedia of Healing Plants*, Piatkus

Neuropsychiatry and Seizure Clinic:University of Birmingham.

anaprodisiac – reduces sexual desire

anti-anaemic – helps with anaemia

anti-arthritic – helps with arthritis

anticatarrhal – helps to remove excessive amounts of catarrh

anticonvulsant – helps to prevent convulsions

anti-emetic – helps to reduce the severity of vomiting

anti-inflammatory – reduces inflammation

antineuralgic – helps with nerve pain

antirheumatic – helps to relieve rheumatism

antisclerotic – reduces hardening of the tissues

antispasmodic – eases spasms (muscles) or convulsions

anti-tubercular – helps to alleviate tubercular infections

aphrodisiac – increases sexual desire

astringent – contracts tissues/skin

bactericidal – destroys bacteria

balsamic – soothing

carminative – helps to settle the digestive system

cephalic – relates to stress disorders in the head

choleretic – stimulate the flow of bile

cicatrisant – helps to form scar tissue

cytophylactic – supports the immune system

decongestive – helps to relieve congestion

diaphoretic – increases sweating

disinfectant – helps to stop the spread of germs

emmenagogue – assists menstruation

expectorant – assists with the removal of mucus

febrifuge – helps to lower fevers

fungicidal – helps to prevent fungal infection

haemostatic – stops bleeding

hallucinogenic – causes visions or delusions

hepatic – aids the liver

hypertensive – raises blood pressure

hypnotic – induces sleep

hypotensive – lowers blood pressure

immuo-stimulant – stimulates the immune system

insecticidal – helps to discourage insects in the home (keeps spiders out)

laxative – loosens the bowel and aids constipation

nervine – strengthens or tones the nerves

parasticide – helps to remove head lice

rubefacient – reddens the skin

soporific – induces sleep

stimulant – increases activity (body systems)

stomachic Taids the digestion

styptic – stops external bleeding

sudorific – increases sweating

vaso-constrictive – constricts blood flow

vermifuge – helps with internal worms

vulnerary – helps to heal wounds and sores

Indian head massage

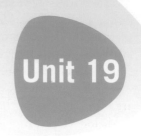

Unit 19

This unit is designed to integrate the skills you have gained from body massage and tailor them to fit a specialised approach to help deal with the stress that is part of twenty-first century living.

You will use several massage movements you are already familiar with.

» effleurage
» petrissage – kneading, rolling, wringing
» friction
» tapotement – tapping, hacking.

Indian head massage, with its eastern cultural values, has been westernised, enabling this form of massage to be used in a variety of settings on a wide range of clients. This unit will introduce you to a selection of oils used for Indian head massage, the benefits of each oil and the reasons for choosing a particular oil. The consultation process will give you an understanding of contra-indications and contra-actions from this approach to massage.

In order to achieve Unit 19 in Indian head massage you must complete the following learning outcomes:

LEARNING OUTCOMES

1 Explain the theory and functions of Indian head massage.
2 Demonstrate an Indian head massage.
3 Evaluate Indian head massage through case studies.
4 Identify professional ethics and safety procedures.

Theory and functions of Indian head massage

Origins: the eastern approach

Eastern approaches to healing adopt a more integrated concept of how a body maintains a healthy state and how it becomes traumatised into a state of 'dis-ease'. Many ancient forms of healing see each person as unique and two people displaying the same symptoms will not necessarily be treated in the same way. Great emphasis is placed on the balance of body, mind and spirit.

» Practice point: Everything exists in relation to something else, not in isolation.

The flow of prana (energy) around the body is an important aspect to both diagnosing and treating illness. Re-balancing the patterns of energy flow is part of Ayurvedic medicine, which is thought to be the oldest medical system known and is widely used in India and other Eastern countries.

Ayurveda is a Sanskrit word meaning 'wisdom or science of life', and massage, including the form known as Indian head massage, has its roots in this complex, holistic approach to well-being.

In the initial stages of diagnosing 'dis-ease' there are similarities in both Eastern and Western medicine. A health practitioner will assess lifestyle, diet, levels of stress and genetic pre-dispositions to certain illnesses. In Ayurvedic medicine the process will also include ancient principles to determine the flow of energy.

Doshas

Doshas are bio-energies that determine body shape, size and certain other physical, mental and emotional characteristics. They are organised into three essential principles:

1   Vata Dosha – movement and change.

2   Pitta Dosha – transformation and metabolism.

3   Kapha Dosha – structure and fluidity.

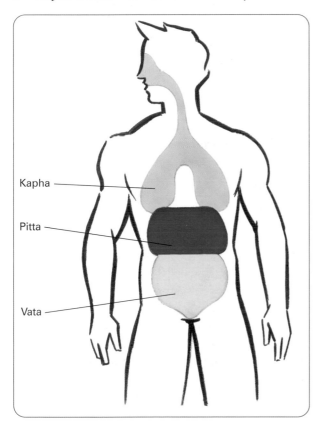

Kapha

Pitta

Vata

Doshas.

We all have a balance of the three doshas in our mind/body make-up, but one may be more dominant than the others. When your 'prakruti' – the natural proportion of the doshas in your system

– is well maintained, you are physically and mentally in balance. The purpose of Ayurveda is to encourage balance by living in harmony with our environment, ourselves and by taking control of every aspect of our lives; putting the body 'at ease'.

'Vikruit' describes when things are out of control; it is the Sanskrit word for 'deviations from one's true nature'.

Marmas

Marmas are points of concentrated energy that are located at the junctions where two or more systems meet, e.g. nerves/blood vessels, nerves/bone, muscles/joints/ligaments.

In traditional Chinese medicine these locations are called *acupoints,* a term you may be more familiar with, and there are many similarities between these two ancient systems of healing.

There are three main marma centres – the head, the heart and the bladder – with a further 107 marma points, some of which are located along the stress areas worked during an Indian head massage routine. Massaging the marma points can influence the Dosha bio-energies.

Chakras

The chakras are seven energy centres that are aligned along the spine. During a head massage you will interact with what are known as the 'higher' chakras:

1   the Crown (Sahasrara)

2   the Third Eye (Anja)

3   the Throat (Vishuddha).

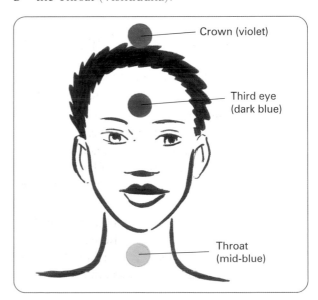

Crown (violet)

Third eye (dark blue)

Throat (mid-blue)

Position of higher chakras.

The chakras in turn are thought to influence the body's endocrine system.

The Crown chakra influences the pineal gland, the body's bio-clock. The importance of this small gland is not, as yet, fully understood, but it is involved in the sleep–wake cycle. It produces a hormone that encourages sleep in response to darkness. In medieval times, the pineal gland was thought to be the 'seat of the soul'.

➤ **Practice point:** An over-production of this hormone from the pineal gland is thought to be responsible for SAD (Seasonal Affective Disorder). People who suffer from this disorder use light boxes to help them deal with the dark gloomy days of winter.

The Third Eye chakra influences the pituitary gland, also known as the master gland. This gland is responsible for the balance of all the chemical messengers that interact with all the other organs of the body. It can be thought of as the conductor of an orchestra, keeping everything in tune.

The Throat chakra influences the thyroid and parathyroids. The thyroid gland controls the body's metabolism.

Balancing the energy patterns in the body is one aspect of encouraging healing. The commitment of the client to look at lifestyle choices and lifestyle changes is equally important. This is sometimes the most difficult aspect of a practitioner/client relationship, making the client aware that, to a great extent, he or she is responsible for his or her own state of health.

The Western approach

It may be difficult to reconcile how we view healing and illness with the Eastern approach, but as our understanding of physiology grows are we really that far apart?

Psychoneuroimmunology is an applied science researching the mind/body link:

➤ psycho = psyche
➤ neuro = mind
➤ immunology = immune response.

How does the body deal with environmental and external input? What are the major causes of many common ailments? Some of the answers may lie in lifestyle choices, which will include diet, smoking,

passive smoking, levels of drinking and levels of stress experienced in both the home and work environment. In an office full of people breathing the same re-circulated air, why is it that some people will catch everything that goes round and yet others never seem to have a day off sick?

The Western experience of resolving health problems is when we find ourselves in a state of 'dis-ease,' we may visit the doctor expecting a 'prescriptive panacea' that will cure what ails us, or purchasing an across the counter medicine, believing the advertising claims of its ability to relieve the symptoms with which we are afflicted. Should our health deteriorate further, the doctor will send us to a specialist, who will deal with the particular part of the body that has the problem.

In these scenarios there is nothing or very little about our uniqueness and no approach that looks at levels of energy. Yet we use the descriptive phrases of 'being run down', 'lacking in energy', 'not feeling ourselves', which is something akin to understanding that we are more than physical beings.

The Eastern approach seems to be very person-centred and 'hands on'. The Western approach to healing adopts an 'umbrella approach' and is very 'hands off': even a visit to a physiotherapist usually entails being wired up to a machine that performs a similar function to a massage.

Assessment task 19.1

The following is a suggested scenario that can be used to cover all your assessment criteria.

Mrs Vitak is finding it hard to concentrate at work. She complains of regular headaches and is finding it difficult to sleep. She has a very small frame and because she is worried about her husband's health (see page 276) she is losing weight.

With attention to detail, explain the culture of Indian head massage and how this form of massage has been altered to be more acceptable to Western tastes. (M)

Define, in detail, the history and culture of Indian head massage. Compare and contrast the approaches of using massage to achieve a balanced state of health. (D)

Any form of massage impacts directly with the skin, the largest organ of the body. This intelligent covering receives and interprets touch via the touch receptors located just under the surface of the skin in the epidermis and deeper into the dermis. The Meissners corpuscles respond to light repetitive touch and the Pacinian corpuscles respond to deep pressure. The brain converts this sensory information, which in turn interacts with the body's internal pharmacy.

In the 1960s it was discovered that the brain had the ability to produce endorphins, the body's own pain killer, which are 10 times stronger than many of the modern analgesics. Since then many different types of neuro-transmitters have been discovered. These neuropeptides have the ability to change how the body will react in certain circumstances:

»» they help the body to deal with pain
»» they can enhance mood, which can influence behavioural patterns
»» they can influence cardiovascular regulation
»» they can control temperature, respiration and immunological processes
»» they help to control food consumption
»» they help to deal with stress and improve motivation.

Theory into practice

How do you think the body would respond to the nurture of touch? What difference do you feel this approach might make to how someone feels? Discuss this in a group.

Further research has revealed that it is not only the brain that produces these amazing hormones, but they can be found in other parts of the body.

Rubbing the skin also produces an internal natural antibiotic that protects against infection and encourages healing, which means the old wives tale of 'rubbing it better' was true.

It is now believed that you cannot have a thought without a physical outcome. Try the activity below to see how important our state of mind is and how this influences physical responses.

The mind/body link

There is another aspect that plays a significant part in the Eastern approach to healing and that is the spirit. How do we in the West equate the spirit in

Theory into practice

Sit and think of a time/place/occasion when you experienced a deep sense of calm or peace. How does your body feel?

Now try the same exercise when you were bubbling over with happiness. How does your body feel?

If it is not too upsetting, remember a sad occasion. How does your body feel?

These exercises will help you begin to understand how interconnected we are and that we cannot treat the body in separate parts. The way we are feeling has definite physical outcomes.

our approach to medicine and health? It is often this mystical ingredient that causes a disbelief in alternative approaches to healthcare. However, if you re-do the exercise when you imagined a place of calm and peace, it is the need for a sense of silence and an awareness of a place away from the 'hurly burly' of everyday living which is missing from our attempt to adopt a more holistic approach. This is a spiritual requirement we all need: a sense of peace and a quiet mind.

Meditation and yoga are the two practices used in Ayurvedic medicine to achieve this deep sense of peace. These practices are becoming more a part of a Western lifestyle, which is what might be called an integrated approach to healthcare, 'using the best of both worlds'.

As we incorporate more from other cultural approaches into how we deal with the stresses and strains of modern life, there are benefits to achieve:

»» Touch in the form of massage nurtures us both physically and emotionally.
»» The physical act of massage nourishes the body by releasing a chemical cascade of hormones, encouraging all the body's systems to function at normal levels, healing and repairing damage.
»» It gives us the ability to relax on all levels, physically, mentally and emotionally. People leading busy lifestyles need to allocate time when they can forget their stresses and problems.

Understanding the theory behind complementary approaches to health enables you to discuss your client's expectations of treatment.

Stress

What is stress? Use a dictionary to see how it defines the word. This will help you to understand the impact it has on the whole person.

The Anatomy and Physiology units will have helped you to understand how the body systems work in conjunction with each other. For stress to happen there has to be a cause – a stress factor called a stressor. This can be either a person or a situation.

Theory into practice

Think of person and/or a situation that 'winds you up' then write down the physical symptoms you felt during that time.

Having the ability to control the amount of stress that occurs is dependent on you being able to recognise the outcomes of stress.

Factors that exacerbate stress:

▸▸ Not being able to release feelings of frustration and anger.
▸▸ Not having control over situations both in the home or work environment.
▸▸ Fear of the unknown.

The causes of stress can be divided into life changing events and constant niggling events over which you have little or no control.

Major stressors:

▸▸ bereavement
▸▸ moving house
▸▸ ill health
▸▸ difficult relationships
▸▸ debt
▸▸ work situations
▸▸ family problems.

Constant stressors

These vary according to personality and situations.

Theory into practice

In a group, make a list of small things that cause you to become either frustrated or angry. Think about one particular situation and make a note of how this makes you feel.

What happens to the body when it starts to experience continual stress? The chemical messengers in the body will trigger the adrenals to release powerful stress receptors – adrenaline, noradrenaline and cortisol. These will speed up the heart rate and raise the blood pressure. The liver converts glycogen to glucose for energy. Other body systems go into a 'tick-over' mode, as nutrients, blood, oxygen and hormones are re-directed in larger amounts to the muscles. Immune responses are suppressed.

'Fight or flight' is the terminology used to explain this state of mental and physical readiness. It means that you will either stand your ground (fight) or run away (flight). There are positive aspects to stress because it gives us a means of survival, enabling us to react positively to challenges; however, it is when the body begins to experience the fight and flight state continuously that serious health problems begin to manifest themselves.

Levels of stress

Level one:
▸▸ broken sleep patterns
▸▸ always feeling tired
▸▸ being bad tempered
▸▸ headaches

We can all find excuses as to why we might feel the way we do.

Theory into practice

List the excuses you might use to explain away the above symptoms.

Level two:
▸▸ feeling anxious
▸▸ feeling depressed
▸▸ experiencing aches and pains
▸▸ continually picking up minor infections (always having a cold)
▸▸ feeling helpless, with unexplained feelings of guilt.

Level three:
▸▸ feelings of persecution
▸▸ not wanting to go out
▸▸ not being able to cope with crowds and confined spaces
▸▸ feelings of despair
▸▸ the body begins to lose its ability to deal with bactcrial invasions.

At what stage would you decide to seek help?

Stress and health

There are many long-term health problems the medical profession recognise as having a 'stressor' factor. Statistics show than an estimated 80 per cent of modern diseases may have their beginnings in stress. Major health issues can include heart problems and irritable or spastic bowel problems.

List the reasons why you feel these two areas might be affected by on-going stress. Are there other health problems you feel may have a 'stressor' involvement?

Further health problems:

- acid problems in stomach
- indigestion
- constipation/diarrhoea
- constant headaches
- backache
- prolonged episodes of fatigue.

Describe the symptoms of stress, with attention to detail. Incorporating the known facts of your client, Mrs Vitak, explain how the use of Indian head massage could help to alleviate some of the symptoms. (M)

Illustrate a comprehensive knowledge of the symptoms of stress and the impact on the overall state of health of the client. Evaluate the use of the massage techniques in Indian head massage routine, analysing the potential outcomes. (D)

Controlling stress

What steps can we take to control stress?

- **Diet:** good nutrition enables the body to function well. Fad diets, too much fat, sugar and processed foods are physical stressors, which impair the heart, digestive system, the immune function and endocrine responses.
- **Exercise:** an excellent outlet for feelings of frustration and anger, it also gives you a 'space' away from stressful situations.

- **Change of lifestyle:** often the most difficult if the stress is caused by a personal relationship. Work-related stress could mean changing jobs, which can be difficult.
- **Change of approach:** this often entails a change of mind set – not allowing people and situations to dis-empower you.
- **Using touch:** massage is a powerful de-stressor. Massage is an interactive process, with the giver receiving similar physical and psychological benefits. Working the shoulders, neck and head – areas of the body where we hold an enormous amount of stress – has an immediate and long-term effect on the body's ability to cope with stressful situations.

Understanding how you arrived at a situation often helps you to understand what is required to make the changes and move away from destructive situations. Also understanding the positive aspects of stress enables you to deal with difficult issues we all have to deal with on a daily basis.

Massage benefits

The best way to remember the beneficial outcomes of Indian head massage is the three 'P's:

- Physical
- Physiological
- Psychological.

Physical benefits

These include: improved circulation, improved immune response, better sleep patterns, better muscle tone, better heart function, improved lymph flow, reduced tension in the muscles and stimulated nerve ends.

Physiological benefits

Heart and circulation: improved circulation will carry all the required nutrients to every cell in the body.

Immune system: an improved immune response will give the body all it requires to fight external infections and to monitor and regulate internal malfunctions, e.g. cancer cells. The immune response is activated by the action of massage. The epidermis produces a substance similar to thymopoietin. This hormone produced by the thymus activates 'T' cell differentiation, meaning the thymus has the ability to instruct different 'T' cells to recognise a different antigen and destroy it. 'T' cells are also called killer cells.

Sleep patterns: While most systems in the body slow down as we sleep, the digestive system stimulates the pancreas, salivary and gastric glands to secrete. There is increased peristalsis and the uretural sphincter also relaxes. As the majority of growth spurts happen at night, deep relaxed sleep is very important for young children and young adults.

Theory into practice

In a group, list any other physiological benefits of sleep you can think of.

By looking at the physiological outcomes of massage you can begin to see how massage, a simple form of touch, can activate the body's internal pharmacy.

Psychological benefits

The psychological effects of massage are both short-term and long-term. Just being able to take time out of a very busy schedule allows both the mind and body to achieve a state of relaxation by switching off.

A relaxed state of mind reduces anxiety, which in turn increases positive feelings, lifting emotions, increasing energy levels and helping to reduce fatigue. Long-term benefits include a sustained sense of well-being and improved body image, awareness and self-esteem. Increased relaxation means the body is not held in a tense state, which depletes energy levels.

Emotional and mental responses

When using 'touch therapies' you interact with your clients on two levels – physically and energetically. As the massage encourages the body to achieve a state of homeostasis, sometimes your clients may cry or disclose very personal and intimate details of past traumas in their lives, which is why confidentiality is so very important. These issues need to be addressed since they are often the reason why the body is in a state of physical 'dis-ease'. Clients soon become aware of the benefits of the 'therapeutic space' that regular treatments offer.

More companies are beginning to realise that their employees work more efficiently when stress levels are kept to a minimum. It may be an excellent business opportunity to introduce Indian head massage into the office environment. It is not essential to have specialist equipment: a chair, a quiet room and excellent skills are all that are required.

Indian head massage treatment

Preparation

Before treatment starts you need to prepare a safe space for you and your client. It is often called a 'therapeutic space'.

Part of the treatment process will involve:

▶ an in-depth consultation, which will require the use of a confidential record system, either record card or computer database

▶ an explanation of expectations and outcomes

▶ an explanation of contra-indications and how they might relate to a client's state of health.

Consultation

Consultation involves talking to and listening to your client. More importantly, it means observing and engaging with your client. Remember that communication is both verbal and visual!

When your client walks into the salon/clinic the communication process has already begun. This is called 'body language'. Observation is very important; for example, noticing that a client is out of breath when no stairs are involved and the client has not had to rush. Why might the person be out of breath? What other observations might give you clues as to your client's present state of health? It is important to observe eyes, skin, hair and body posture.

Communication also involves listening

Many therapists dis-empower their clients by not listening to or engaging with them. The consultation is not about asking a series of questions and ticking the boxes just to cover a legal requirement. It is a process of asking a question then listening to what your client is telling you.

Some older clients will have long and complex medical histories, but may only tell you about current problems, forgetting some of the past issues, or they may tell you what they think you want to hear.

Always allow sufficient time for the initial consultation. If you have a client who has a lot to say, don't sit displaying a bored silence; acknowledge you are listening by saying 'yes' or 'I understand', **Never** use this interaction to start regaling clients with your own experiences: they are not paying to be your counsellor!

Confidentiality is imperative. A detailed medical history is an important aspect of creating a safe 'therapeutic space'. Difficulties can arise when a client recommends a friend, because it is almost as if the client feels he or she has ownership in this situation. The client may ask you about the problems his or her friend is experiencing and how the person is getting on.

Theory into practice

How would you respond to the situation described above? In pairs, use role-play to show how you would deal with an inquisitive client.

Theory into practice

How difficult is it to listen?
In pairs, do a talk and listen exercise. Then feedback to the rest of the group what you remember being told by your partner. This exercise can be used at the beginning of a short course as an introductory exercise.

Contra-indications

Part of the consultation process is to discuss both contra-indications if applicable and contra-actions (outcomes). Contra-indications can be put into two categories: general or doctor specific.

General contra-indications can include the following:

» **Skin disorders, diseases, infections or irritations:** grazes, sepsis, infected acne, boils/carbuncles, undiagnosed lumps, bumps or swellings, recent scar tissue, bruises, swollen inflamed painful areas, loss of skin sensation, vitiligo or leucoderma, hairy areas, very damp skin, sunburn, crêpey and very fine or very aged skin, moles.

» **Nervous disorders:** claustrophobia, tense disposition, nervous disposition. Circulatory disorders, varicose veins, dilated arterioles, vascular areas.

» **General health problems:** migraine, dizziness, nausea, sinus problems, raised temperature.

Doctor-specific conditions

Medical conditions; ongoing supervision by a doctor, specialist or consultant. Heart disease, pacemaker, pregnancy, high/low blood pressure, epilepsy, severe depression and mental health problems, diabetes, thrombosis, phlebitis, hepatitis, cancer, medical oedema, recent brain surgery.

Looking at both lists you may feel that it would be impossible to treat most clients. With many of the general conditions, contra-indication means to proceed with caution and, as with any massage routine, you would treat each of your clients as an

---

Indian Head   Massage Record Card

For Massage

PERSONAL DETAILS

Name:

Address:

Tel. No:	Date of Birth:
Doctor's Name:	Tel. No:

Address:

Reasons for coming:

Any previous treatment:

GENERAL HEALTH *please tick*

Allergies/skin problems ☐	Lumps/swellings ☐
Menstruation pattern ☐	Digestive/bowel disorders ☐
Epilepsy ☐	Operations ☐
Blood pressure ☐	Hepatitis/HIV ☐
Fluid retention ☐	Headaches/migraine ☐
Respiratory problems ☐	Diabetes ☐
Medication ☐	Metal plates/pacemaker ☐
Pregnancy ☐	Circulatory disorders ☐
Throat/sinus ☐	Bladder/kidney disorders ☐
Back problems ☐	Liver disorders ☐
Nervous conditions ☐	Injuries ☐
Heart conditions ☐	

Details of above:

Are you currently being treated by a Doctor, Chiropractor or other practitioner?

LIFE STYLE

Home involvement:
Work involvement:
Active/Sedentary:
Eating habits:
Drinking/Alcohol/Other:
Smoking:
Sleeping pattern:
Interests:
Stress levels:
Personality:

A consultation form (front).

OBSERVATIONAL		
Skin:		
Hair:		
Body shape/Type:		
Expressions/Body language:		
Posture:		

RELEVANT CASE HISTORY NOTES/CLIENT ASSESSMENT

RECOMMENDED TREATMENT PLAN/TREATMENT OBJECTIVES

I confirm that I understand fully the consultation and treatment proposed and that all the information I have forwarded is accurate. As a trainee giving treatment he/she cannot be held wholly responsible for possible outcomes.

Client's signature		Date	

RECORD OF TREATMENTS

Date	Treatment given	Medium	Home advice

A consultation form (back).

individual – adapting the routine according to his or her needs. This involves the use of a treatment plan, which should always be attached to the record card kept in the salon/clinic. This gives continuity of treatment if another therapist is involved.

Never just read a record card/treatment plan and assume that nothing has changed. It is important to receive feedback from each treatment given.

Working as a group, and using knowledge from your previous massage experience, look at the list of general contra-indications and discuss how you might adapt the treatment to suit.

Contra-actions also need to be discussed with your client before treatment commences. Because you engage with your client physically and energetically, there can be several outcomes.

All holistic therapies aim to help the body to achieve homeostasis: in other words, allowing the body to become aware of the state it is in and seek to rectify the situation. To reach a state of balance, the body may go through a series of 'healing achievements' on both a physical and emotional level. It is important to make your client aware of this. Touch therapies are very powerful tools for healing. (We will look at outcomes in more detail when we prepare an aftercare leaflet.)

Planning your treatment after consultation involves looking at the outcomes of the various massage movements available and the possibility of having to adapt the routine to suit a certain medical condition.

Massage movements and benefits

Massage has four major beneficial effects on the condition of the hair and skin.

1 The stimulation of blood and lymph delivers fresh supplies of nutrients and encourages the removal of waste and excess fluid in the tissues, promoting a healthy environment for cell repair and renewal.

2 The friction movements of the fingers and hands on the skin aids desquamation, improving both the texture and appearance of the skin.

3 The stimulation of the sebaceous glands encourages the production of sebum on both the scalp and the face, keeping the skin and hair supple.

4 Massage cleanses the skin by encouraging the sweat glands to function move efficiently, thereby removing any debris from the surface of the skin.

Below are some of the benefits of the different forms of massage used in Indian head massage.

- **Effleurage** is the stroking movement used to introduce other massage strokes and to link them together. It is used to start and conclude a series of movements or a routine, and is usually a light rhythmic stroke with the pressure applied towards the heart. This movement will bring the client to a state of relaxation.
- **Reinforced (petrissage) movements** include kneading, picking up, wringing and rolling. These movements introduce a deeper pressure and are more stimulating. The trapezius muscle holds the majority of tension experienced in the upper body and these movements can be used to relieve muscular tension and stiffness in this and other muscles.
- **Percussion (tapotement) movements** include tapping, cupping and hacking. These movements are also stimulating and are included in a routine to tone and invigorate. It is very important to regulate the amount of pressure when using these movements, but they are excellent for improving poor circulation.
- **Practice point:**
  Important safety tip: Percussion movements should never be used on the spinal column. Work either side of the spinal vertebrae.

Theory into practice

In which situations would you *not use* percussion movements?

- **Friction** movements are used to concentrate on defined areas within the body. Pressure is a consideration when using this movement.

Theory into practice

Discuss as a group where you feel the use of frictions would be beneficial.

- **Vibrations** interact with the nerve endings of the body and can be used to sedate or stimulate. They are an excellent form of treatment for a facial routine.

Now you have an in-depth consultation from your client, alongside an understanding of the some of the benefits of massage and the different movements you will be using, you can begin to work out your treatment plan.

- **Practice point:** No two clients are alike and your treatment routine should not be by rote but tailored to meet the client's individual needs.

Theory into practice

Working as a group, consider which benefit is linked to which massage movement and how you would use this knowledge to tailor for need?

Product knowledge
Choosing an oil

In Ayurvedic medicine, the oil would be chosen to suit the Dosha type, for example:

- **Vata Dosha type:** lively, energetic, physically and emotionally sensitive. When stressed will suffer from anxiety and broken sleep patterns. Vata-calming oils would include sesame, olive, almond and wheatgerm.
- **Practice point:** Wheatgerm oil is often used in a blend as a preservative, because of its high concentration of Vitamin E. Always check for any wheat allergies.
- **Pitta Dosha type:** friendly and warm, enjoys a lively debate. When stressed can become angry and controlling. Pitta-cooling oils would include coconut, almond and sunflower.
- **Kapha Dosha type:** it takes a lot to upset a person with a dominance of Kapha in their make-up. They are the 'laid back' model.

Kapha-burning/warming oils would include mustard, sesame and safflower.

- **Practice point:** Mustard oil is not used in a 'Westernised' treatment.

In Ayuverda, oils are chosen and used in a special oil therapy. This specialised head massage therapy is called 'shirodhara'.

With the client in a prone position, warm medicated oil is trickled onto the third eye chakra position from a small pot suspended above the couch. The therapist gently strokes the oil through the hair for about 30 minutes. Massage of the scalp enables the oil to permeate the skin, increasing the efficacy of the chosen oil with its blended herbs or essential oils. It is possible to adapt this treatment and introduce oils into a 'Westernised' Indian head massage routine.

These oils can be bought from either Chinese or Indian stores but, because oils are partially absorbed by the skin, it is always best to look for an organic source and oils from the first pressing

The most popular oils used in the West are sweet almond oil and grapeseed oil.

Sweet almond oil

This oil is made from the kernels of the fruit produced by the almond tree. It is very popular with massage therapists because it is light in texture and can be used to blend other vegetable or nut oils, and as a carrier for essential oils. This oil is very rich in protein and contains vitamins A, B1, B2, B6 and E.

Main therapeutic uses:
➤ dry or chapped skin
➤ helps to sooth eczema and psoriasis
➤ suits all skin types.

➤ **Practice point:** Because this oil is extracted from a kernel and there is a growing problem with nut allergies, always check your client does not have a nut allergy. Do not confuse sweet almond oil with the oil made for culinary purposes from bitter almonds.

Grapeseed oil

This oil is a by-product of the wine-making industry. The seeds of grapes are washed, dried, ground and then pressed with the aid of heat. Grapeseed is not available as a cold pressed oil. It is popular because there are no known contra-indications and it is relatively cheap. The only problem is that it will often stain if you use white towels. It is suitable for all skin types and can be used to blend with other carrier oils and essential oils.

Two further oils you can add to your list for use in an Indian head massage routine include sesame and coconut.

Sesame oil

The use of this oil for massage is highly regarded in Ayurvedic medicine for both internal and external uses. It is also used to prevent grey hair.

➤ **Practice point:** do not confuse the massage oil with the dark brown oil used for cooking.

Sesame oil can be used on its own or blended with other vegetable oils or essential oils. It is rich in Vitamin E, iron and phosphorus.

Main therapeutic uses:
➤ it is reputed to ease muscular tension, stiffness and muscular pains.
➤ **Practice point:** sesame oil may irritate sensitive skin: do a patch test before using.

Coconut oil

This oil could be said to be the oil of choice in the southern areas of India for Indian head massage. It is a semi-solid oil made from the dried flesh of the coconut. Because the oil is highly refined many of the original nutrients will have been destroyed. It can be used with other oils or as a carrier for essential oils.

➤ **Practice point:** As with other nut oils, always check with your clients for any sensitivity they may have experienced with nut-based products. It is possible to blend in essential oils for the hair treatment, but only if you are a fully qualified aromatherapist.

In the West we are less inclined to use oil in a hair treatment, especially given that to achieve the best effect it would need to be left on for at least 12 hours. However, if you are able to convince your client, the effect is remarkable – it will leave the hair feeling like silk.

Hair types and choice of oil
Normal hair
Oil of choice for this type of hair would be coconut oil.

Dry hair
If the hair is dry the causes are usually over-exposure to chemical irritants found in certain shampoos and hair treatments, or in the environment. Oil of choice for this hair type would be either coconut or sweet almond.

➤ **Practice point:** if your choice of oil is nut based, and your client has a nut sensitivity, you would have to use grapeseed oil.

Greasy hair
Diet, hormonal imbalance and diet can contribute to greasy hair. Oil of choice for this hair type would be either sesame or sweet almond oil. (Check for allergies.)

Dandruff
Poor diet, stress, fatigue and incorrect hair care, can contribute to the embarrassment of dandruff. Oil of choice for this hair type would be either coconut or sweet almond oil. (Check for allergies.)

Greying hair
Prolonged stress and a poor diet is thought to contribute to the hair turning grey, although genetic considerations and ageing have to be taken into

consideration. Oil of choice for this type of hair would be sesame oil. (Check for allergies.)

Hair loss

➤ **Practice point:** avoid vigorous movements if your client's hair is very thin, and do not use the 'tug, lift and let go' movement.

High levels of stress which increases muscular tension on the scalp is thought to hinder the supply of blood, which may contribute to early hair loss.

➤ **Practice point:** Two major muscles, the frontalis and the occipitalis, are joined by a tendon called epicranial aponeurois, covering the skull like a cap. It is tension in these muscles that can cause the feeling of wearing something tight over the head.

The oil of choice for this hair type would be sesame oil, but check for any nut allergy and change to a vegetable-based oil if necessary.

Removing oil from the hair after treatment

Use a shampoo without an inclusive conditioner. Apply neat to the oiled hair and work in until it looks like clotted cream, then rinse and shampoo in the normal way.

Preparing the 'therapeutic space'

Preparing a therapeutic space involves:

➤ the treatment area
➤ you as the practitioner
➤ your client.

To create the right impression, hygiene is very important. During an Indian head treatment you are in very close proximity to your client, so personal hygiene will include regular bathing, checking for body odour and using deodorants. Make sure your uniform is laundered regularly. Beware of your breath and do not eat heavily-spiced food or salads laced with garlic if you have treatments booked the next day. Take care to ensure the space you use for treatment is kept clean. Any towels used need to be laundered on the hot wash cycle and clean towels provided for each client.

➤ **Practice point:** the need for a hot wash cycle. If you use a folded towel as a mat under a client's feet, or as a neck roll, you must be careful not to transmit any infections via the towel.

Assessment task 19.3

Using the scenario on page 306, set out clear and concise recommendations for the use of Indian head massage and the requirements for aftercare and home-care. (M)

Evaluate the information from the suggested scenario to justify the decision for using this type of massage routine. Illustrate a comprehensive knowledge to justify the need for aftercare and home-care. (D)

Procedure

Delivering the treatment

Make sure that you have everything you need close to hand, and that you have washed your hands.

Invite your client to remove all jewellery – necklaces, earrings, glasses, hair-combs and hair pins. Use a small pot with a lid for safekeeping, and place it under the chair.

Use a chair with a low back. The back of the chair should be no higher than the lower end of the shoulder blades (the bra-line).

A small soft pillow in the client's lap provides a comfortable platform on which the client can place his or her hands. Invite the client to turn the palms upwards, as if to receive a gift.

If the client is agreeable, ask him or her to remove the shoes. If the floor is cold, place a small mat or folded towel under his or her feet. If you use a mat, cover it with a piece of couch roll. The temperature

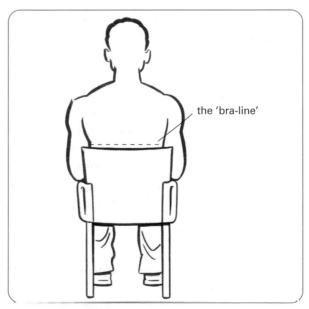

the 'bra-line'

Positioning the client on a chair.

of the working area must be warm, since when the body relaxes your client may feel cold.

Check your posture. Relax your shoulders and make sure you pull them slightly backwards; we spend so much of our time with 'rounded shoulders'. Keep your hips and knees level with your feet slightly apart.

It is also best to allow yourself a little time to relax your body and clear your mind before you touch your client.

▶ **Practice point**: any tension in your body will transfer to your client.

Centre yourself on the client you are working with. Breathing with your client at the beginning of the treatment helps you to engage wholly with the process and the client. When you feel ready, stand behind your client and move your feet to a hip-width apart. Make sure your client's spine is straight, then ask the client to relax the shoulders and so begin the process of relaxation.

Place both hands gently on your client's head. With your client, take three deep breaths, inhaling and exhaling slowly, letting any tension go.

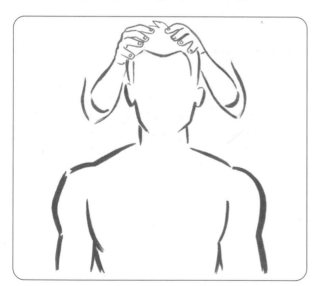

Hands placed on head, standing behind client.

▶ **Practice point**: Do not overdo this stage. Because we tend to shallow breathe, breathing at this level tends to have the same effect as fine wine – it goes straight to the head.

Relaxing the neck
Move to the side of your client; do not lose contact as you change position. Place your left hand on the forehead so it rests just below the hairline. With the other hand, support the back of the head so this hand covers the occipital region of the skull.

▶ **Practice point**: any movement of the head should be slow and gentle, exerting no force.

Encourage the client to breathe slowly and regularly, letting any tension go on the 'out' breath.

Taking care not to over-extend the neck in either direction, move the head back and forwards and then from side to side.

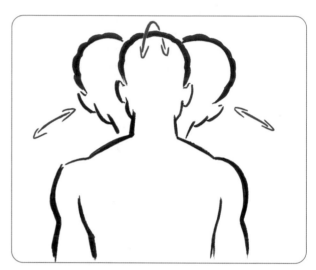

Moving the head backwards and forwards and then from side to side.

Smoothing down
Stand behind the client and introduce the massage with a relaxing movement before starting work in specific areas. Place both hands on the head, then move down either side of the head, encasing the neck; rest the hands on the shoulders and sweep

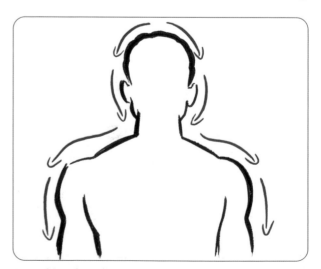

Smoothing down.

down the arms, ending at the elbows. Repeat this movement three times, slowly and gently but deliberately.

Back routine

This is where the stress route begins. Place both hands on the back, with thumbs positioned either side of the spine and resting under the shoulder blades (scapulae).

▸▸ **Practice point:** always work alongside the spine – never on the spinal cord.

Using both hands, and working either side of the spine starting at the lower back, move your thumbs up towards the shoulders, increasing the pressure with each movement. Repeat three times.

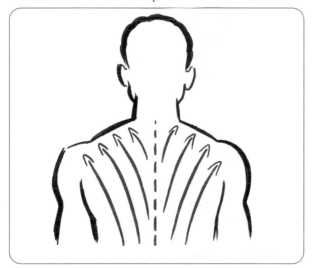

Whole back massage.

To finish the movement, work across the shoulders and down the arms to the elbows.

Effleurage the neck and shoulders.

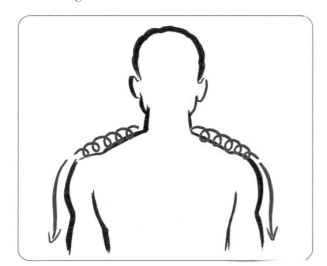

Work across the shoulders and down the arms.

Using one hand only, balance the second hand on your client's shoulder and rub the heel of your hand along the outline of the shoulder blade, starting at the base of the scapula and moving up to the base of the neck. Sweep your hand over the shoulder back to your starting position and repeat these movements twice more. Then repeat on the other side of the back.

▸▸ **Practice point:** remember not to lean down on your client with the 'resting' hand.

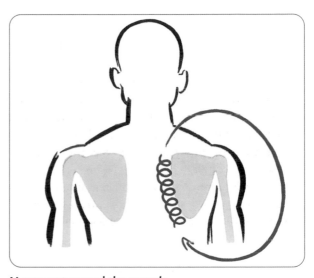

Movement around the scapula.

Repeat this movement using your fingers and work into the shoulder blade, starting at the base of the scapula towards the shoulder. Sweep back down and repeat the movement three times each side.

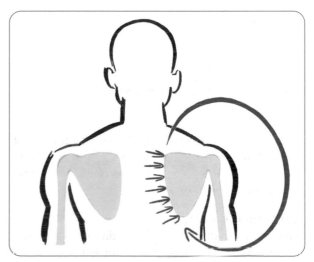

Finger friction towards scapula.

Practice point: the second major stress area is along the shoulders towards the base of the neck. Located midpoint between the spinal cord and shoulder acromion is an energy point which should be avoided, especially if your client is pregnant. (The acromion is where the scapula articulates with the collarbone and major energy centres are located in the joints.)

Thumb rolls

If working through the client's clothes, use the top seam of the garment as a guide.

Place both hands at the outer each of each shoulder. Using the thumb and index finger, roll the flesh forward (you will find flesh quite limited in this area). Repeat three times and then move to the midpoint of the shoulder and repeat three times. The final area is the base of the neck, either side of the spinal cord. Place the hands on the shoulders and, using the thumbs, roll the flesh towards the index finger.

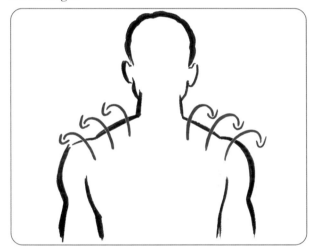

Thumb rolls on shoulder.

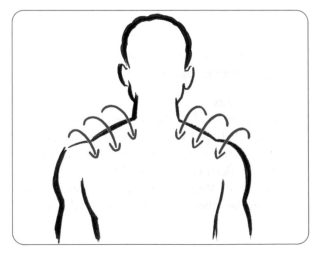

Finger pulls on shoulder.

Finger pulls

Starting at the base of the neck and working outwards towards the outer edge of the shoulders, pull the fingers over the top of the shoulder towards the thumb. Repeat this movement three times in each position.

Hacking across the shoulders

Practice point: It is important when performing any percussion movement to make sure the pressure is correct and that you use the right portion of your hands. Only use the outer edge of the little fingers to strike the areas across the shoulders.

Work across the shoulder area, lifting the hands to cross the spine. The number of times you repeat this movement will depend on client type and constitution.

Move lower down the back to cover the scapula areas of the back. Always lift the hands to move across the spinal vertebrae. Cupping these areas can help with any congestion found in the chest.

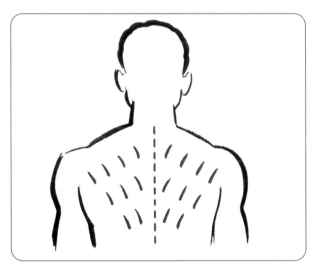

Hacking on the back.

If the client is frail, elderly or very slightly built, you can use a sawing movement across the shoulders and the back. This is also a stimulating movement, but not as 'forceful' as hacking.

Practice point: effleurage is used to co-ordinate the routine and to move from one part of the body to another.

Using both hands, sweep from the outer edge of the shoulders up the neck to just under the ears, then sweep back down to the outer edge of the shoulder and down the arms to the elbows. Repeat three times.

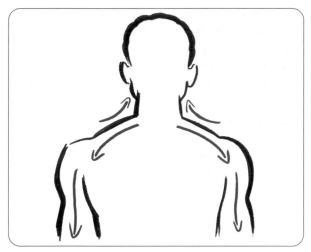

Effleurage on arms and shoulders.

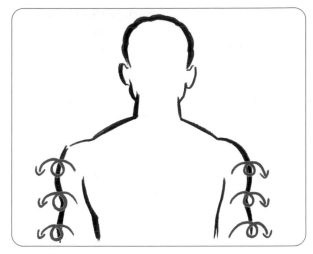

Lift and squeeze muscle.

Arm roll

Using both hands at the same time, roll the heels of your hands down to the elbow line. Repeat the movement three times.

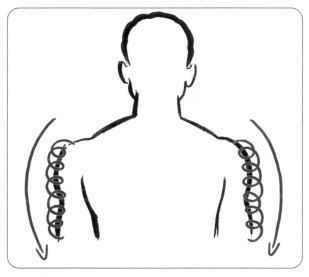

Arm rolls.

Squeeze and lift

Using both hands, place your hands on the top of the deltoid muscle, squeeze firmly and pull away. Work down to the elbow line. Once you are in this position, hold the forearms with your hands under the elbow, lift the arms up and then return them to the original position.

This movement helps to release tension that builds up in the joints of the shoulders.

Lift shoulder joints.

▸▸ **Practice point:** you may find that some elderly clients do not like this movement. Remember: always adapt the routine to the client's needs.

Neck squeezes

Support the front of the head with one hand and tilt the head slightly forward. Start just under the occipital bone. Using index finger and thumb, squeeze the flesh on one side of the spinal column and pull away. Work down the neck three times. Repeat on the other side of the spinal column.

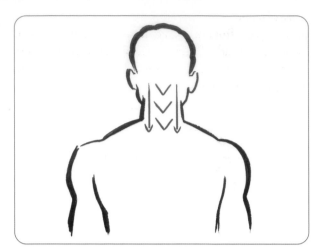

Neck work either side.

Heel rub the occipital bone

With the head in the same position, use the heel of the hand to create a friction movement along the occipital bone.

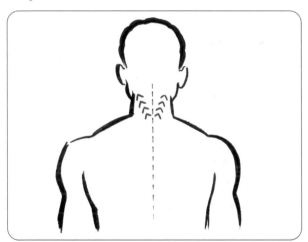

Occipital rub.

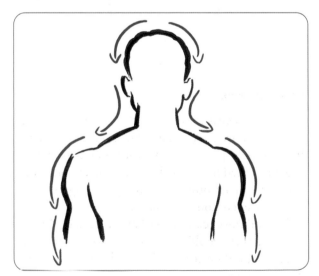

Linking movement before head routine.

Before moving onto the head, use a linking routine similar to the introduction movements.

Making waves

If oil is to be used during the hair routine, rest one hand on your client's shoulder to retain contact and add the oil to the palm of this hand. Place the other hand on top of this hand, and move the hands together to sufficiently distribute the oil over both hands. Snake your hands through the hair, going in deeper with a shampoo movement, kneading and distributing the oil over the whole scalp.

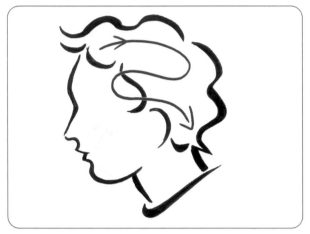

Adding oil.

Heel of hand rub

Support one side of the head by placing one hand just above the ear, allowing the head to rest in this position. Using the heel of the other hand, start in front of the ear and work in a shallow arc to the back of the head. Repeat three times. Move the hand to the front of the head again at the hairline, level with the middle of the eye, and work in an arc towards the back of the neck, repeating the movement three

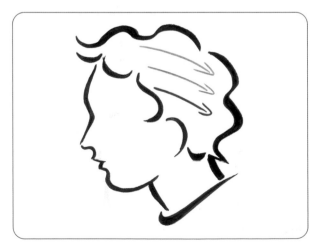

Heel of hand rub on head.

times. Finally, with the hand just slightly to one side of the centre of the head at the hairline, work from the front of the head to the occipital bone at the back. Repeat this movement three times.

Change hands and repeat all these movements on the other side of the head.

Finger friction rub

To deepen the pressure, these movements can be repeated using the fingertips and friction circles, working along the same pathways.

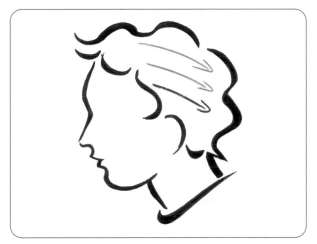

Finger friction.

Tug, lift and let go

Using both hands, thread your fingers through the hair and lift the hair in a short tug and then let go. Work the whole head. If your client has very short hair, use your fingers to pluck the hair.

This stimulating movement encourages blood supply to the scalp. It is also a great tension release.

➤ **Practice point:** do not use this movement for clients with thinning hair.

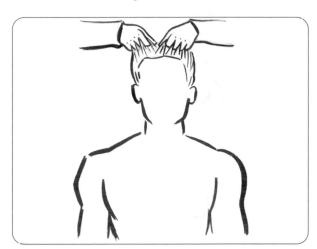

Tug, lift and let go.

Raindrops

Using your fingers, make raindrop movements all over the head. Starting with rapid movements, gradually slow the pace until the fingers are gently dropping onto the scalp.

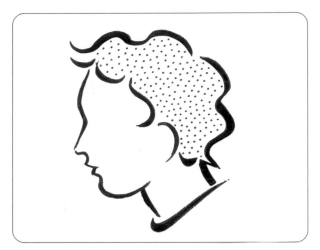

Raindrop movements.

Raking the hair

Starting from the hairline, rake your fingers through the hair in a slow languid movement. Rake towards the crown of the head.

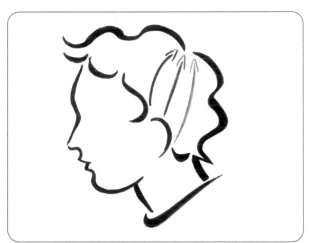

Raking the hair.

To enable access to the face, the client's head needs to rest against your chest. The head should remain in an upright position, not bent backwards and with the chin tilted upwards. This position enables you to trace the facial outlines, using your fingers to 'see' around the contours of the face.

A rolled towel can be used at the back of the neck for support: Fold a hand towel into three lengthways, then turn and roll. This makes an ideal neck support.

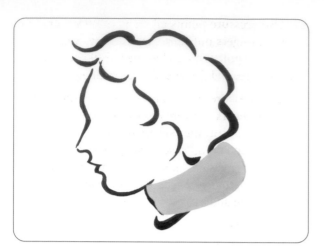

Position of towel on neck.

At this point of the treatment it is sometimes beneficial to use a drop of lavender in the palm of your hands.

▸ **Practice point:** Lavender can be used neat on the skin.

If your client does not like lavender, tangerine has an amazing effect on an over-active nervous system, but would need to be blended with a carrier before being used on the skin. The warmth of the skin in the palms of the hands helps to vaporise the oil, and your client can breathe in the aroma as your hands move in front of the face.

After placing the towel roll behind the neck, and checking that your client is comfortable, link your hands together. Starting at the base of the neck, just under the chin, move your hands up towards the top of the head. Make sure you are not too close to the face. Return your hands to the starting position and repeat once more.

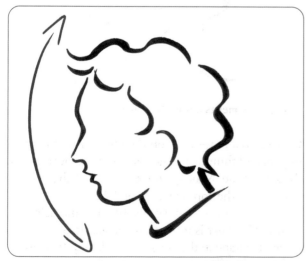

Chakra basket.

With this movement you will interact with the higher chakras.

Facial effleurage

Start by cupping the chin with one hand at a time and stroke upwards towards the ear on each side of the face. Stroke the forehead and cheeks to familiarise yourself with the contours of the client's face.

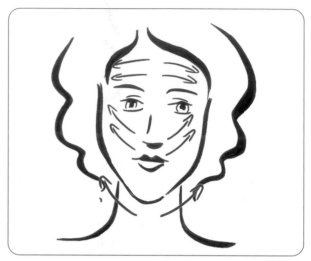

Facial effleurage.

Place the palms of your hands over the temples either side of the face. Using a firm pressure so that tissue movement can be seen, move the hands in a circular motion.

▸ **Practice point:** The two main muscles that hold tension in the face are the temporalis and masseter. Stress can cause these muscles to contract, causing severe bi-temporal headaches.

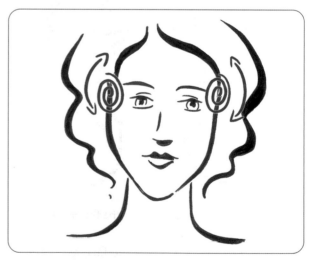

Circular temple movements.

Lightly tap the whole face avoiding the eyes. Vary the rhythm of this movement, ending with slow gentle tapping.

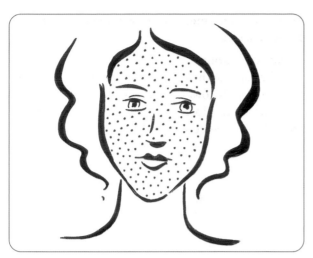

Tapping on face.

Using both hands and the middle fingers, and starting between the eyebrows, use small circular movements to work:

1   From the eyebrow up to the hairline, then follow this pathway out to the temples.

2   From the eyebrow up to the middle of the forehead, then follow this pathway out to the temples.

3   For the final movement, place your middle fingers just above the eyebrows and move along the brow towards the temples.

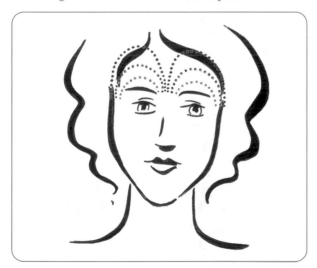

Pressure points above the eyes on the forehead.

The following movements on the face are excellent for sinus problems and for removing any excess tissue fluid.

Now using both hands and your middle fingers, start between the eyebrows.

1   Use pressure points all along the brow and pull both fingers outwards towards the ears.

▸▸ **Practice point:** remember the link between the ears, nose, and throat and sinus drainage.

2   Use pressure points under the eyes then pull both fingers outwards towards the ears.

▸▸ **Practice point:** the skin around the eyes is very delicate and prone to stretching: be very careful with your pressures in this area of the face. Also make sure that you work along the top of the cheekbone and not inside the eye socket.

3   Use pressure points starting mid-way either side of the nose, then move under the cheekbones and drain towards the ears.

4   Use pressure points starting either side of the base of the nose, then move under the cheekbones and drain towards the ears.

5   Place both thumbs at the point of the chin and curl the index fingers towards the palm of the hand. Place the knuckles of the index fingers under the jaw line and massage towards the ears.

Repeat all these movements three times.

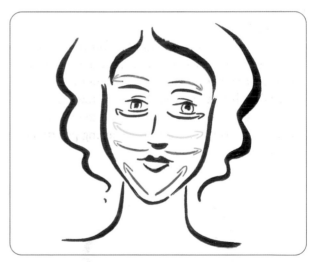

Finger movements across the face.

On the final movement on the chin, bring the index fingers and thumbs up the ears, working both ears at the same time. Massage the outer rim of the ear (the helix) from the top down to the lobe.

▸▸ **Practice point:** in Auricular Therapy, the helix area of the ear is manipulated to alleviate inflammation in the body. Manipulating the apex (top) of the ear can help with hay fever.

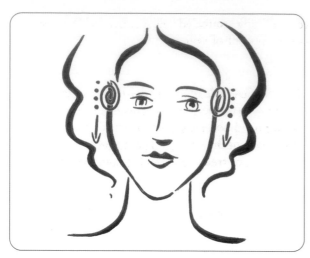

Pulling the ears.

Finger feather the whole face.

Link your hands in front of the face just below the chin and repeat the movements used at the start of the facial routine.

End the treatment by placing your hands on both shoulders. Then hold your client's head with one hand and remove the rolled towel from the back of the neck.

Ask your client to keep his or her eyes closed for a few seconds more, and then ask the client to slowly open the eyes and become aware of the surroundings.

Do not let the client get up for a few minutes. Ask him or her to stay seated while you pour a glass of water.

➨ **Practice point:** do not use very cold water because the body would have to waste energy to bring the water to blood heat before it can utilise the water efficiently.

Home-care and aftercare

Although outcomes are discussed with your clients before the treatment starts, it is essential that these are reiterated at the end of the treatments. They should also be given to the client as part of the information that you include on your aftercare leaflet.

Aftercare leaflet

List the possible outcomes but emphasise the healing achievements. Do not use the terminology 'healing crisis': although crisis signifies change, it may also cause your clients unnecessary worry.

Possible reactions:
➨ feeling weepy or unusually tired

➨ unexplained headache or slight dizziness
➨ nausea or slight stomach upset
➨ broken sleep patterns
➨ an awareness or re-occurrence of symptoms related to present or previous health issues.

Aftercare instructions:
➨ Try to avoid any stressful situations at home or at work.
➨ Increase the intake of water or herbal teas to help flush toxins out the system.
➨ Avoid alcohol, heavy meals or processed foods.
➨ Eat light, easily-digested food.
➨ Aim for an early night.

Theory into practice

What else would you need to include on your aftercare leaflet? Design your own leaflet, using a personal logo and company name.

Professional ethics

In any professional discipline, it is important to have a standard of acceptable behaviour. Once qualified, it is advisable to become a member of a professional association or governing body, all of which will have a code of ethics that members are expected to adhere to. The following bullet points are what is expected of a student during training and will form the basic guidelines for acceptable professional standards once qualified.

➨ Therapists must conduct themselves in a professional manner at all times.
➨ Respect the religious, spiritual, social and political views of your clients irrespective of creed, race, colour or sex.
➨ Never abuse the relationship between yourself and your client.
➨ Always co-operate with other health care professionals, referring cases outside your skill range or therapeutic knowledge to those with the relevant qualifications.
➨ Always explain the services you offer and discuss fees with your client before any treatment starts.
➨ Keep accurate, up-to-date, confidential records of treatment.
➨ Never disclose client information without the prior written permission of the client, except when required to do so by law.

- Never claim to cure, diagnose a medical condition, or give unqualified advice.
- Ensure that all marketing material represents your practice professionally.
- Ensure that your working environment complies with all current health, safety and hygiene legislation.
- Ensure that you have insurance from a recognised professional body.
- Endeavour to become a member of a professional association which sets high standards for the industry.
- Continue with your professional development.
- Keep personal and professional life separate.

Health, safety and hygiene for the therapeutic space

All forms of complementary treatments require the same high standards of client care.

To avoid cross-infection, consideration must be given to the following:

- the treatment area
- the equipment
- the client
- the therapist.

(Refer to the standards laid out in the Aromatherapy Module, page 280.)

Consultation aims

Consultation aims for any form of massage would include the following:

- evaluating client expectations
- ensuring the client's suitability for treatment
- establishing a good rapport
- answering client queries
- agreeing a treatment plan.

It is important that all consultations have these criteria irrespective of the treatment a client has chosen.

It can be very tempting in a busy clinic to have a routine that fits all requirements. Always refer back to the original concept that each of your future clients will be a unique individual requiring a routine that will meet their particular needs. A lifestyle profile as part of your consultation will give

you a more rounded perspective of the person sitting in front of you.

Theory into practice

Design a consultation form with questions that are not too probing that will give you the background and lifestyle choices of each client. Also put together a record card that is more than a list of treatments and appointments.

Having a more rounded view of each client will help you in your choice of oil and, if you are a qualified aromatherapist, in choosing the blend of oils that may enhance the treatment.

Observation

Indian head massage gives you, the therapist, an opportunity to gauge your client's reactions to the routine as a whole and to specific moves within the routine.

- **Practice point:** adapt the routine according to your client's preference and needs.

Evaluating treatments

It is important to have feedback from your clients. It makes your clients feel valued and will enable you to develop your treatment plan.

Testimonials

During your case studies it helps to have a checklist of the whole treatment. It provides a self-assessment critique by building on your strengths and pointing out the areas requiring attention.

Assessment task 19.4

Demonstrate an awareness of the potential hazards with Indian head massage. Describe, with attention to detail, the procedures you would use to reduce any risk. (M)

Identify potential problems in relation to the hazards associated with Indian head massage. Evaluate the required safety procedures and need to adapt your approach to the massage procedure. (D)

1 What are the names of the three Doshas?

2 Where are the concentrated areas of energy that relate to the marma points?

3 What are the names of the higher charkas you interact with during your facial massage?

4 What is the terminology for the mind/body link?

5 What impact will long-term stress have on sleeping patterns?

6 Name three health problems that have been linked to stress.

7 What do you need to check with your client before using a nut oil?

8 Why is it important for a therapist to de-stress with relaxed breathing before starting a treatment?

9 Where is the point located on the shoulder that should not be used with a client who is pregnant?

10 When would you not use the 'tug, lift and let go', movement?

11 List the five aims that a good consultation will help you achieve?

12 Why are testimonials important?

References and bibliography for Unit 19: Indian head massage

Bird, J. (1990) *Understanding Diseases*, The C. W. Daniel Company Limited.

Bloom, W. (2001) *The Endorphin Effects*, Piatkus

Burnham-Ariey, M. & O'Keefe, A. (2001) *Indian Head Massages*, Thomson

Godagama, Dr. S. (2001) *The Handbook of Ayurveda: A Practical Guide to India's Medical Wisdoms*, Kyle Cathie

Methta, N. (1999) *Indian Head Massages*, Thorsons

Simon, D. (1997) *The Wisdom of Healings*, Rider

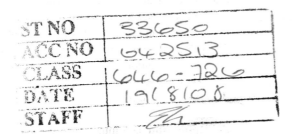

Glossary

acid mantle balance of acid and alkaline on the skin's surface which protects against bacterial infection

acne vulgaris skin disorder caused by inflammation of the sebaceous glands

actin muscle protein

adipose fatty tissue which insulates the body and internal organs

adrenal gland endocrine gland which secretes adrenalin

aerobic chemical reaction involving oxygen

afferent towards the brain

agonist prime muscle responsible for a movement

alimentary canal alternative name for the digestive system

amino acid chemical produced by the digestion of protein

anabolism 'building up' process involved in metabolism

anaerobic chemical reaction which does not involve oxygen

anion negatively-charged ion which is attracted to the anode

anode positive electrode or pole in electrotherapy

antagonists muscles that have opposing actions, e.g. biceps and triceps

anti-bacterial chemical which destroys bacteria

aorta largest artery; leads from the left ventricle of the heart

apocrine sweat glands found in axilla and genital areas

appendicular part of the skeleton consisting of the upper and lower limbs

aponeurosis sheet-like connective tissue

atom smallest particle of an element

ATP adenosine triphosphate, unit of energy in cells

atrium upper chambers of the heart which receive blood from veins

autoclave method of sterilisation for metal implements, similar in appearance and action to a pressure cooker

axial skeleton consists of the skull, thoracic cage and vertebral column

axon conducts nervous impulses from the body of a nerve cell

bacteria single cell organism, the simplest of all living micro-organisms

basal cell layer lowest of five layers of the epidermis (also called **stratum germinativum**)

benign non-malignant

Breslow thickness medical measure used to analyse moles

blood pressure pressure applied by blood to the artery walls

bronchi tubes which carry air from the trachea to the lungs

calcification method of formation of bone tissue

callous area of thickened skin usually on the foot

cancellous spongy bone tissue found on the inside of most bones

capillary small blood vessels that form a network which links arteries and veins

carbohydrate essential nutrient which provides the body with energy

cartilage type of strong connective tissue

catabolism 'breaking down' process involved in metabolism

cathode negatively-charged electrode or pole used in electrotherapy

cation positively-charged ion which is attracted to the cathode

cellulite polarity electrotherapy for treatment of cellulite, also called body galvanism

chloasma skin disorder characterised by patches of hyperpigmentation

clinical waste waste substances contaminated with body fluid

collagen fibrous connective tissue of the skin

comedone core of sebum in a follicle, also known as a blackhead

compact tissue hard bone tissue which surrounds spongy tissue

consultation dialogue between a client and a therapist prior to treatment which forms the basis of the professional relationship

contra-indication any condition which prevents treatment taking place

cosine law states that the intensity of radiation at a surface varies according to the cosine of the angle between the incident ray and the normal ray

COSHH Control of Substances Hazardous to Health, 2003: legislation concerned with the safe handling of hazardous substances

dermis largest layer of the skin, located under the epidermis

desquamation continual process of natural skin shedding

diastolic part of a heartbeat in which the heart relaxes and the ventricles fill with blood

digestion process of breaking down food to supply the body with energy and raw materials

disincrustation facial electrotherapy using galvanic current for a deep cleansing treatment

dowager's hump postural abnormality, also called kyphosis

ectomorph slim body shape lacking natural curves and muscle, often underweight

effleurage stroking massage movement used to start, end and link procedures

efferent away from the brain or other organ

elastin stretchy connective tissue which gives skin its elastic quality

electrolyte charged ions in a solution, capable of conducting electricity, e.g. saline

electrotherapy facial or body therapy performed using specialised electrical equipment

endocrine ductless gland that secretes hormones directly into the bloodstream, e.g. thyroid, ovary, testes

endomorph rounded body shape with padded contours, prone to weight gain

enzyme molecules of protein which act as catalysts in chemical processes

ephilide freckle

epidermis upper layer of skin containing five sub-layers or strata

epiphyses end part of a long bone

epithelial group of connective tissue consising of various types which differ in shape to suit their function, e.g. squamous, cuboidal, columnar

erythema reddening of the skin due to dilation of capillaries

erythrocytes red blood cells

exocrine gland that secretes through a duct, e.g. salivary gland

expiration breathing out

extracellular outside of a cell

faeces waste product of digestion consisting of fluid, cellulose and dead bacteria

facultative micro-organism that can survive with or without oxygen

fungus larger micro-organism that can cause infections such as ringworm

gamete mature sex cell that takes part in fertilisation

gastric juice secretions from the stomach involved in digestion

haem- prefix that indicates something related to blood

haemoglobin substance which gives blood its red colour and transports oxygen

hamstrings collective name for the group of muscles at the back of the thigh: biceps femoris, semitendinosus, semimembranosus

herpes simplex viral condition known as a cold sore

hirsuitism masculine hair growth pattern in women

holistic the 'whole'; to treat holistically is to consider physical, physiological and psychological aspects of the client

homeostasis biological processes which are self-regulating and therefore maintain a state of optimum stability, e.g. temperature control

hormone chemical messenger transported in the bloodstream to target organ

hyper- prefix indicating higher or too much

hyperaemia increased blood flow to an area

hypertension alternative name for high blood pressure

hypertrichosis general overgrowth of hair in males or females

hypo- prefix indicating lower, less than or not enough

hypoglycaemia low blood sugar associated with diabetes mellitus

impetigo bacterial skin infection

indication reason that a treatment is recommended

indifferent inactive electrode used in electrotherapy to complete an electrical circuit

inguinal relates to the groin area, e.g. inguinal ligament, inguinal node

infra-red electromagnetic rays with wavelengths of 70–400,000nm

insertion part of the muscle which moves towards the origin during an activity

interstitial located between the tissues, e.g. interstitial fluid

intracellular within a cell

inverse square law the intensity from a source of radiation will vary inversely with the square of the distance from the source of radiation

ion charged atom

iontophoresis electrotherapy using galvanic current which works on the principle that like repels like and opposite poles attract

isometric static muscle movement or contraction without movement

isotonic muscle action resulting in active movement

IUD intraurinary device, e.g. contraceptive coil

IVA integrated vocational assessment

keratin protein found in skin, hair and nails

keratinocytes cells which produce keratin

kyphosis postural abnormality charcterised by a humped back

lactation breastfeeding

lactic acid by-product of energy production in muscles; build-up causes fatigue

leucocytes white blood cells

lordosis postural abnormality charcterised by a hollow lower back

luminous radiant heat lamps which penetrate deeper than non-luminous lamps

lymph straw-coloured fluid which carries waste and helps to fight infection

malignant life-threatening condition such as cancer

melanin colour pigment found in skin and hair

melanocyte cell which produces melanin

mesomorph muscular body shape found on an active individual, usually with no weight problems

metabolism chemical reactions within cells

muscle fatigue following vigorous or prolonged activity, caused by build-up of **lactic acid**

micro-lance disposable, sterile lance used for removal of milia

micro-organism living organisms only visible through a microscope

milia core of hard sebum, also called whiteheads

MLD manual lymph drainage, massage technique which stimulates lymph flow

myosin muscle protein

nerve bundle of neurones

neurone nerve cell

non-luminous infra-red lamps with longer waves that penetrate the skin superficially

obligate organism that requires oxygen in order to survive

oedema swelling or fluid retention

oestrogen female hormone

onychocryptosis ingrowing nail, usually found on the big toe

onychogryphosis nail disorder characterised by thickening and excessive ridges

onycholysis nail disorder characterised by separation from the nail bed

onychomycosis ringworm of the nails

onychophagy bitten nails

oocyte reproductive cell in the ovary

organ combination of tissues responsible for particular functions, e.g. liver

organic containing carbon

origin part of the muscle which remains fixed during movement

osmosis movement of molecules through a semi-permeable membrane

ossification method of bone formation, also known as calcification

osteoblast cell responsible for the formation of bone tissue

osteoclast cell responsible for the breakdown of damaged or worn bone tissue

osteoporosis condition resulting in brittle bones

ova unfertilised female reproductive cells, single-ovum

ovary female reproductive organ

oxidisation chemical process of breaking down substances in the presence of oxygen

ozone produced by passing oxygen through ultra-violet; has anti-bacterial and therapeutic qualities

pancreas large endocrine and exocrine gland located behind the stomach

papillary layer uppermost layer of the dermis

papule small raised skin lesion, may contain pus

paronychia bacterial infection of the nail

pathogen micro-organism that causes disease, usually a virus or bacteria

pediculosis capitis parasitic infection known as head lice

peristalsis reflex, wave-like contraction of muscles in the alimentary canal

petrissage deep manual massage movements including kneading

phagocyte cell which destroys harmful bacteria

plasma liquid part of blood

platelet disc-shaped structure in blood which causes clotting

prickle cell layer part of epidermis, also known as stratum spinosum

pterygium nail disorder characterised by overgrowth of cuticle

pustule raised skin lesion around hair follicle containing pus

reticular layer deepest layer of the dermis

sanitation method of cleaning which only partially destroys harmful bacteria

scoliosis spinal abnormality charcterised by 'C'- or 'S'-shaped lateral curves

seborrhoea condition resulting from over-active sebaceous glands

sebum natural, oily substance produced by sebaceous glands

scabies skin disorder caused by the parasitic itch mite

shiatsu form of manual massage focusing on pressure points

sphygmomanometer instrument used for measuring blood pressure

sterilisation total destruction of harmful micro-organisms

systolic part of a heart beat where blood pressure peaks

tapotement tapping movements performed in manual massage

tendon tough cord of collagen which attaches muscle to bone

tinea fungal infection also known as ringworm

tissue collection of cells with similar structure and function, e.g. connective tissue

ultraviolet rays of the electromagnetic spectrum with wavelengths of 10–400 nm

varicose vein distended and painful veins caused by excessive pressure

vena cava largest veins – inferior and superior, which carry blood to right atrium of the heart

ventricle lower chambers of the heart

virus micro-organism which causes disease, e.g. common cold

vitiligo skin disorder charcterised by lack of pigmentation

Index